a LANGE medical book

Radiology On Call
A Case-Based Manual

Roland Talanow, MD, PhD
Department of Radiology
Cleveland Clinic
Cleveland, Ohio

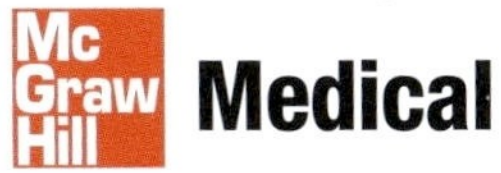

New York   Chicago   San Francisco   Lisbon   London   Madrid   Mexico City
Milan   New Delhi   San Juan   Seoul   Singapore   Sydney   Toronto

Radiology On Call: A Case-Based Manual

1 2 3 4 5 6 7 8 9 0   CTP/CTP   15 14 13 12 11

ISBN 978-0-07-163797-8
MHID 0-07-163797-4

Notice

Medicine is an ever-changing science. As new research and clinical experience broaden our knowledge, changes in treatment and drug therapy are required. The authors and the publisher of this work have checked with sources believed to be reliable in their efforts to provide information that is complete and generally in accord with the standards accepted at the time of publication. However, in view of the possibility of human error or changes in medical sciences, neither the authors nor the publisher nor any other party who has been involved in the preparation or publication of this work warrants that the information contained herein is in every respect accurate or complete, and they disclaim all responsibility for any errors or omissions or for the results obtained from use of the information contained in this work. Readers are encouraged to confirm the information contained herein with other sources. For example and in particular, readers are advised to check the product information sheet included in the package of each drug they plan to administer to be certain that the information contained in this work is accurate and that changes have not been made in the recommended dose or in the contraindications for administration. This recommendation is of particular importance in connection with new or infrequently used drugs.

This book was set in Helvetica by Thomson Digital.
The editors were Michael Weitz and Brian Kearns.
The production supervisor was Sherri Souffrance.
Project management was provided by Aakriti Kathuria, Thomson Digital.
The design was adapted by Mary McKeon; the cover designer was Thomas De Pierro.
China Translation & Printing, Ltd., was printer and binder.

Library of Congress Cataloging-in-Publication Data

Talanow, Roland.
  Radiology on-call : a case-based manual / Roland Talanow.
      p. ; cm.
  Includes bibliographical references.
  ISBN-13: 978-0-07-163797-8 (pbk. : alk. paper)
  ISBN-10: 0-07-163797-4 (pbk. : alk. paper)
  1. Diagnosis, Radioscopic—Case studies. 2. Radiology, Medical—Case studies. I. Title.
  [DNLM: 1. Radiography—methods—Case Reports. 2. Radiography—methods—Handbooks.
WN 39]
  RC78.T119 2011
  616.07'57—dc22

                                                                    2011008221

*Dedicated to all radiology students
who will find this text helpful to their studies.*

CONTENTS

III. NEURO

IV. MUSCULOSKELETAL

PREFACE

This reference book provides the most common entities a radiologist, emergency physician, and resident might encounter during the day in the emergency room or during in-house call. It also serves medical students and clinical residents preparing for their ER rotation. It is not intended to be a textbook for emergency radiology. The author kept the text to a minimum, only providing pertinent facts and short descriptions to make the reader familiar with each respective entity. On the other hand, the author provided a large collection of pertinent references in case the reader wants to learn more about specific topics. There are many freely available high-quality review articles on specific topics discussed in this book. To avoid spending an extra amount of money on commercial literature, the author provides for each book section a selection of references to high-quality journal articles that are freely and directly available to the reader. All cases are adapted from the author's on-call radiology tutorial (www.oncallradiology.com), which provides the cases also in interactive modes and more imaging material. For this reason, each image is provided with a number in parenthesis that refers to the case ID in the online tutorial.

The book's format has been structured in such a way that physicians and students can comfortably carry this book in his/her lab coat, thus always being at hand when needed.

The numbers featured throughout the book shown next to the following symbol (🖥), refer to the case ID in the interactive online tutorial. Each case can be accessed by this number at the following non-McGraw-Hill Web site: www.oncallradiology. com/#, with "#" being the respective case ID. If you have any questions regarding this Web site, please contact the author directly at roland@talanow.info

- Anatomy
- Technique
- Lungs & Airways
- Pleural Space
- Mediastinum, Heart & Vessels
- Chest Wall & Diaphragm
- Devices
- References

1. Anatomy

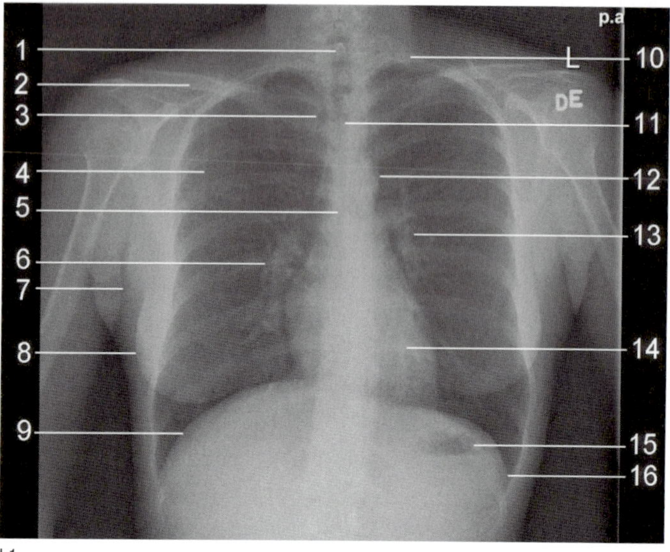

I-1

CHEST RADIOGRAPH – ANATOMY 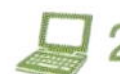 2

 1. Spinous process
 2. Right clavicle
 3. Right sternoclavicular joint
 4. Medial border of right scapula
 5. Carina
 6. Right hilum
 7. Right axillary fold
 8. Lateral breast shadow
 9. Right hemidiaphragm
10. Left first rib
11. Trachea
12. Aortic "knob" (distal arch)
13. Left hilum
14. Heart
15. Stomach bubble
16. Left costophrenic angle

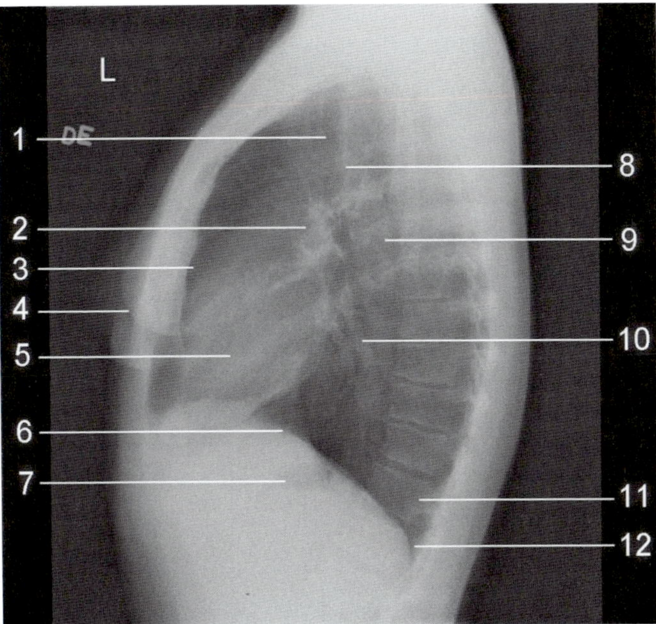

I-2

1. Trachea
2. Hilum
3. Retrosternal space
4. Breast shadow
5. Heart
6. Diaphragm
7. Stomach bubble
8. Aortic arch
9. Descending aorta
10. Pulmonary vessels
11. Vertebral body
12. Posterior costophrenic angle

2. Technique

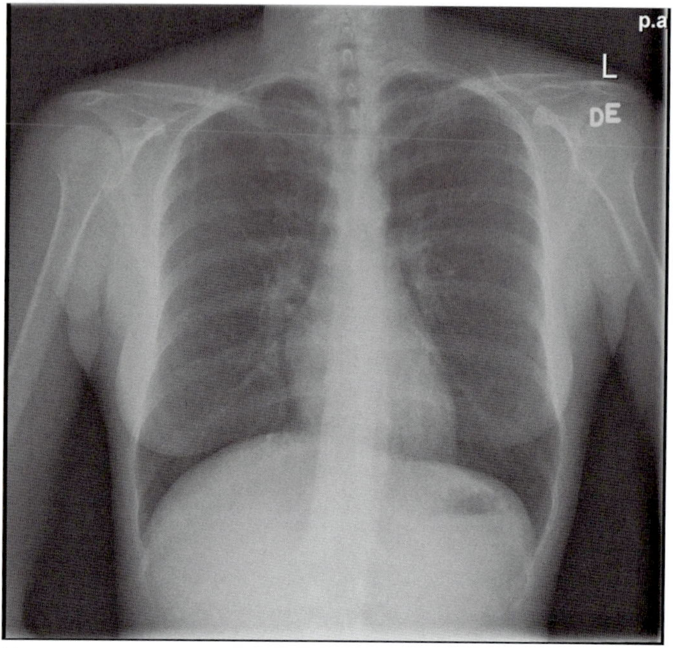

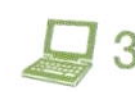

I-3

■ THE RIGHT TECHNIQUE –
POSTEROANTERIOR VIEW

Proper technique important

- Posteroanterior (PA) preferred: Anteroposterior (AP) makes heart larger.
- Portable (ICU) films are AP.
- If possible: second view (lateral) for better localization.
- Erect and good inspiration (to avoid superimposition).
- Check for heart, lungs, upper airways, bones, and soft tissues (don't forget visualized abdomen).
- Look for patient rotation.

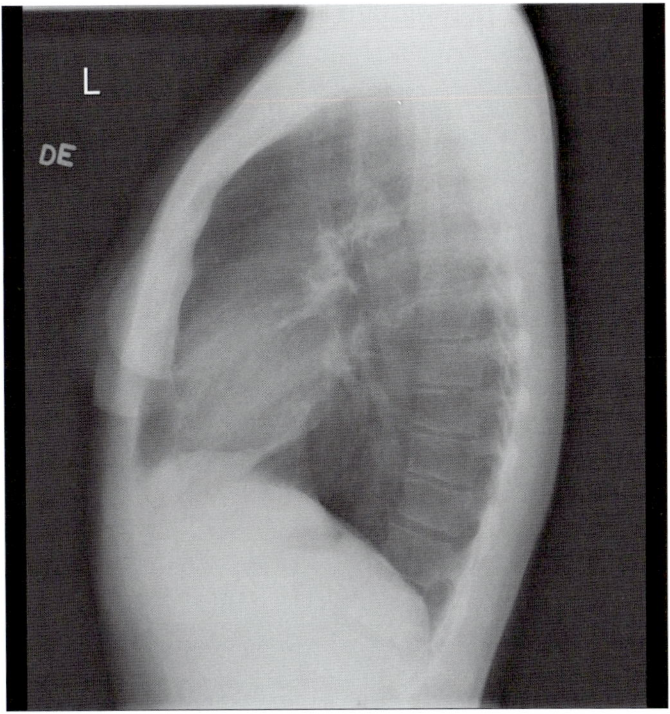

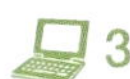

I-4

THE RIGHT TECHNIQUE –
LATERAL VIEW

3

Normal exam
- Both lungs equally translucent
- Heart diameter <1/2 of thorax diameter
- Heart border clearly visible on both sides
- Smooth branching and pruning of pulmonary vasculature
- Trachea midline
- Diaphragms equally shaped (right slightly higher)
- Costophrenic angles clearly visible
- Pleura not visible (if yes – thickening)
- Hila not enlarged (no lymphadenopathy, mass/cancer)
- Skeleton normal (no fractures, dislocations)
- Soft tissues unremarkable (foreign bodies)

■ THE RIGHT TECHNIQUE 2 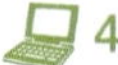 4

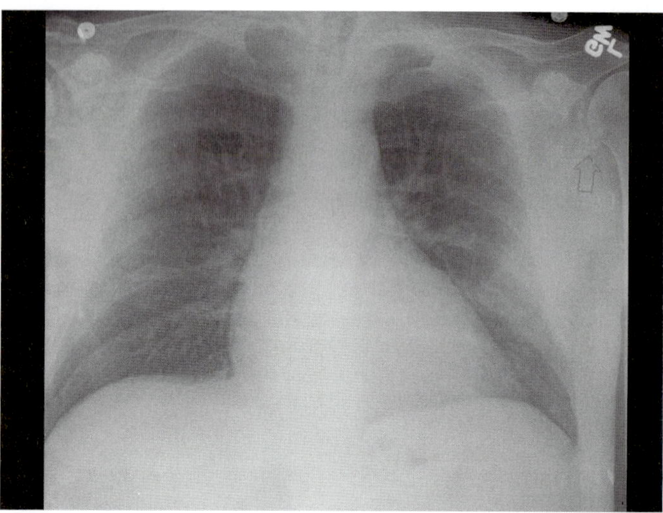

I-5

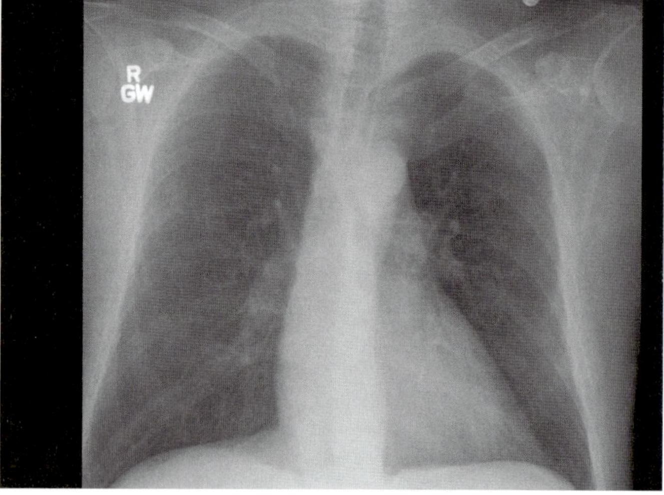

I-6

- Importance of good inspiration and erect technique
- Portable (AP) films
- Lungs under aerated (may mimic tumors or infiltrates)
- Heart larger

This is an example of what can happen when a suboptimal technique is used. The left upper image was taken in poor inspiration, which leads to underaeration and crowding of parenchymal structures/vessels. The arrow points to a vessel that mimics a cavitary lesion that was easily recognized after a repeat radiograph (left bottom image) was performed in better inspiration.

The following are magnified views of the images to the left:

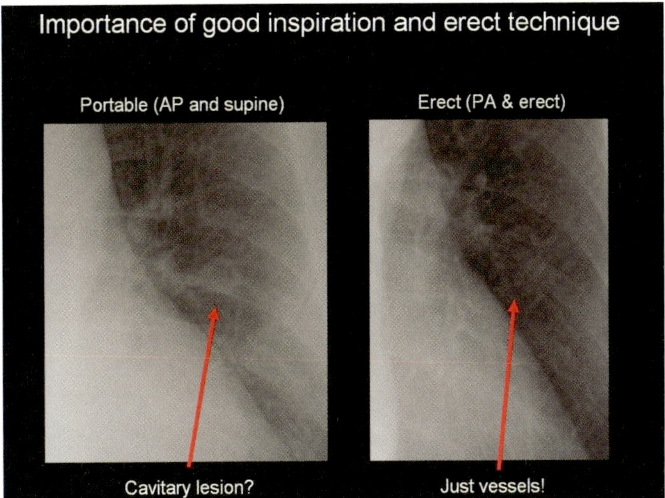

I-7

■ Table I-1. Chest Radiograph Evaluation   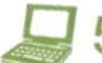 5

Lungs	Opacities with volume loss	Atelectasis
	Opacities without volume loss	Pneumonia Tumor Hemorrhage Pulmonary edema
	Focal hyperlucency	Pneumothorax Bullae/blebs (COPD) Absence of structures (eg mastectomy)
	Shift (toward pathology)	Atelectasis Postoperative volume loss Pneumothorax
	Shift (away from pathology)	Pleural effusion Tension pneumothorax Tumor
Mediastinum	Widening (>8 cm)	Vascular ectasia/aneurysm Tumor Hematoma (post-traumatic) Abscess Lymphadenopathy
Hila	Enlarged	Lymphadenopathy Pulmonary arterial congestion (COPD) Pulmonary venous congestion (congestive heart failure [CHF])
Heart	Enlarged cardiac silhouette	Cardiomegaly Pericardial effusion/tamp.
Pleural space	Blunted costophrenic angles	Pleural effusion Pleural thickening
Chest wall	Fracture, dislocation	
Diaphragm	Elevation	Subpulmonic abscess Atelectasis Diaphragmatic rupture Phrenic nerve paralysis

3. Lungs & Airways

◼ OBSTRUCTIVE LUNG DISEASE – INTRODUCTION

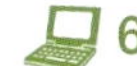 6

- Etiologies: Chronic Obstructive Pulmonary Disease (COPD), asthma, etc.
- Hyperinflated lungs
- Flat diaphragms
- Wide intercostal spaces
- Horizontal oriented ribs
- Wide retrosternal space
- Relatively small heart

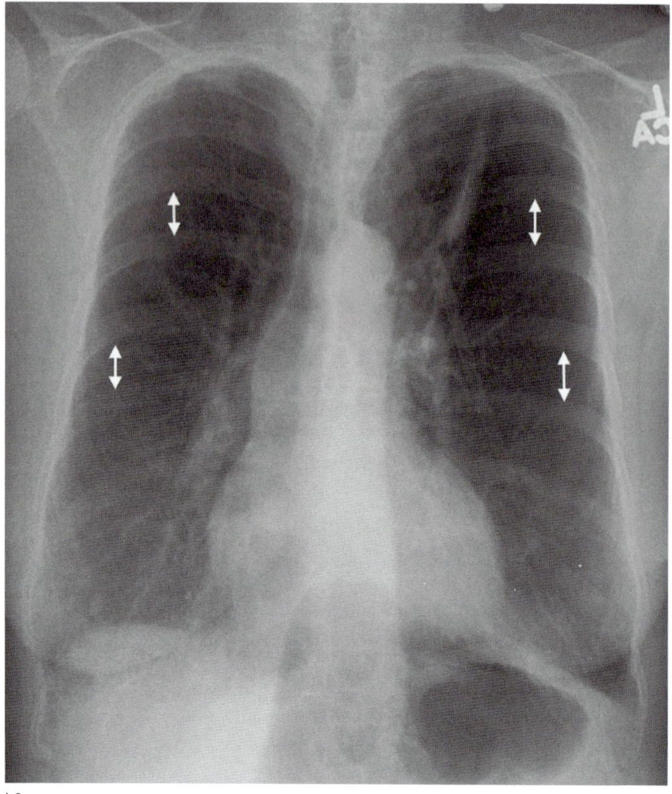

I-8

■ COPD

This patient has:
- hyperinflated lungs
- hyperlucent lungs
- widened retrosternal space (top, double arrow)
- flattened diaphragms (top dashed arrow)
- widened intercostal spaces (left; double arrows)

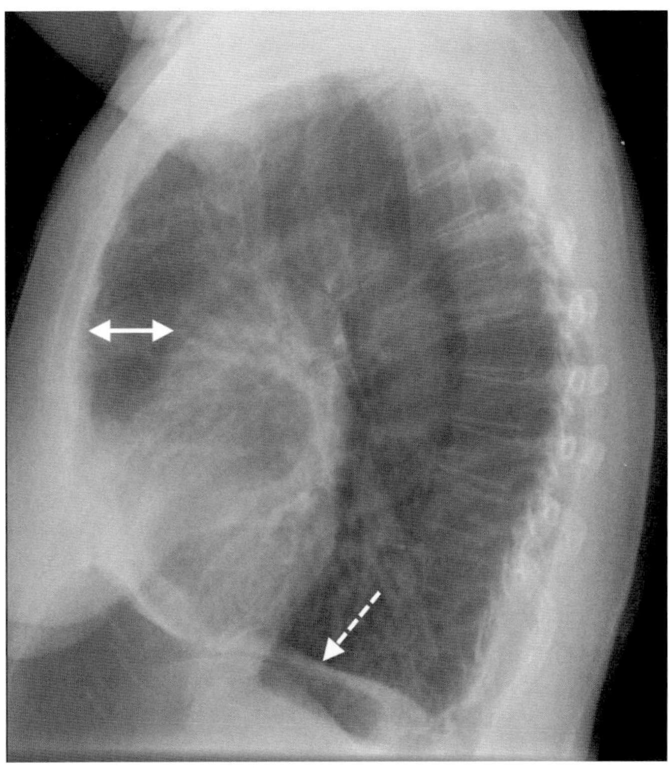

I-9

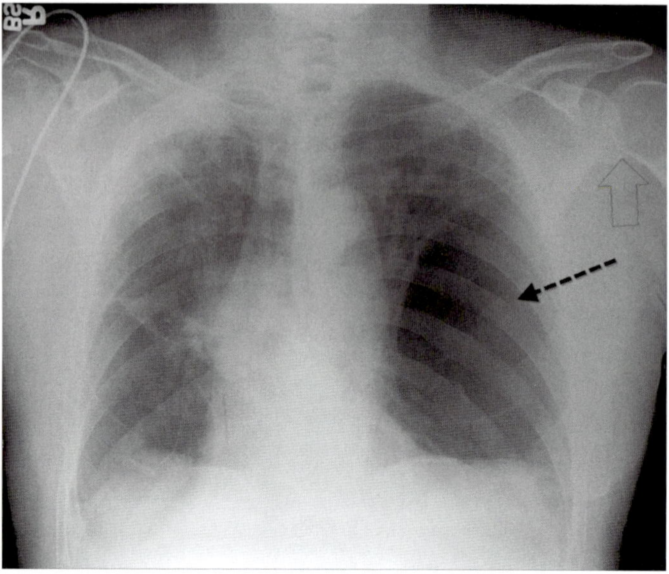

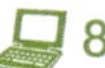

I-10

BULLOUS EMPHYSEMA

Frontal chest radioghraph demonstrates a large lucency in the left lower and mid-lung zones (arrow). Chest CT in lung windows confirms a large bulla (arrow). Multiple smaller bullae are also identified, compatible with bullous emphysema.

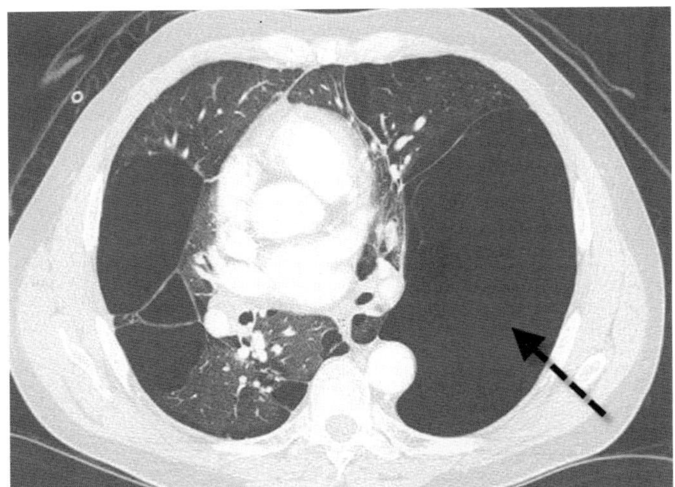

I-11

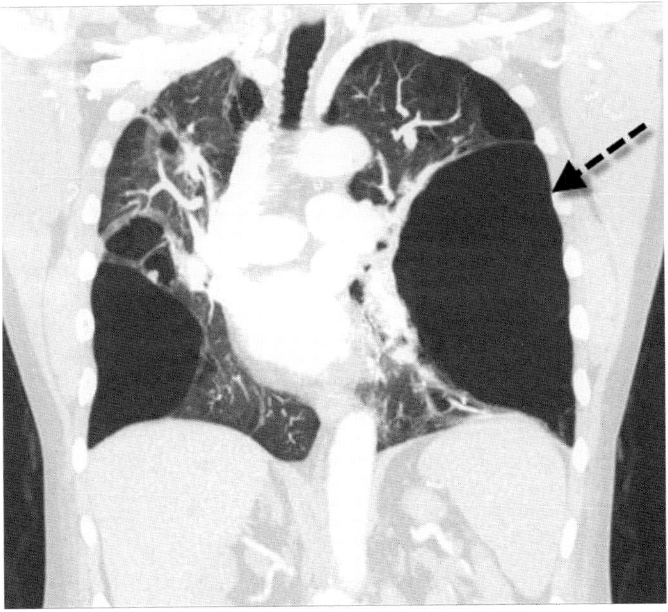

I-12

VOLUME LOSS – INTRODUCTION 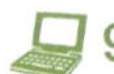 9

- Multiple etiologies (surgical, atelectasis, pneumothorax)
- Mediastinal shift toward the pathology (traction/"sucker")
- Compared to space occupying lesions: mediastinal shift away from lesion (mass effect/"pusher")

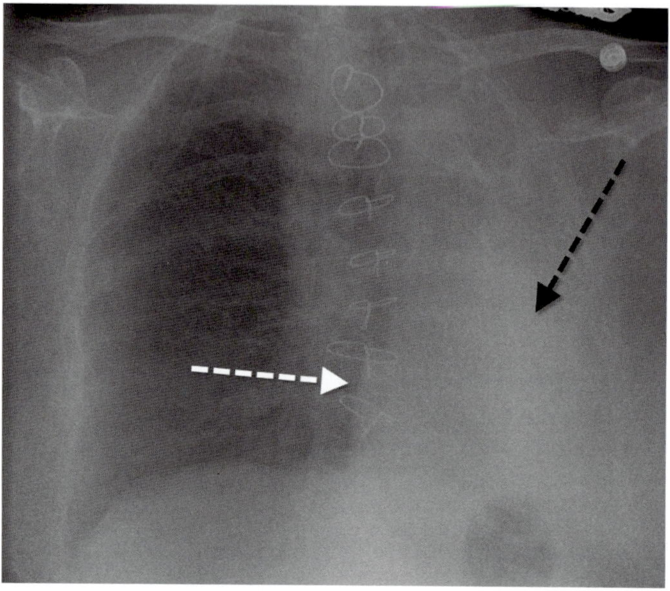

I-13

VOLUME LOSS – PNEUMONECTOMY 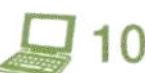 10

Status post-left pneumonectomy

- The entire left hemithorax is opacified (airless; black arrow).
- Mediastinal shift toward area of volume loss, heart in left hemithorax (white arrow).

LUNG LESIONS – INTRODUCTION 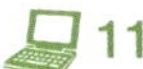 11

Table I-2. Benign Versus Malignant Features

	Benign features	Malignant features
Size	<2 cm	>3 cm
Doubling time	<30 days or >2 years	>30 days and <2 years
Calcification	Popcorn, laminated	Eccentric
Shape/margins	Round, well-defined margins	Lobulated, spiculated, cavitated, indistinct margins
Tissue	Fat (hamartoma)	
Age	<35 years	>35 years
Satelite nodules	+ (granuloma)	
Enhancement	<20 HU difference	>20 HU difference
FDG PET	Norm- or hypometabolic	Hypermetabolic
Other	Feeding/draining vessel (AVM), "Halo" of groundglass (invasive aspergillosis), endemic areas (histoplasmosis, tuberculosis)	Bubbly appearance, air bronchograms, cavitation

Lesions with doubling time
- <30 days: infection, fast-growing metastases (eg choriocarcinoma, seminoma, osteosarcoma)
- >2 years: hamartoma, histoplasmoma

Risk factors for lung cancer
- Smoking (87%)
- Asbestos exposure
- Radon exposure
- Prior radiation (eg Hodgkin's lymphoma, breast cancer)
- Diffuse interstitial lung fibrosis

■ LUNG CANCER – INTRODUCTION   🖥 12

- Poorly (if not) calcified
- Poor margins (but can be also well marginated)
- Size >1 cm
- History (smoker, asbestos exposure)
- Central: small cell, squamous, carcinoid
- Peripheral: large cell, bronchioalveolar (BAC)

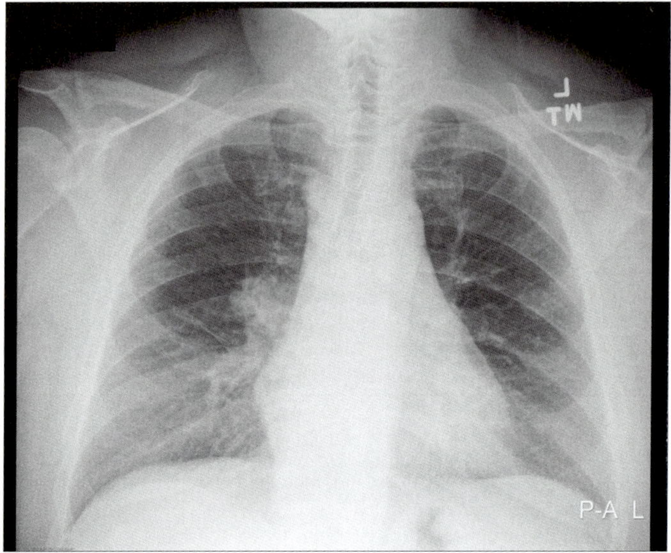

I-14

■ RIGHT LOWER LUNG TUMOR –
SQUAMOUS CELL CARCINOMA   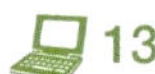 13

A round mass is seen projecting over the right hilum. However, the lateral
view confirms its position in the right lower lobe!

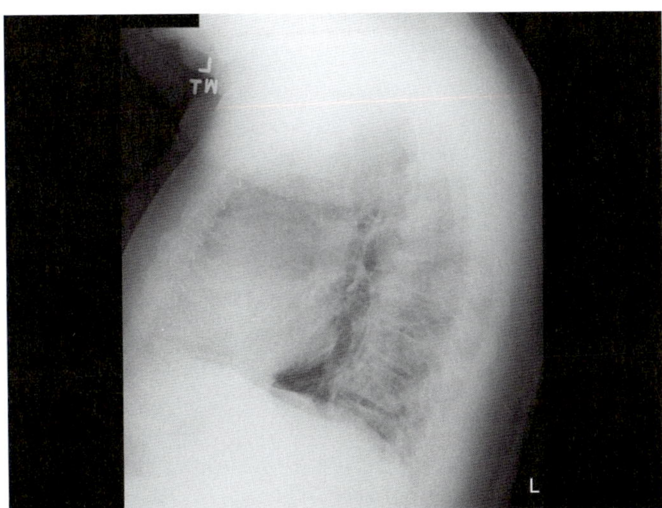

I-15

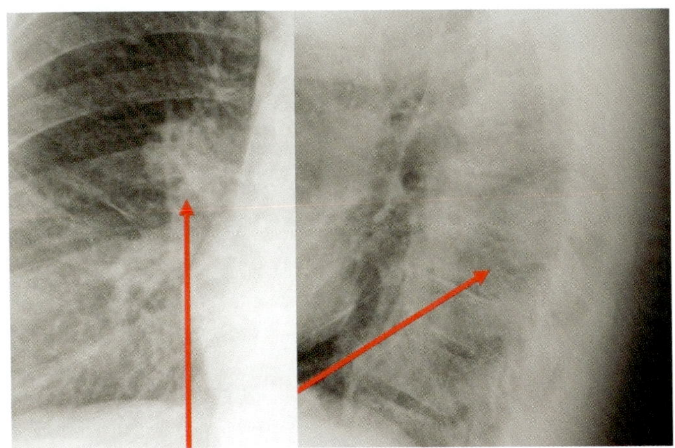

I-16

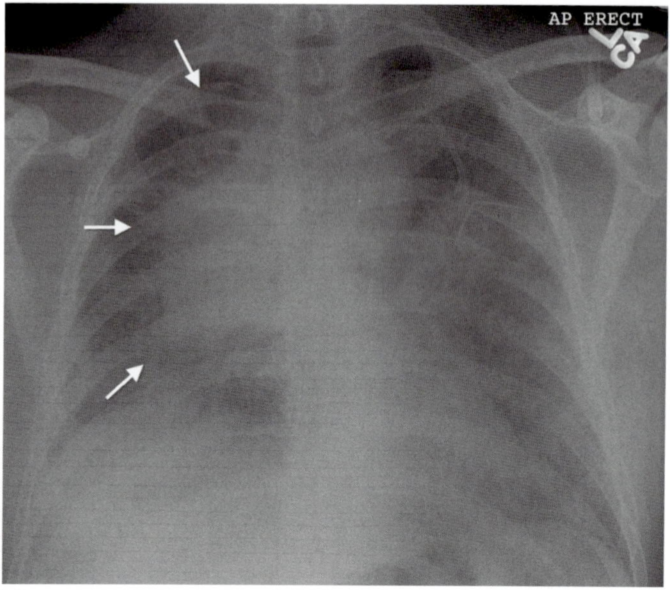

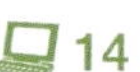

I-17

NON-SMALL CELL LUNG CANCER 14

Frontal chest radiograph demonstrates a large right hilar mass with poor margination (arrows). A contrast-enhanced CT (next page) better demonstrates its extension into the right middle and upper lobes (white arrows).

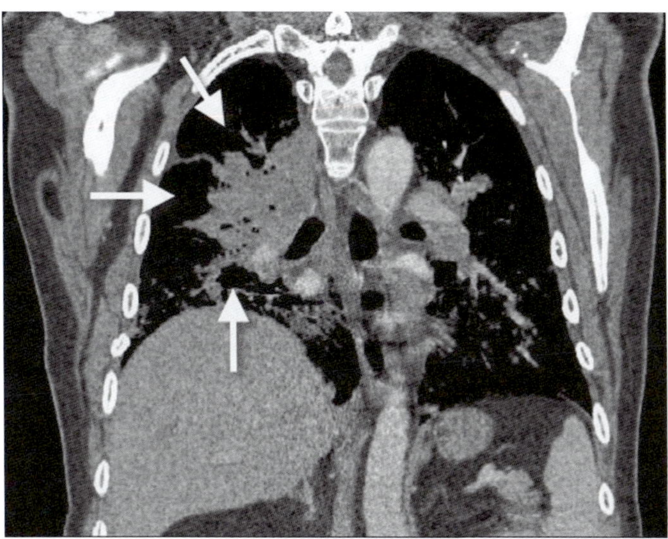

I-18

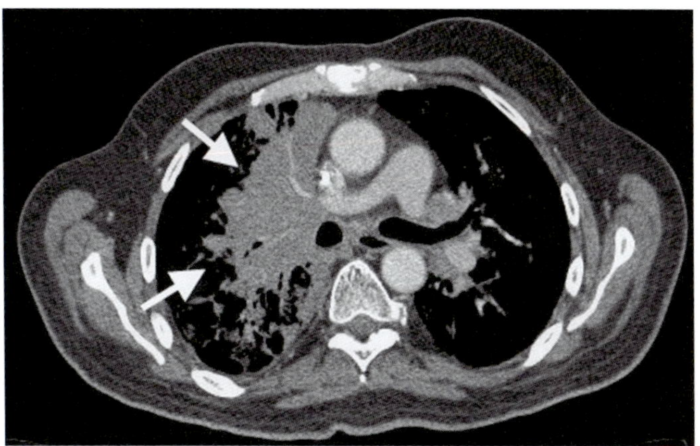

I-19

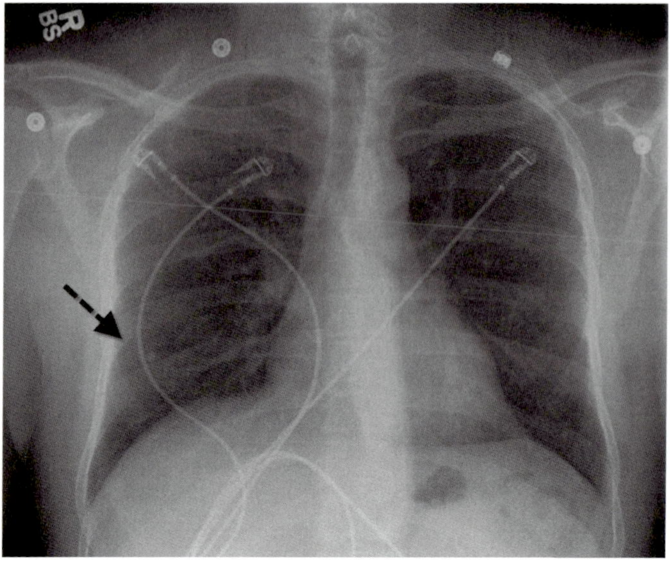

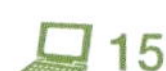

I-20

■ "HARMLESS" LESIONS MIMICKING CANCER – CALCIFIED GRANULOMA

15

Calcified granuloma

- Dense calcification
- Well defined
- Sharp margins
- Size <1 cm

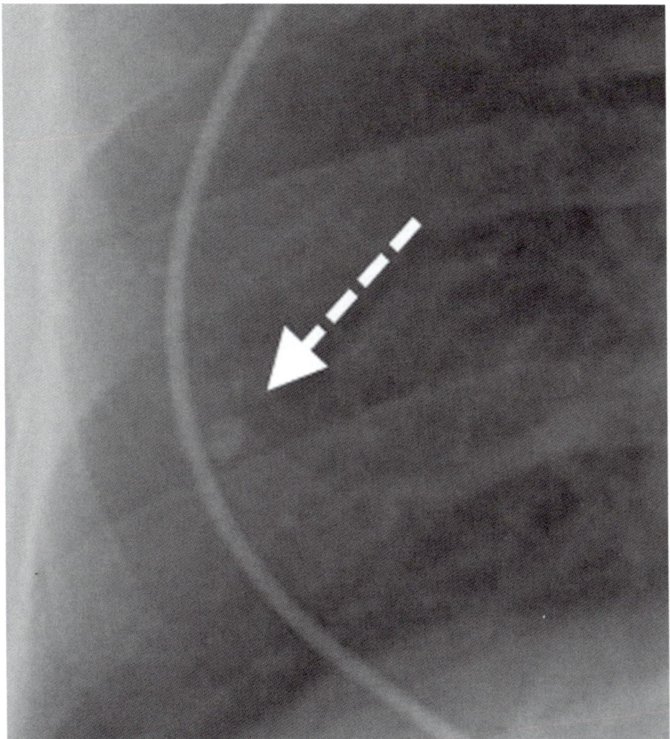

I-21

Calcified Granuloma

Magnified view from the prior image. There is a subcentimeter, well defined dense calcified nodule in the right lower lung zone, compatible with a calcified granuloma.

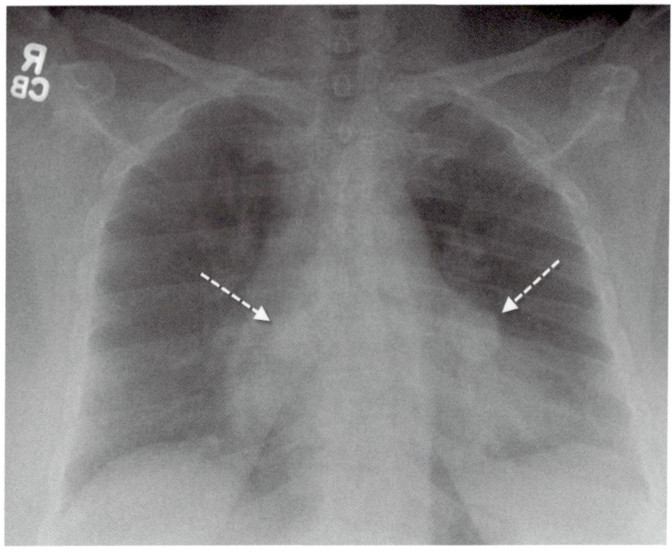

I-22

"HARMLESS" LESIONS MIMICKING CANCER – CALCIFIED LYMPH NODES

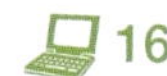 16

Calcified lymph nodes

- Calcified lymph nodes (from histoplasmosis)
- (Bi)hilar calcifications
- Sometimes "lymph node" shaped
- History helpful (histoplasmosis, sarcoidosis, tuberculosis, etc.)

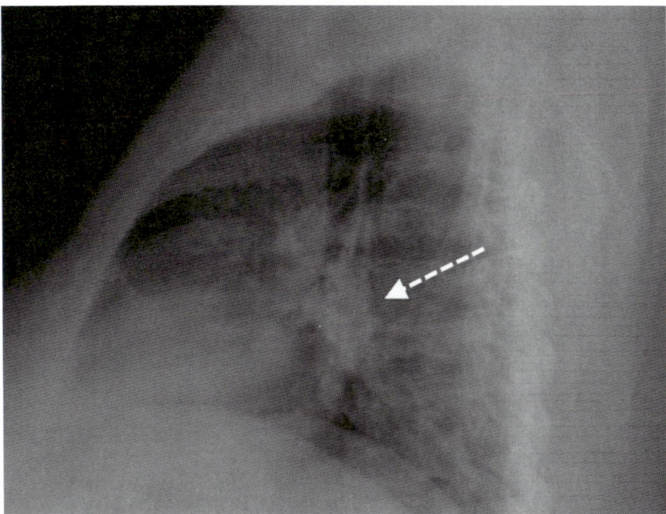

I-23

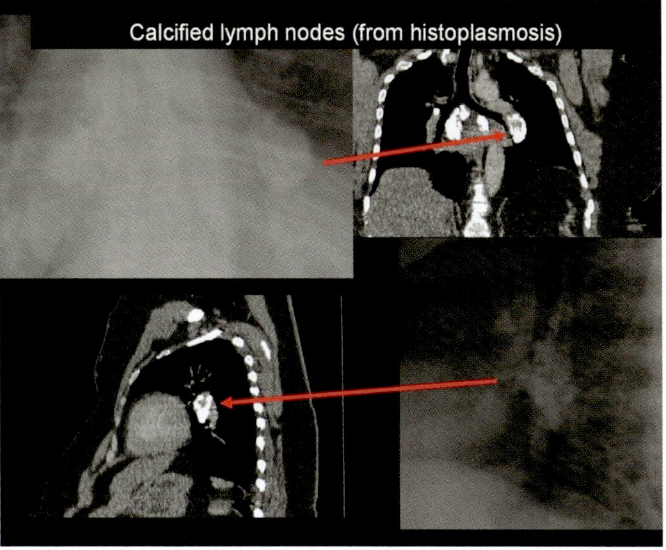

I-24

▪ PNEUMONIA – INTRODUCTION   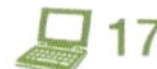 17

- Lung infiltrate (airspace process)
- Air bronchogram (patent airways crossing the infiltrate)
- Clinical correlation important (fever, leucocytosis, cough)
- Lower lungs more frequently affected due to aspiration
- Right lower lobe more frequent than left lower lobe due to steeper course of right main stem bronchus

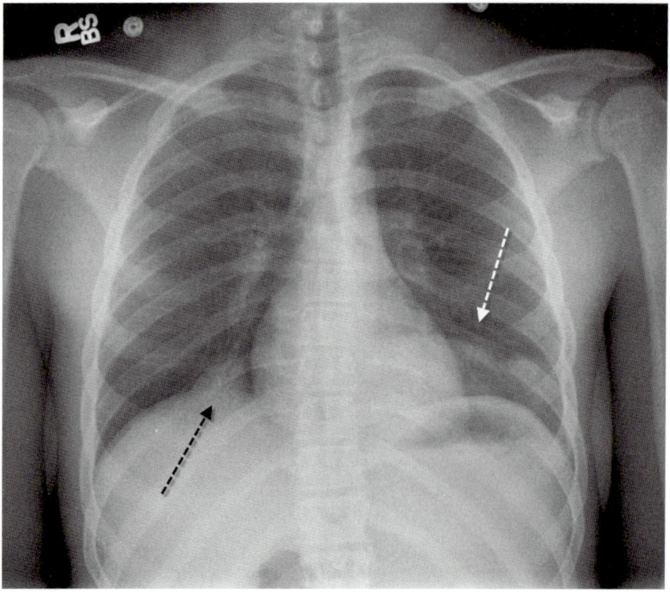

I-25

▪ BILATERAL LOWER LOBE PNEUMONIA   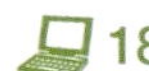 18

- Lateral view confirms lower lobe location.
- Both infiltrates are located below the major fissures.

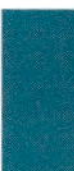

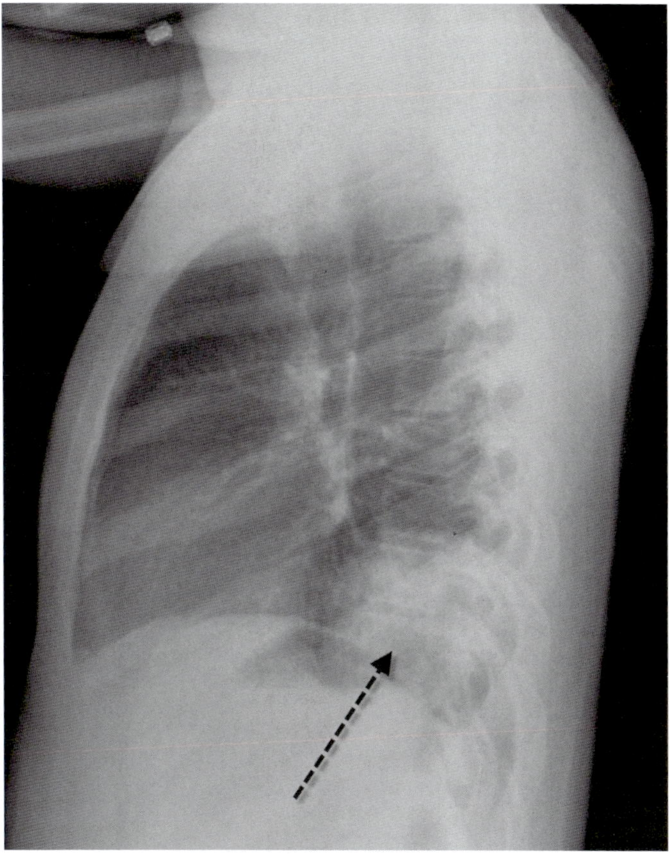

I-26

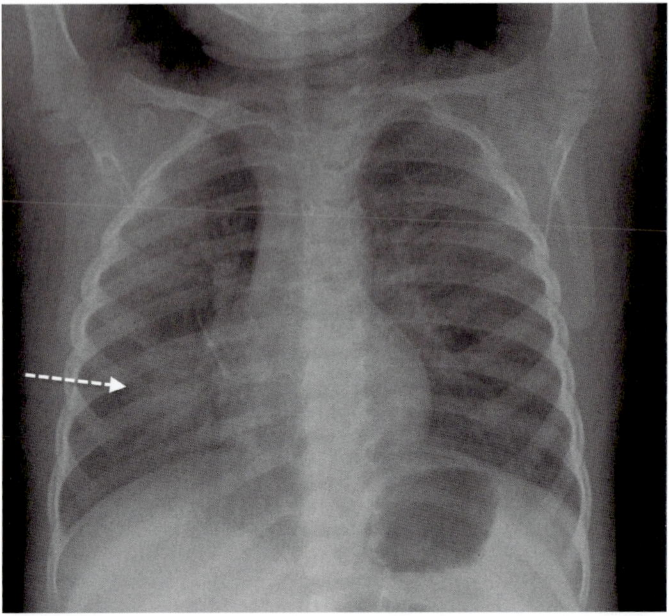

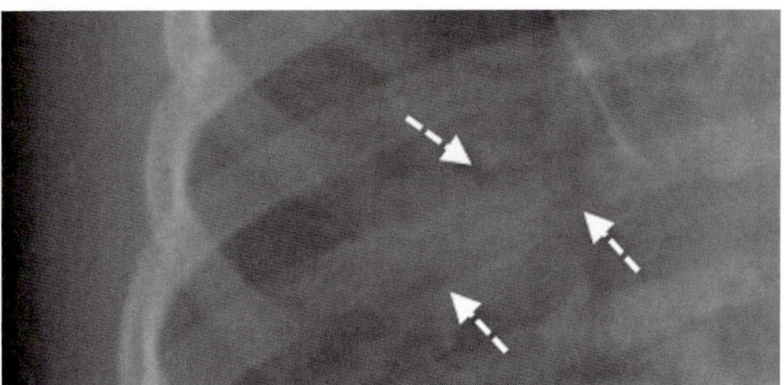

I-27

I-28

◼ RIGHT MIDDLE LOBE PNEUMONIA 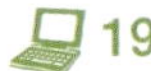 19

- Infiltrate is located above the right major fissure.
- Left lower image demonstrates air bronchograms within the infiltrate – a typical feature of an airspace process.

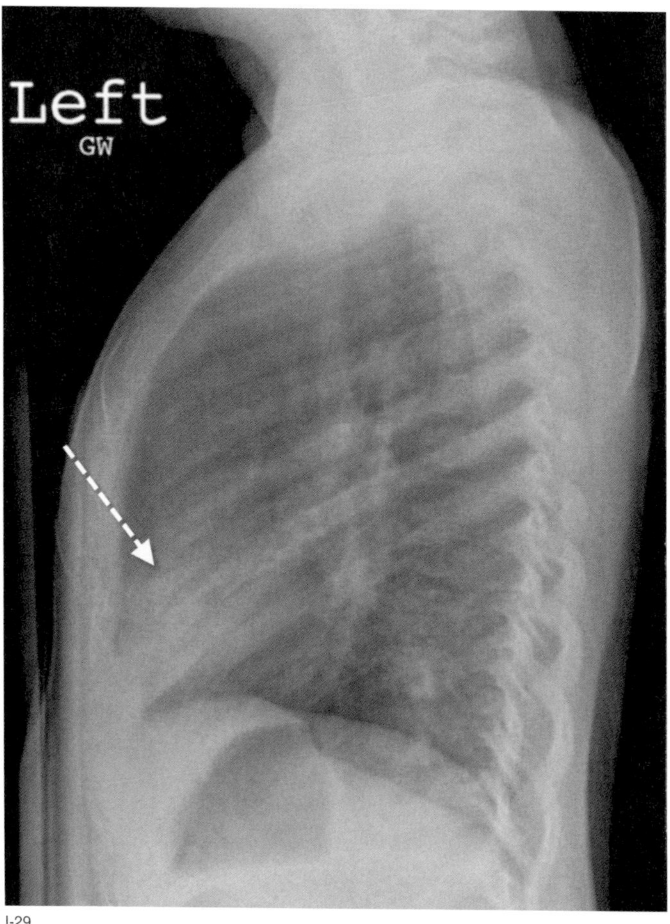

I-29

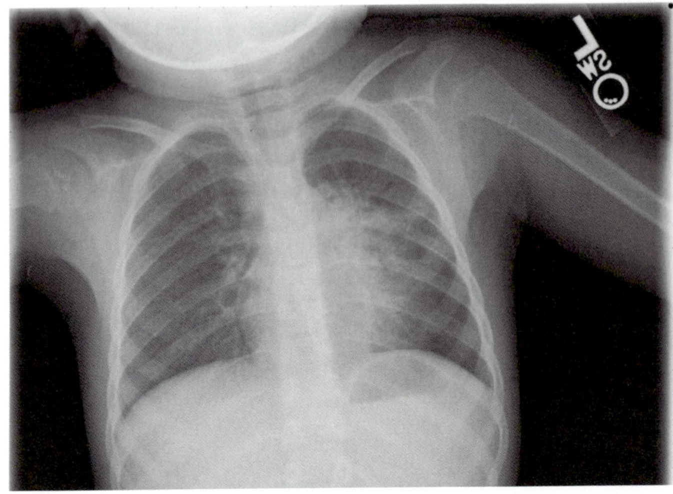

I-30

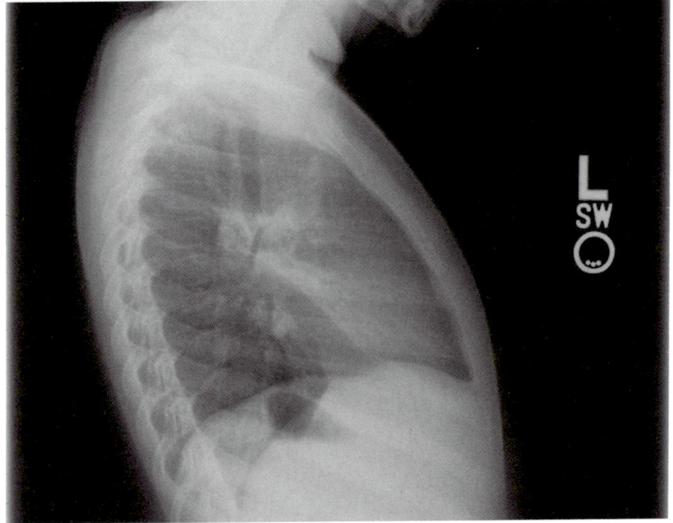

I-31

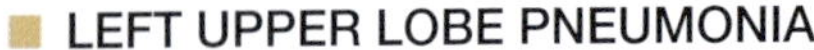 **LEFT UPPER LOBE PNEUMONIA**   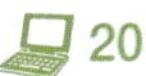 20

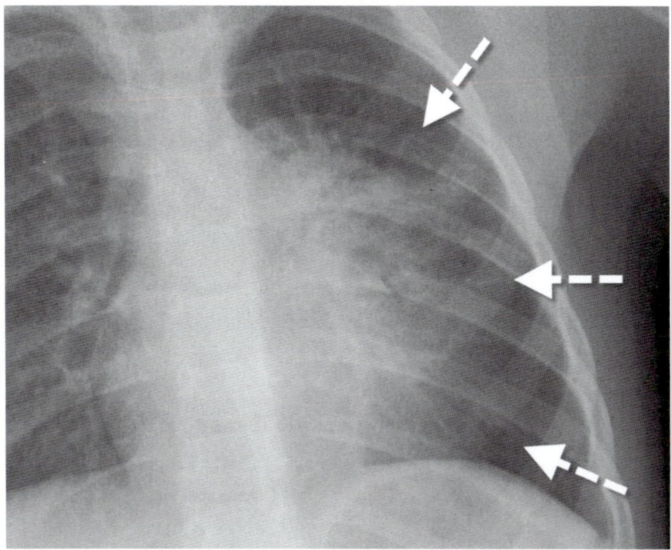

I-32

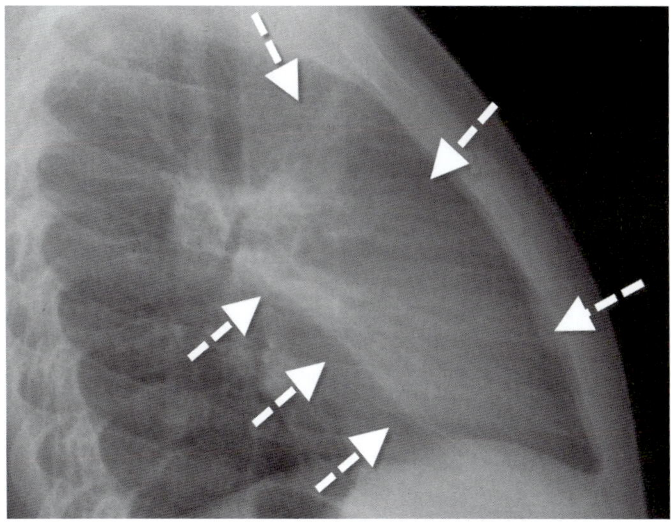

I-33

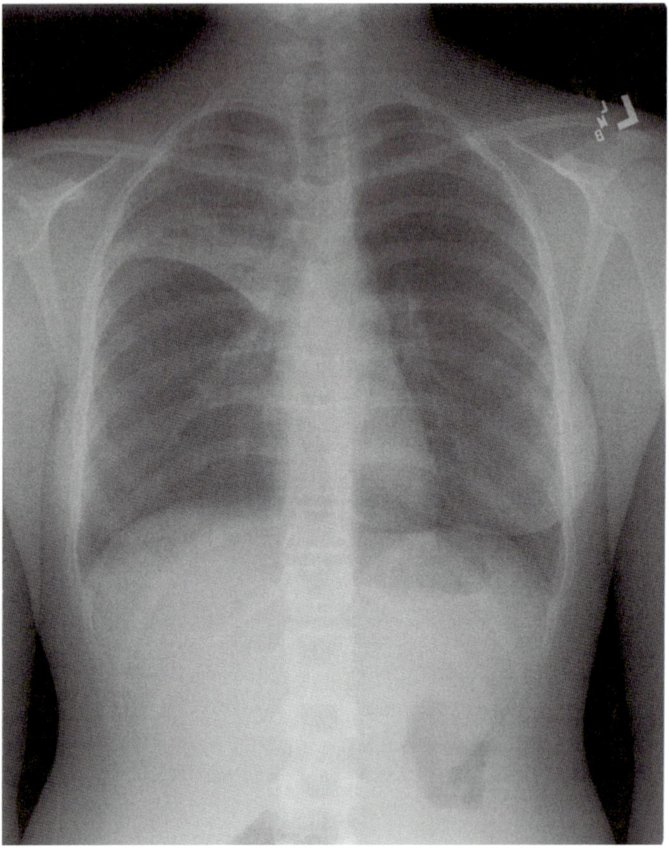

I-34

■ RIGHT UPPER LOBE PNEUMONIA 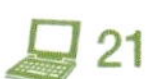 21

Right upper lobe (RUL) pneumonia and partial RUL atelectasis
There is partial collapse of the right upper lobe, causing elevation of the minor fissure (first image, white arrows), obscuring the right paratracheal border (black arrow). In addition, this patient has a right upper lobe pneumonia (see air bronchograms, black dashed arrow). An underlying, centrally located, and obstructing lesion should be excluded.

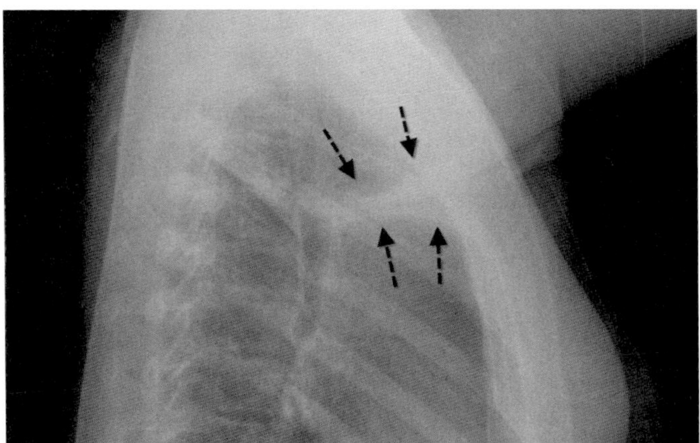

I-35

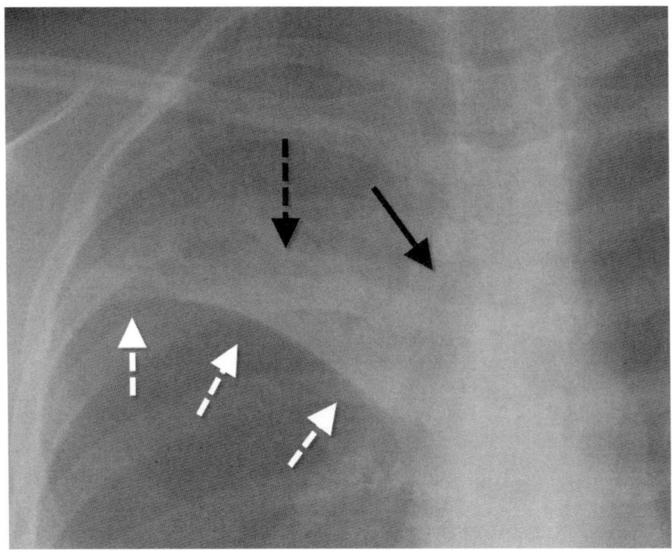

I-36

ATELECTASIS – PATTERN   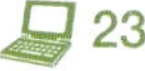 22

Pattern of collapse
- Right and left upper lobes: anterior-superior-medial
- Right and left lower lobes: posterior-inferior-medial
- Right middle lobe: anterior-inferior-medial

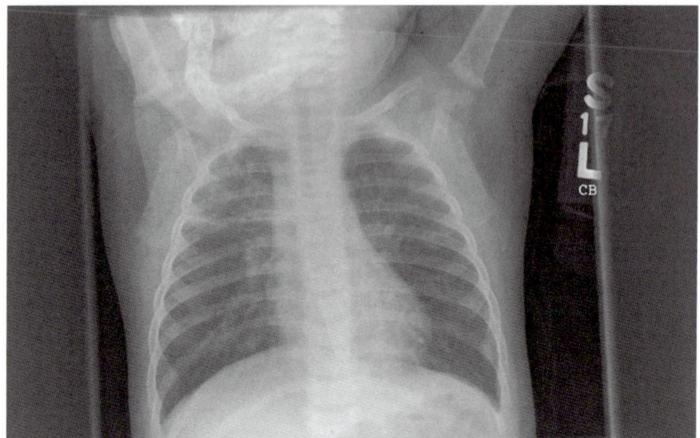

I-37

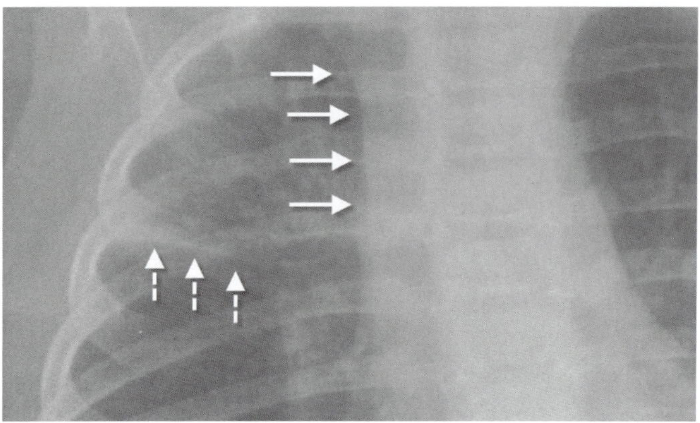

I-38

RIGHT UPPER LOBE ATELECTASIS   23

Right upper lobe collapses: anterior-superior-medial

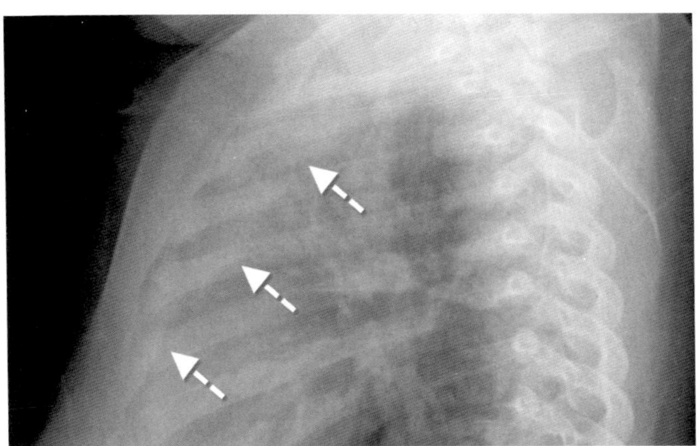

I-39

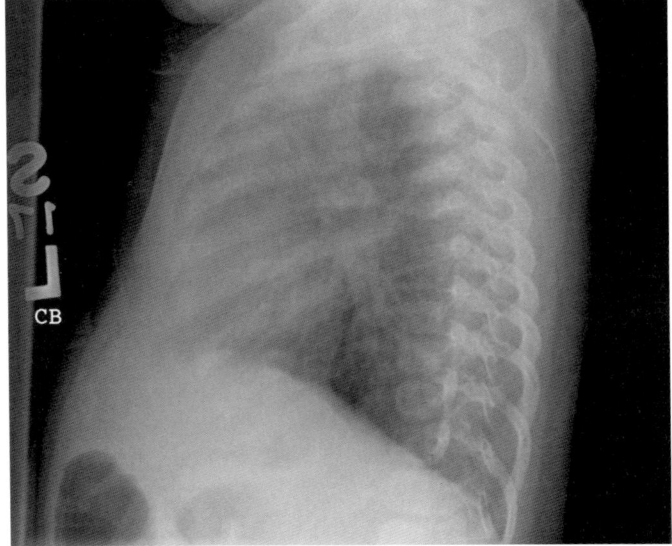

I-40

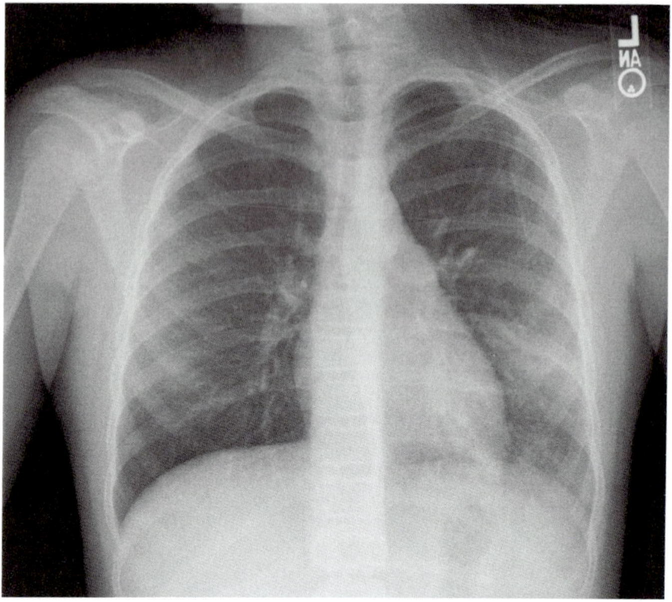

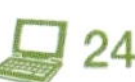

I-41

LEFT LOWER LOBE ATELECTASIS   24

There is a segmental collapse in the anterior aspect of the left lower lobe (black arrow, white arrows). There is obscuring of the left hemidiaphragm (dashed black arrows) – compare to the well delineation of the right hemi-diaphragm (white dashed arrow left image).

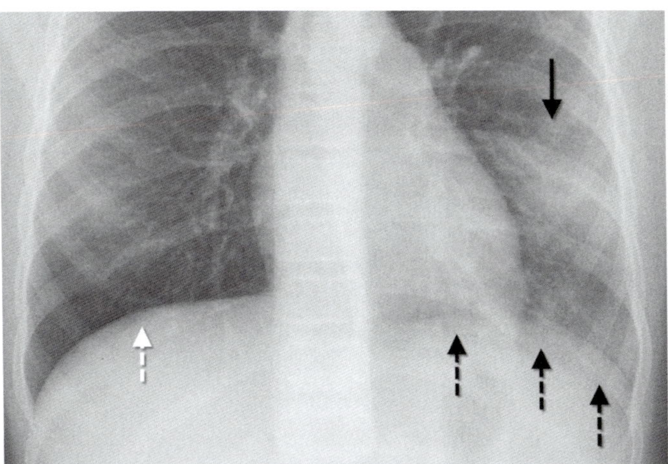

I-42

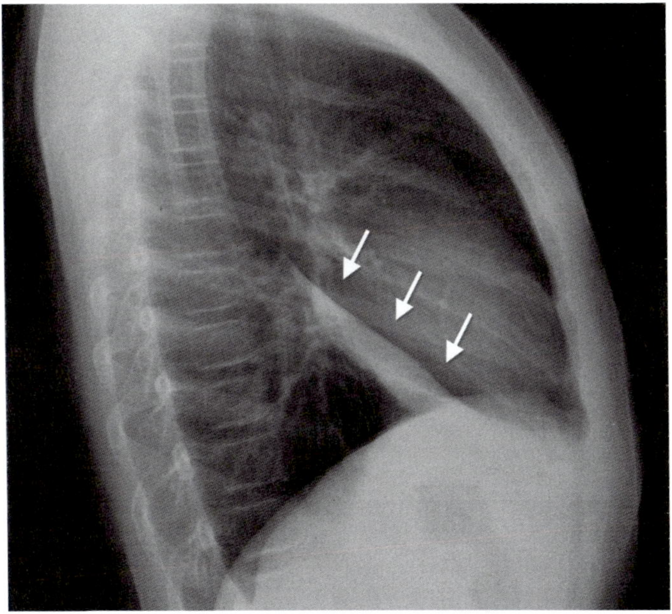

I-43

▪ SMALL AIRWAY DISEASE – INTRODUCTION 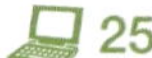 25

- Due to viral infection or reactive airway disease
- Peribronchial cuffing
- Air trapping

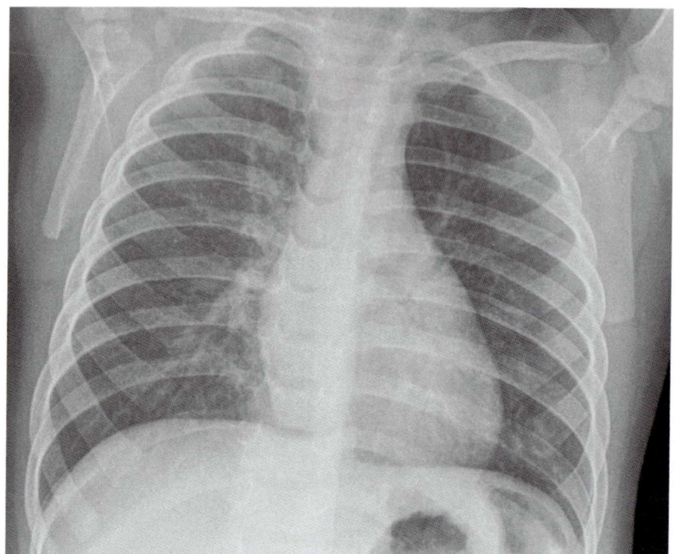

I-44

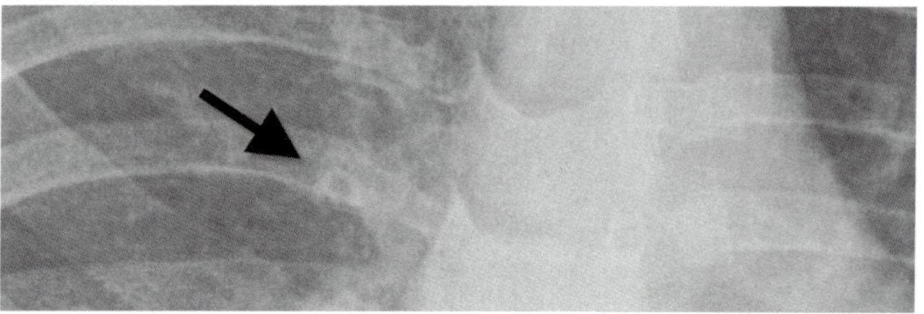

I-45

▪ VIRAL BRONCHIOLITIS 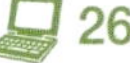 26

Small airway disease – viral bronchiolitis
Frontal and lateral chest radiographs show mild peribronchial cuffing (arrows), which is typical for small airways disease.

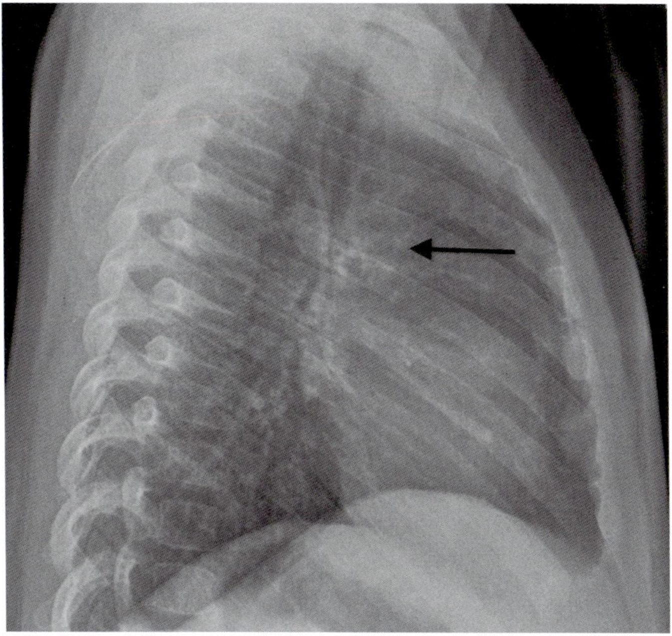

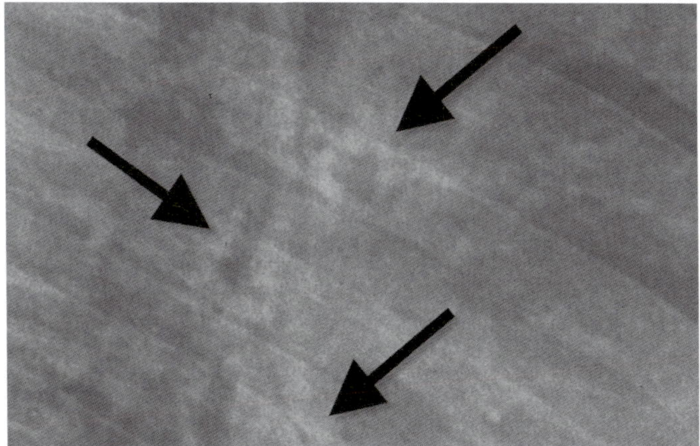

I-46

I-47

4. Pleural Space

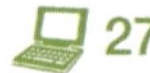 PNEUMOTHORAX – INTRODUCTION   27

Pneumothorax

- History (central-line placement, emphysema, trauma, tumor)
- No vascular markings beyond pleural line.
- Ipsilateral lung collapsed/more dense (depends on size).
- Elevation of ipsilateral hemidiaphragm (depends on size).
- Can hide behind ribs.
- Look for tension pneumothorax (mediastinal shift away from pneumothorax).

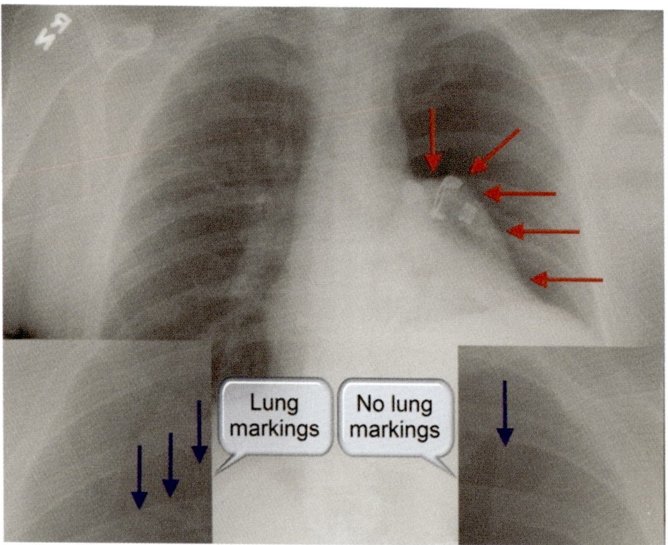

I-48

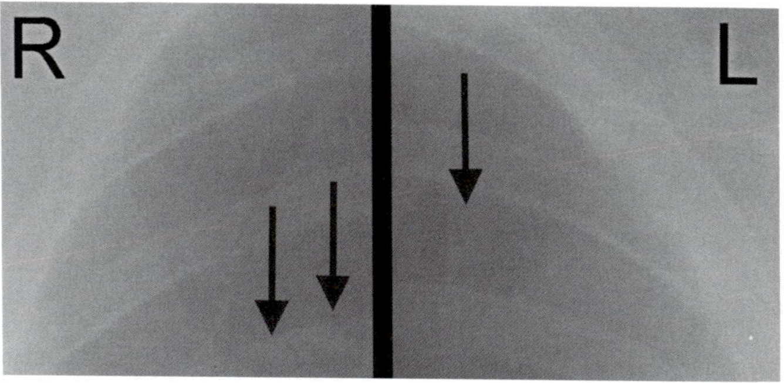

I-49

LARGE PNEUMOTHORAX 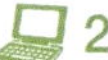 28

A single AP upright view of chest shows a large left pneumothorax with associated advanced collapse of left lung (left image red arrows). Absent lung markings on the left compared to the right (see magnified view on top image).

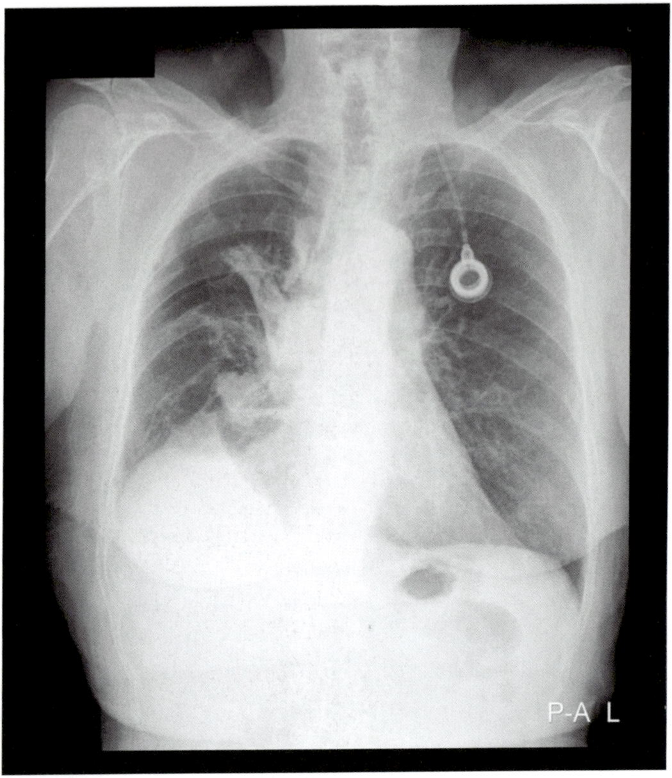

I-50

■ LARGE RIGHT PNEUMOTHORAX   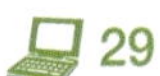 29

- Look along the pleural margins (arrows)!
- No vascular markings beyond pleural line.
- Ipsilateral lung is collapsed and more dense.
- Ipsilateral hemidiaphragm is elevated.

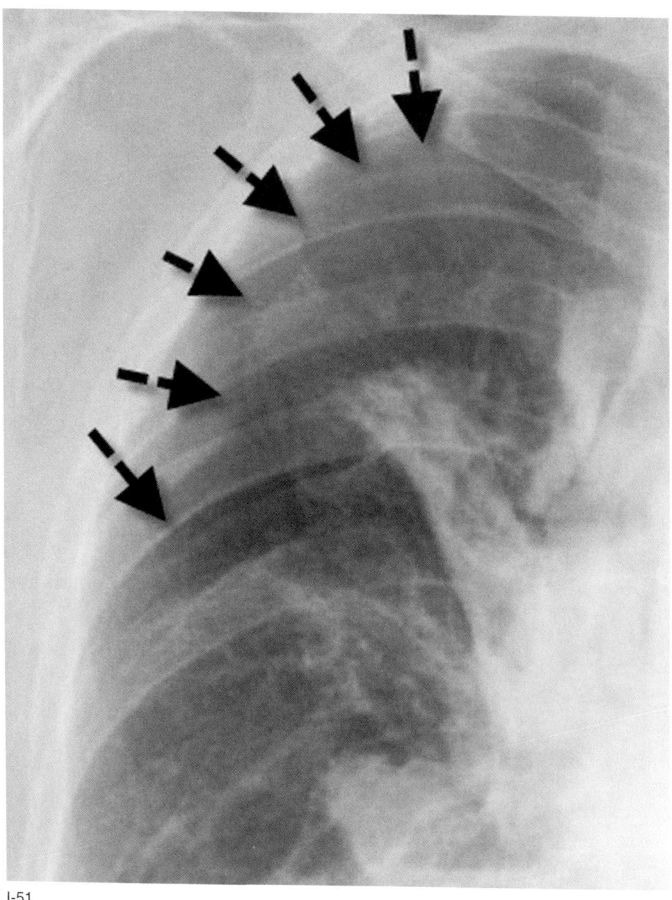

I-51

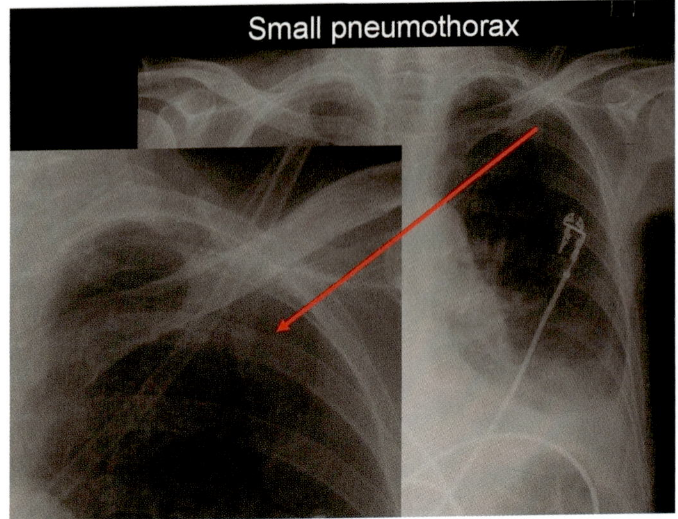

I-52

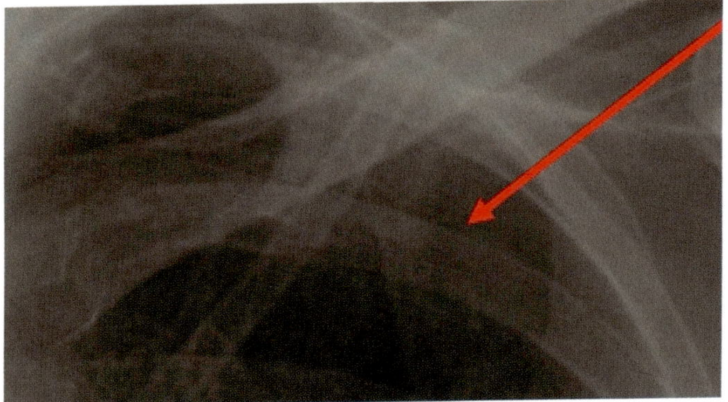

I-53

■ SMALL PNEUMOTHORAX   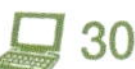 30

- Can hide behind ribs.
- Pleura may run parallel to ribs and may be misinterpreted as rib margin (arrow).

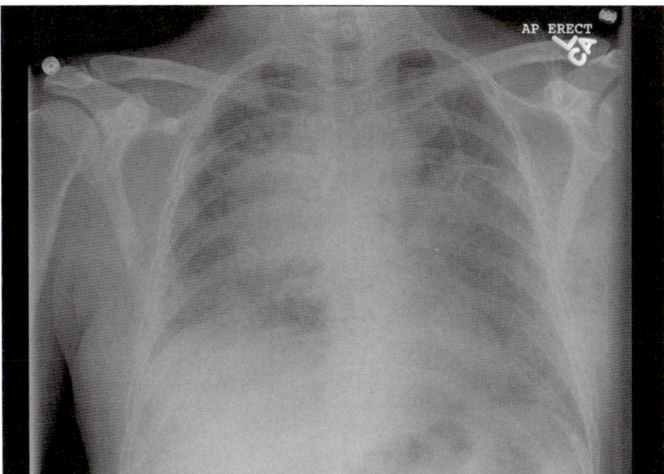

I-54

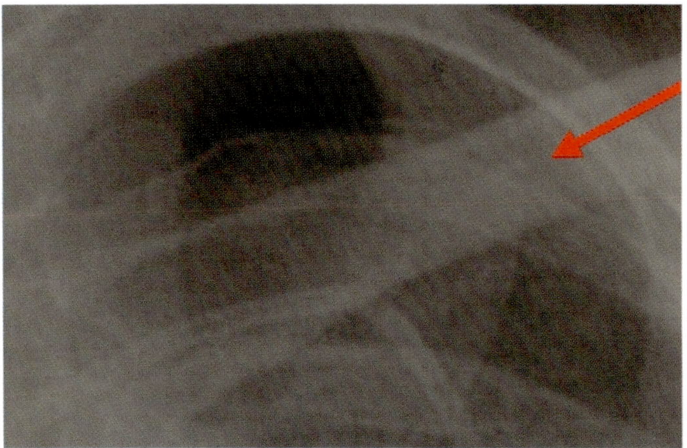

I-55

■ SMALL PNEUMOTHORAX 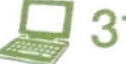 31

- Can hide behind ribs.
- Pleura may run parallel to ribs and may be misinterpreted as rib margin (arrow).

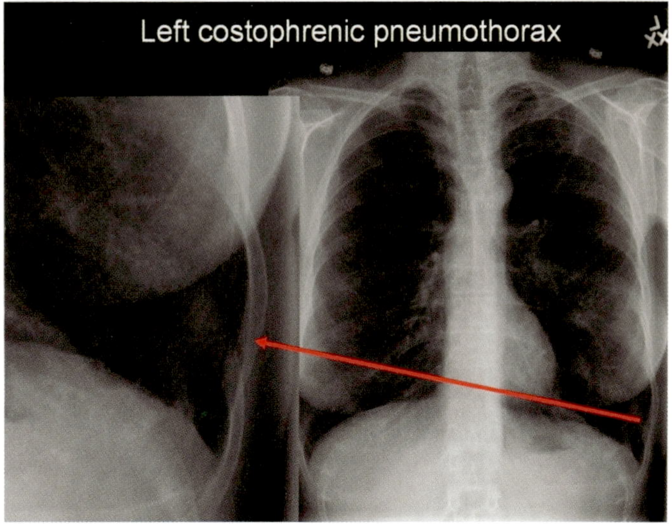

I-56

COSTOPHRENIC PNEUMOTHORAX 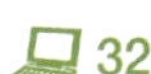 32

Small costophrenic pneumothorax

- Can hide behind ribs.
- Pleura may run parallel to ribs and may be misinterpreted as rib margin (arrow).

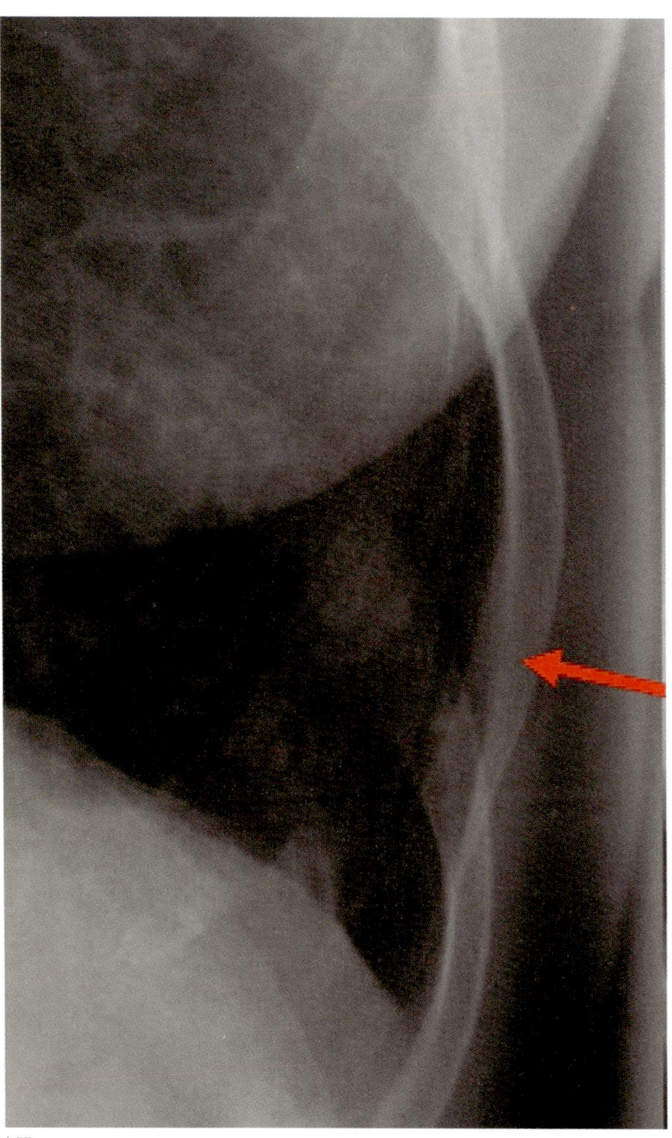

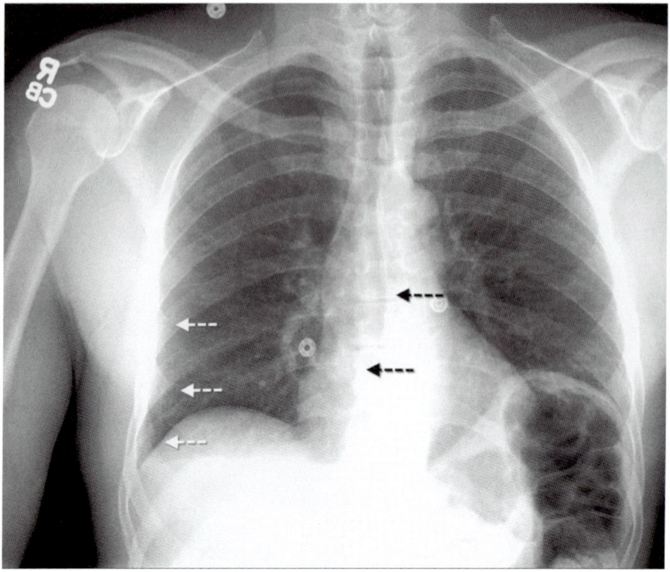

I-58

■ LOCULATED RETROSTERNAL PNEUMOTHORAX 💻 33

This patient was involved in an Motor Vehicle Accident (MVA) and suffered serial rib fractures (left image, white arrows). In addition he developed a loculated, retrosternal pneumothorax (black arrows, left images; white arrows, top image).

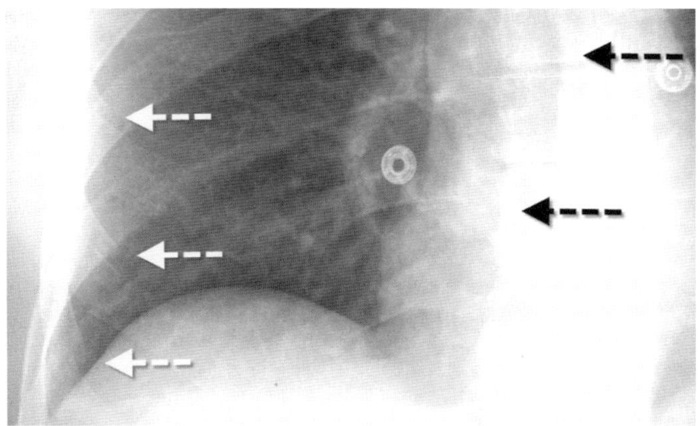

I-59

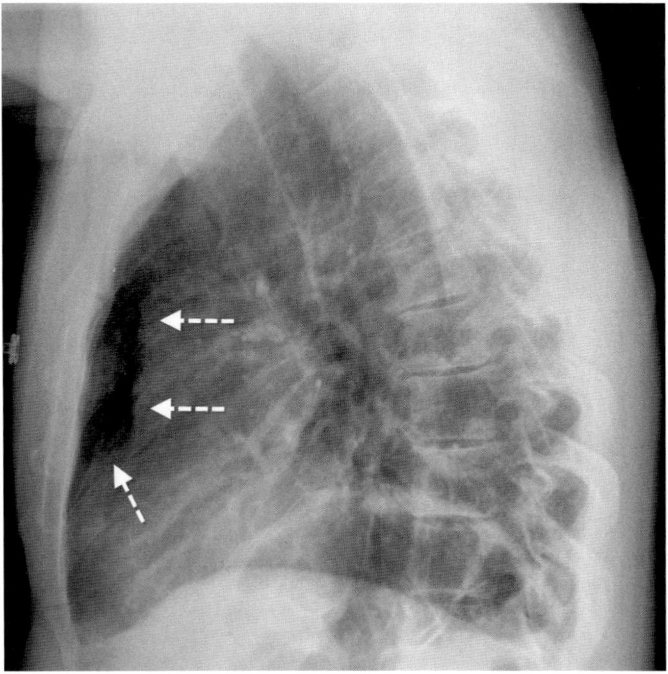

I-60

■ PLEURAL EFFUSION – INTRODUCTION 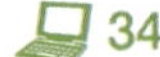 34

Pleural effusion

- Small (blunting of costophrenic angle)
- Large (partial/complete opacification of the lung)
- Multiple etiologies (CHF, trauma, postoperative, malignant, infectious)
- If unsure, do decubitus view (fluid moves – solid lesions don't!).

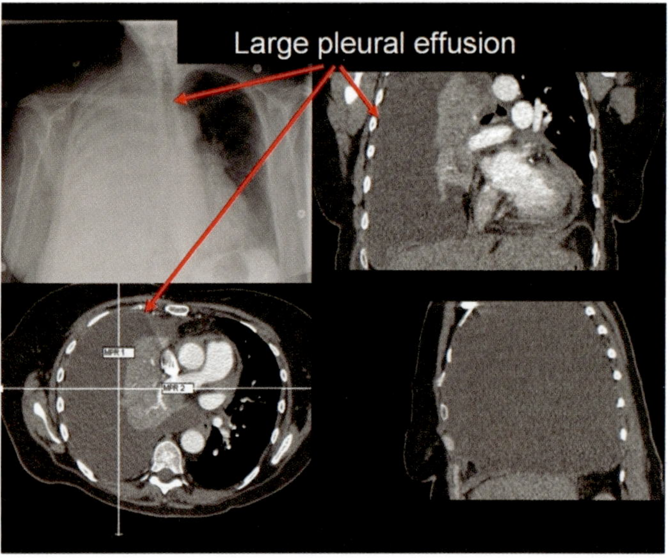

I-61

■ LARGE PLEURAL EFFUSION 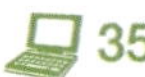 35

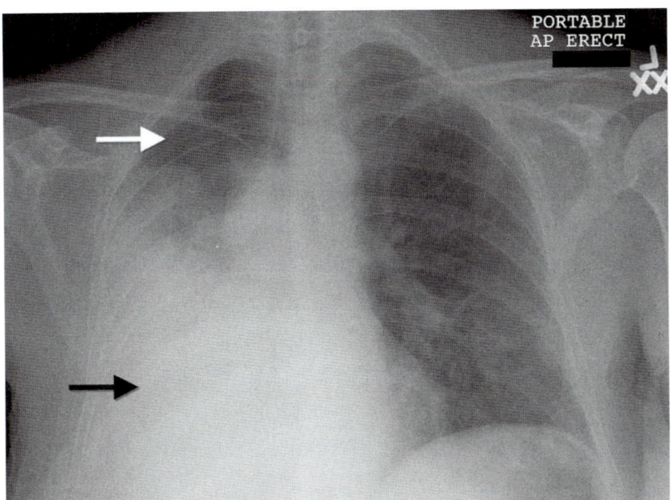

I-62

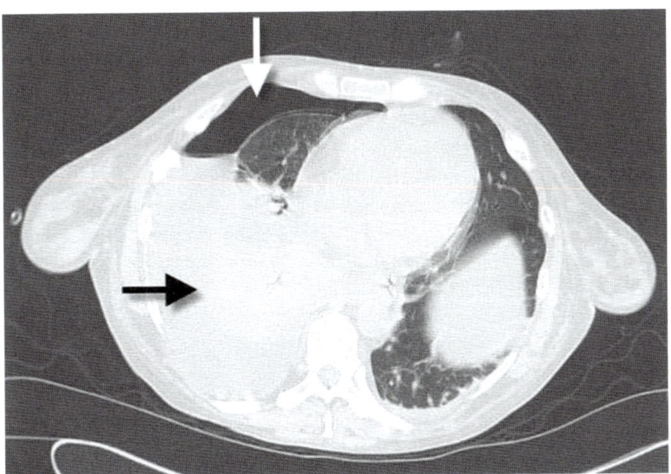

I-63

HYDROPNEUMOTHORAX 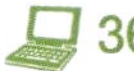 36

Frontal chest radiograph and CT show a right pleural effusion (black arrows) and a right pneumothorax (white arrows).

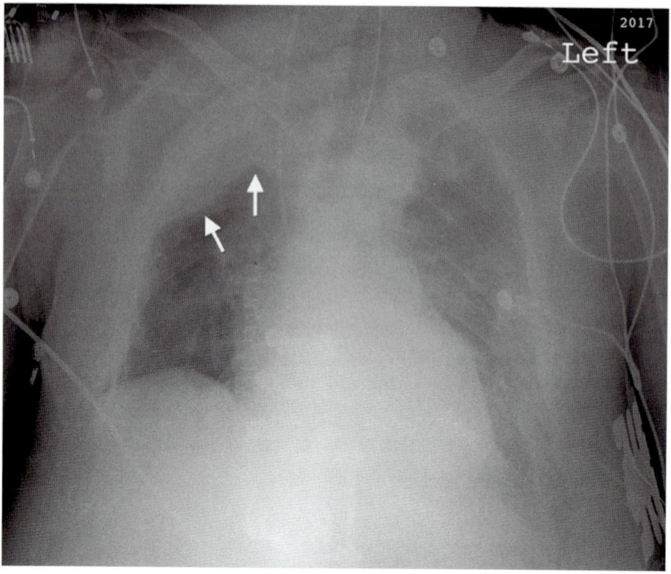

I-64

PLEURAL CAP

37

"Pleural cap"

There is a pleural effusion in the right lung apex. Fluid in the apex of the hemithorax is recognized as a pleural or apical cap. A comparison image from the day before (second image) did not reveal the pleural cap, excluding a chronic pleural process (neoplasm, pleural fibrosis/thickening, etc.).

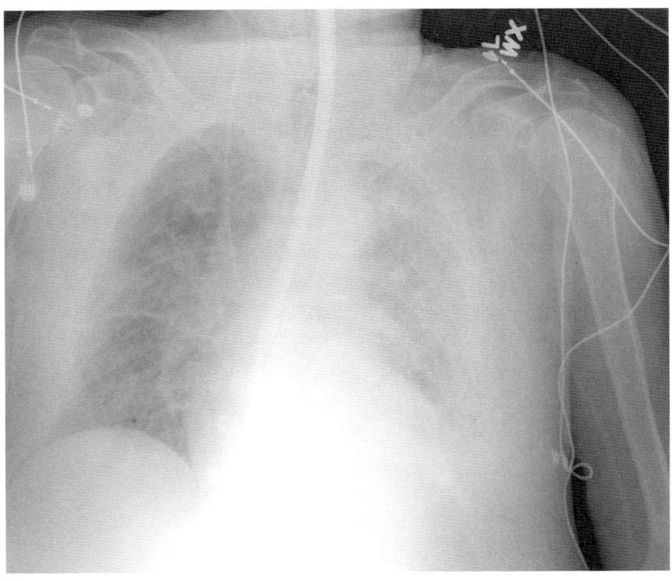

I-65

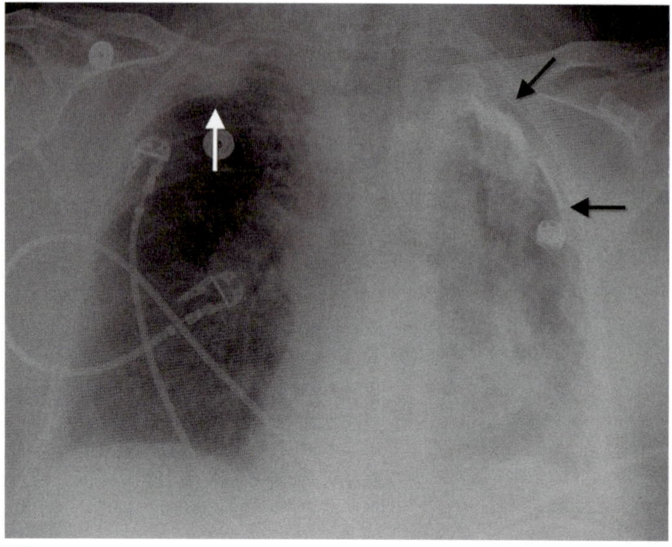

▩ TUBERCULOSIS (TB) – TUBERCULOMA AND CALCIFIC FIBROTHORAX

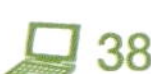 38

Tuberculosis (TB)

Incidence of TB is increasing (especially due to increased global travel). TB can present in multiple ways:

Primary TB

- Homogeneous consolidation (no cavitation)
- In upper or lower lobes
- With/without associated lymphadenopathy

Reactivation TB

- Typically in lung apices (white arrow in top first image).
- TB pleural empyema might lead to calcific fibrothorax (black arrows).

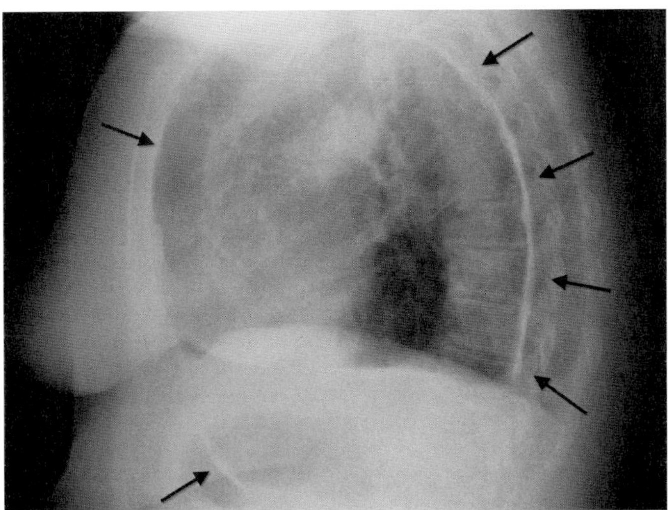

I-67

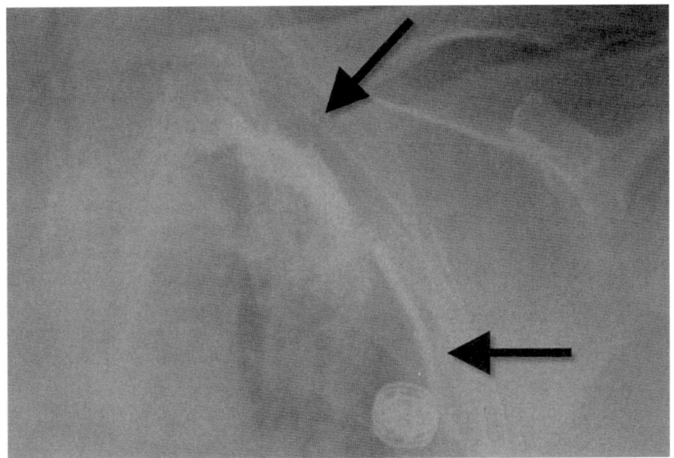

I-68

5. Mediastinum, Heart & Vessels

◼ CONGESTIVE HEART FAILURE (CHF) – INTRODUCTION

Congestive heart failure (CHF)

Multiple causes
- Coronary artery disease
- High blood pressure
- Cardiomyopathy (dilated, hypertropic, restrictive)
- Congenital heart disease
- Heart valve disease
- Heart tumor
- Lung disease
- Volume overload (renal disease)

Imaging findings
- Enlarged heart
- Prominent central vessels
- Kerley B lines
- Patchy lung opacifications
- Cephalization (upper vessels prominent)

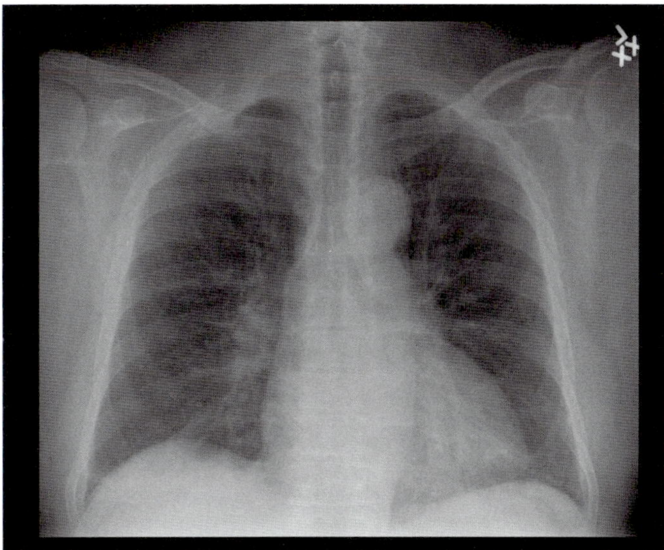

I-69

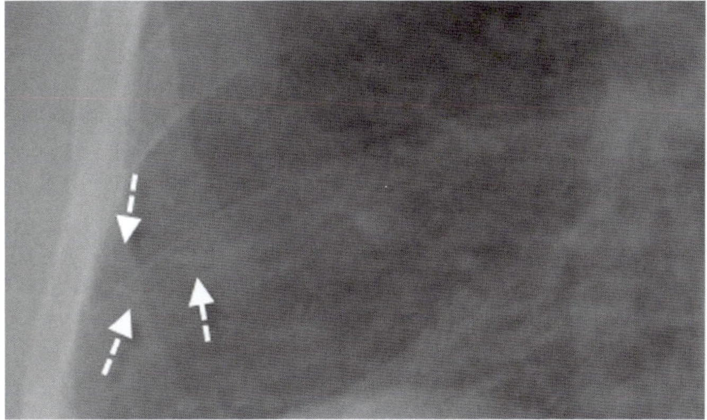

I-70

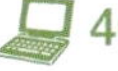 MILD CHF   40

- Mild CHF – Kerley B lines (arrows)

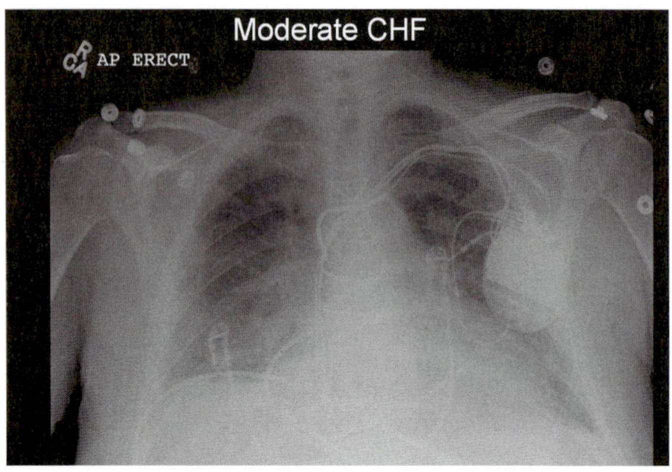

I-71

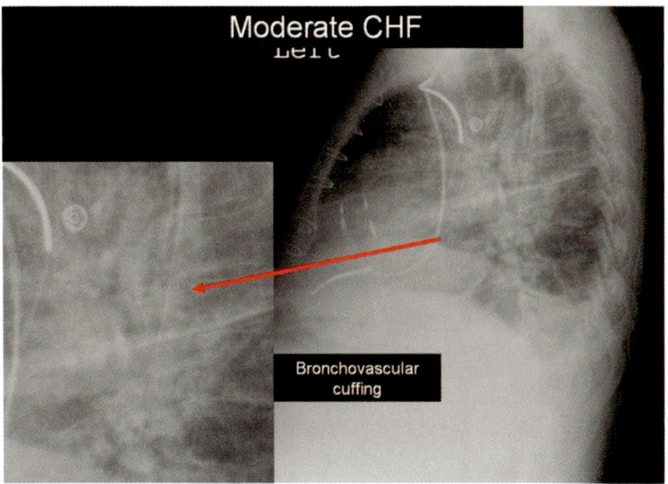

I-72

MODERATE CHF – BRONCHOVASCULAR CUFFING

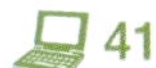 41

- Moderate CHF – bronchovascular cuffing (arrows)

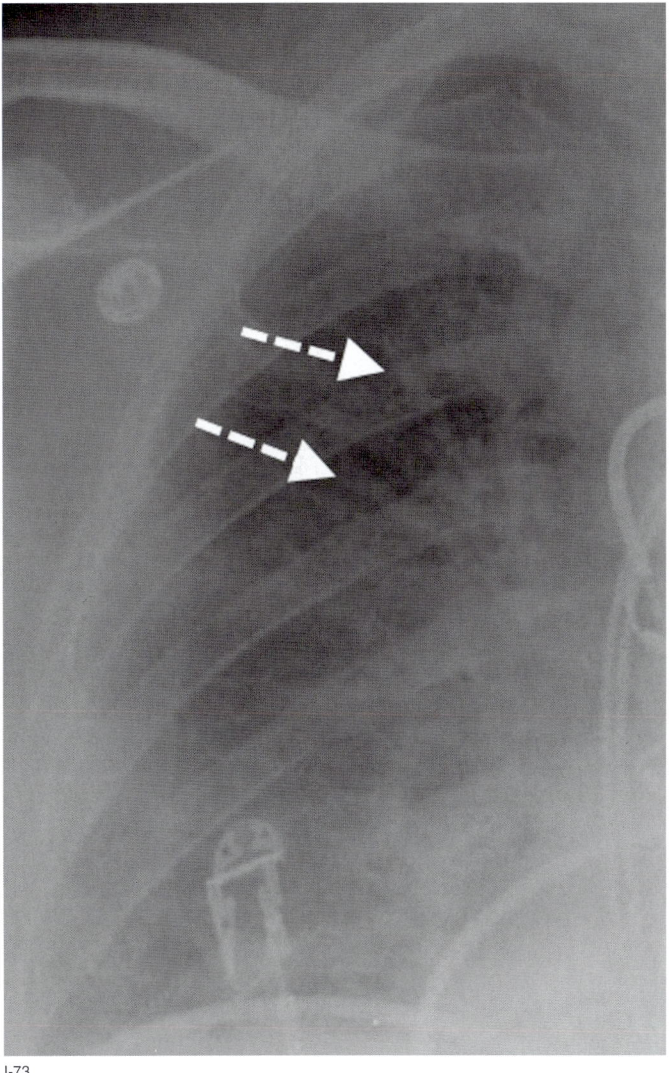

I-73

MODERATE CHF – CEPHALIZATION 42

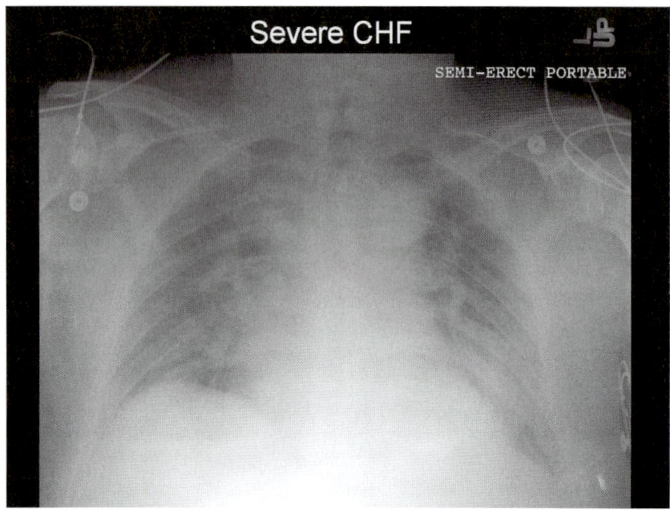

I-74

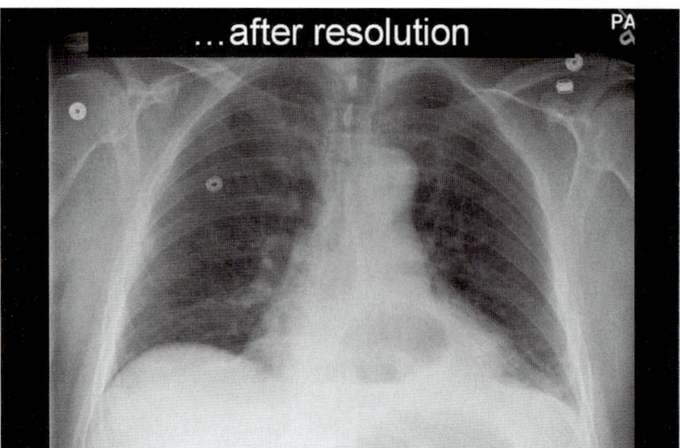

I-75

■ SEVERE CHF – PATCHY INFILTRATES 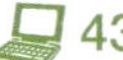 43

- Severe CHF – patchy infiltrates (upper image) and after resolution (bottom image)

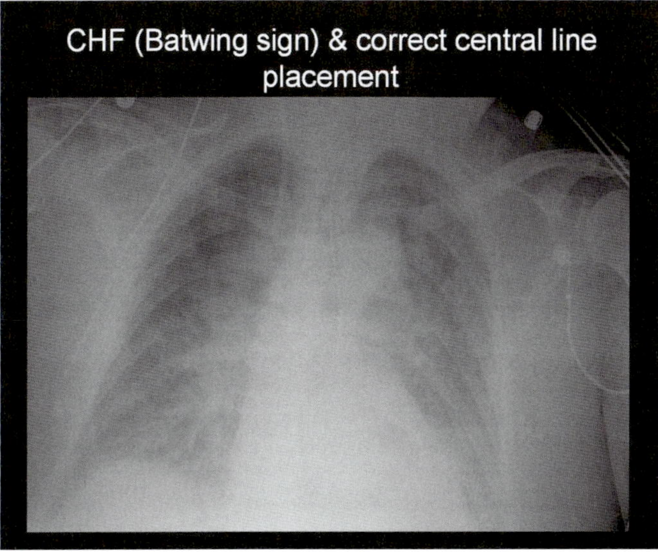

I-76

SEVERE CHF – BATWING SIGN 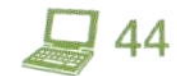 44

■ PULMONARY EDEMA – INTRODUCTION

 45

Pulmonary edema

Cardiogenic causes
- Heart failure
- Cardiac arrhythmias
- Fluid overload (eg renal failure)
- Cardiomyopathy
- Obstructing valvular disease (eg mitral stenosis)
- Myocarditis and infectious endocarditis

Non-cardiogenic causes
- Smoke inhalation
- Head trauma
- Sepsis
- Hypovolemic shock
- High altitude
- Disseminated intravascular coagulopathy (DIC)
- Near-drowning
- Massive aspiration
- Heroin overdose

Imaging findings
Cardiogenic (see CHF)

Non-cardiogenic:
- Ground glass opacification
- Air bronchograms

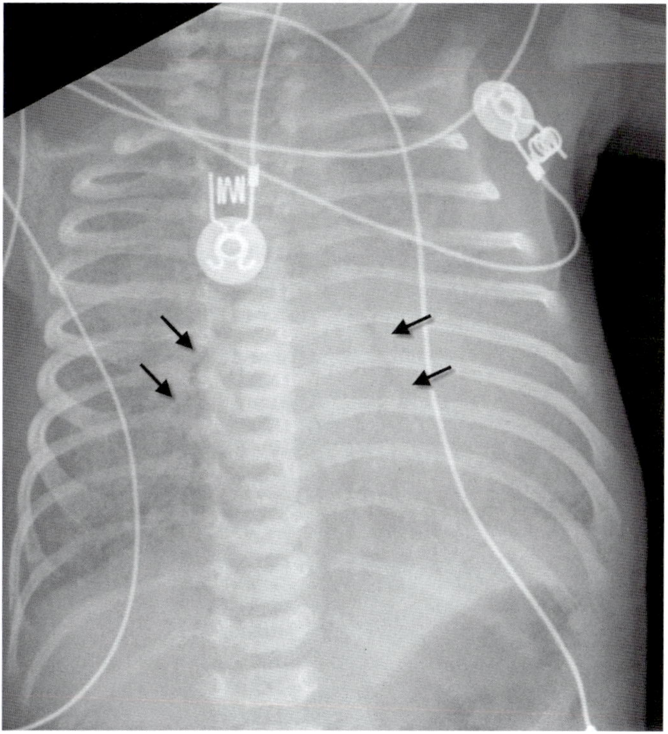

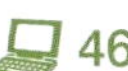

I-77

■ PULMONARY EDEMA 📖 46

Frontal chest radiograph of this infant with IRDS shows diffuse ground glass opacified lungs with air bronchograms (arrows).

■ PULMONARY HYPERTENSION – INTRODUCTION

▭ 47

Pulmonary hypertension

Multiple etiologies
- Chronic thrombotic/embolic disease
- COPD, ILD
- Sleep apnea
- Chronic exposure to high altitude
- Developmental lung abnormalities
- Cardiac/valvular disease
- Familial
- Idiopathic

Imaging findings
- Enlarged pulmonary artery (>30-mm diameter)
- Large right and left pulmonary arteries
- Abrupt tapering of right and left pulmonary arteries
- Tiny peripheral pulmonary artery branches
- Diffuse oligemia throughout lungs

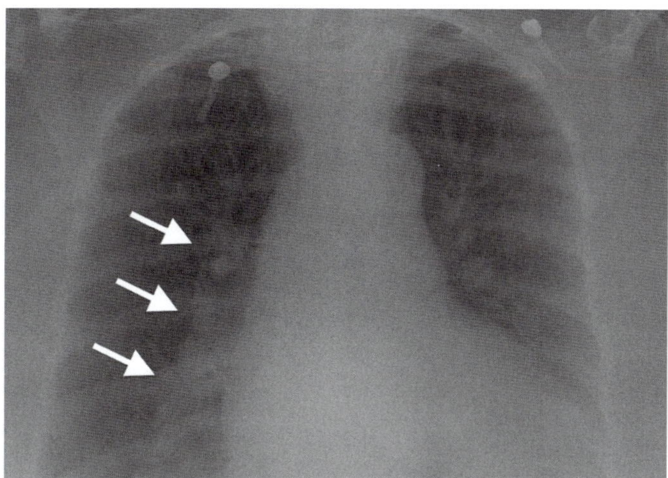

I-78

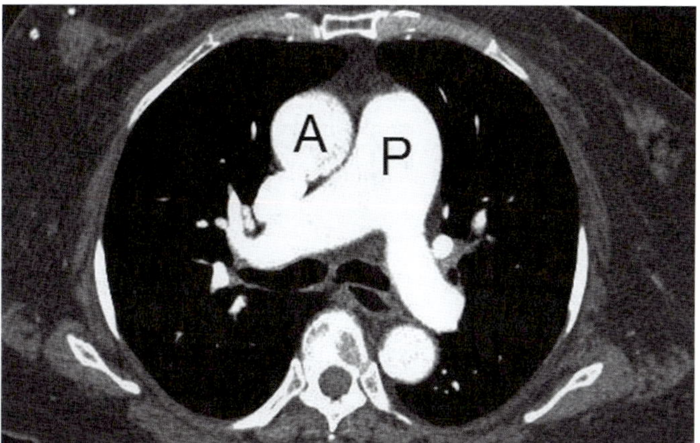

I-79

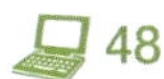 48

■ PULMONARY HYPERTENSION

First image shows the frontal radiograph of a patient who developed pulmonary hypertension secondary to COPD. There is enlargement and abrupt tapering of the right and left pulmonary arteries (arrows). Axial contrast-enhanced CT (second image) shows enlargement of the main pulmonary artery (P), which has a larger diameter than the ascending aorta (A).

■ PULMONARY EMBOLISM (PE) – INTRODUCTION

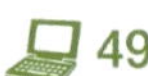 49

Pulmonary embolism (PE)

- Common and potentially lethal condition that can cause death in all age groups.
- Complication of underlying venous thrombosis (usually lower extremities).
- Patients at risk: previous gynecologic surgery, major trauma, indwelling venous catheters.
- D-Dimer has a very high negative predictive but low positive predictive value.
- Usually starts in calf veins, and propagates to popliteal vessels before going to lungs – ultrasound essential to rule out DVT.
- In two-thirds of patients with PE the site of DVT cannot be visualized by ultrasound; thus a negative duplex ultrasound does not markedly reduce the likelihood of PE.

Imaging modalities

- Chest radiograph is virtually always negative.
- Angiogram is still "gold standard" but practically replaced by multidetector CT (MDCT), which has comparable sensitivity and specificity to pulmonary angiography.
- Benefit of MDCT: fast, can also detect other underlying causes of the patient's symptoms.
- V/Q (ventilation/perfusion) scanning is indicated when other modalities are not possible (contrast allergy, renal failure, etc.)

Imaging findings (PE)

Pulmonary angiogram

- (Wedge shaped) absent perfusion distal to the embolus

MDCT

- Filling defect in pulmonary artery and/or branches
- Acute PE: more central filling defect (within the center of vessel lumen)
- Chronic PE: more wall adherent filling defect

V/Q scan Prospective Investigation of Pulmonary Embolism Diagnosis (PIOPED) criteria

Normal V/Q scan: No perfusion defects are seen.

High-probability V/Q scan:

- Two or more segmental or larger perfusion defects with normal chest radiographs and normal ventilation
- Two or more segmental or larger perfusion defects where chest radiographic abnormalities and ventilation defects are substantially smaller than the perfusion defects
- Two or more subsegmental and one segmental perfusion defect with normal chest radiograph and normal ventilation
- Four or more subsegmental perfusion defects with normal chest radiograph and normal ventilation
- In most clinical settings, high-probability scan pattern considered positive for PE

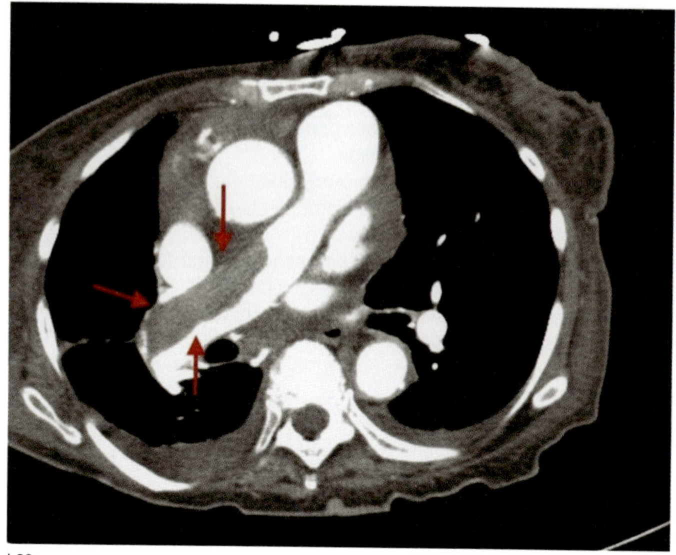

I-80

PULMONARY EMBOLUS IN RIGHT PULMONARY ARTERY

 50

This pulmonary embolus has a more chronic appearance, since it is wall adherent. Acute emboli are more centrally located within the vessel lumen. This patient has also a right atrial thrombus (arrow, right image). Atrial thrombi may not cause symptoms by itself (sometimes arrhythmia) but pose the risk of dislodging and causing pulmonary embolism.

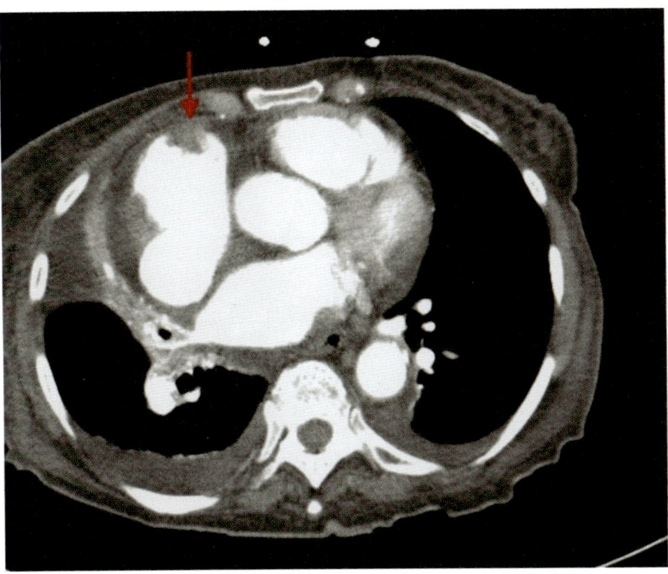

I-81

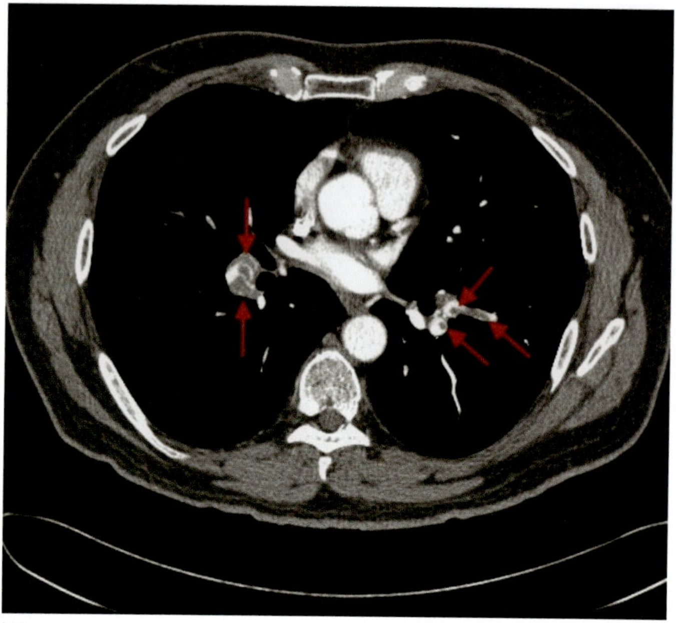

I-82

SHOWER OF PULMONARY EMBOLI  51

Multiple luminal filling defects are seen in the segmental and subsegmental branches of bilateral pulmonary arteries (arrows), consistent with a shower of acute pulmonary emboli. The more central luminal location of the emboli speaks more for an acute event.

Second image is a coronal reformatted image of the same patient.

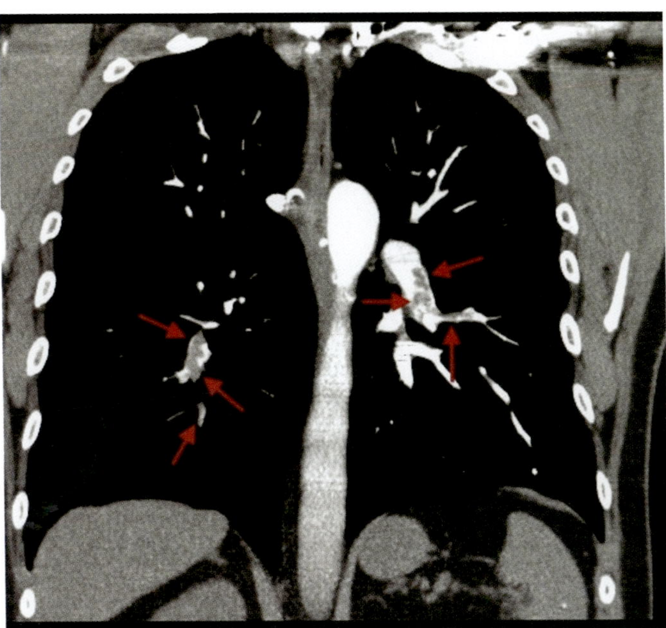

I-83

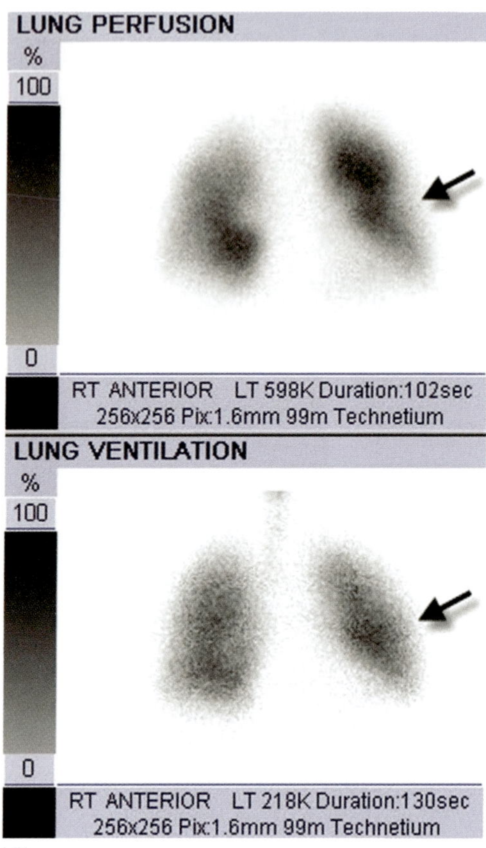

I-84

PULMONARY EMBOLISM – HIGH PROBABILITY ON V/Q SCAN 52

Mismatched perfusion abnormalities are identified in both lungs, specifically in the superior and inferior lingular segments within the left lung (arrow).

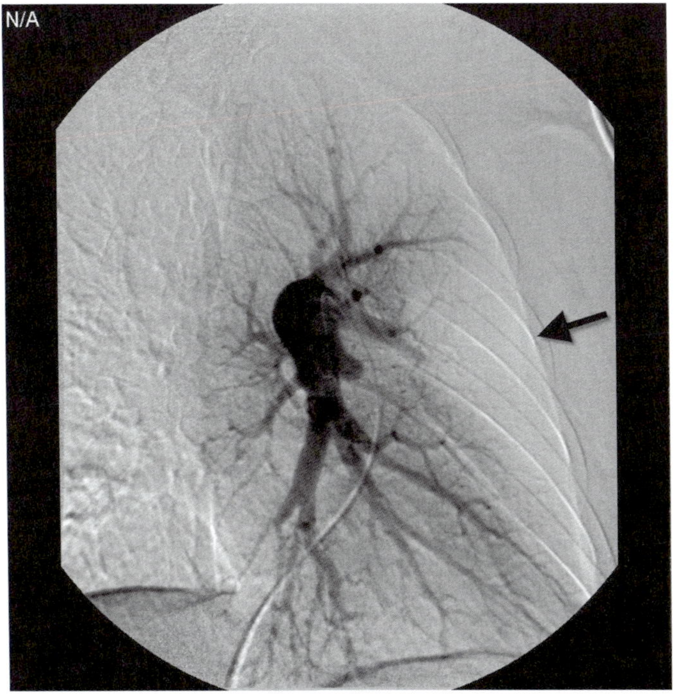

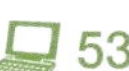

PULMONARY EMBOLISM – PULMONARY ANGIOGRAM 53

Angiogram of the left pulmonary artery demonstrates an abrupt contrast stop in several segmental artery branches, causing a wedge-shaped defect (arrow). This area corresponds to the mismatched defect seen on the V/Q scan (see first image).

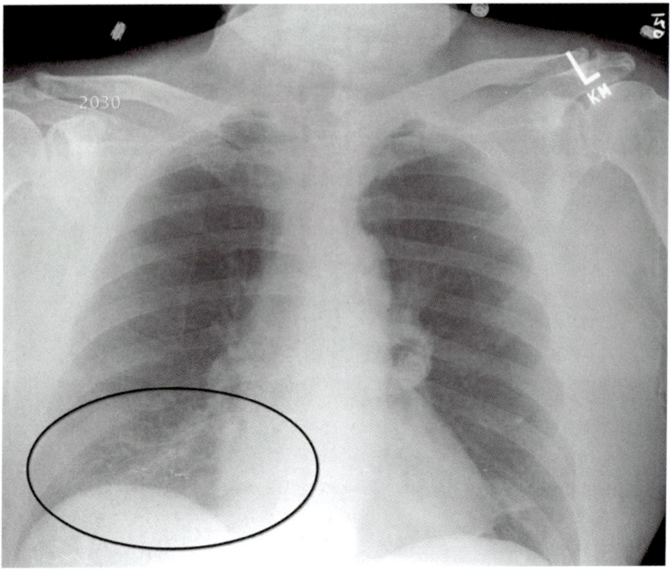

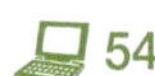

I-86

PULMONARY EMBOLISM – INTERMEDIATE PROBABILITY ON V/Q SCAN

54

Pulmonary embolism

Frontal chest radiograph (top image) demonstrates an opacity project-ing over the medial right lung base. The patient presented with acute chest pain, and a V/Q scan was ordered to rule out pulmonary embolism (see right image).

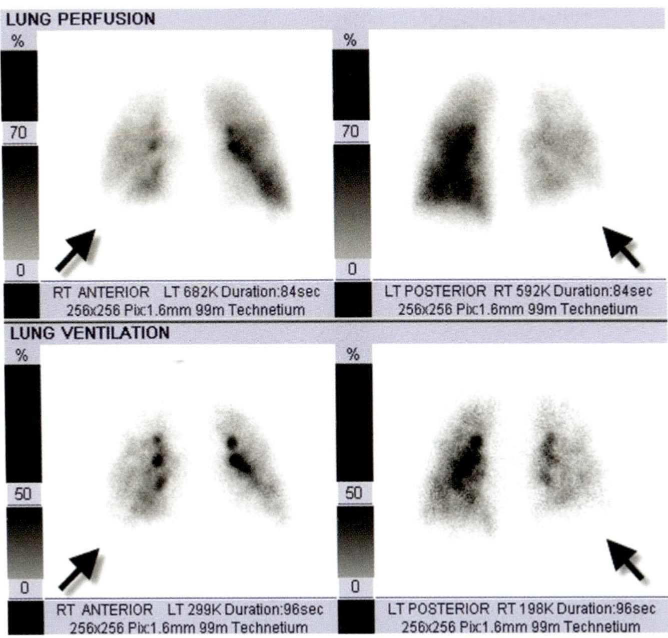

I-87

Intermediate probability for PE on V/Q scan

This V/Q scan demonstrates multiple nonsegmental matched ventilation/ perfusion abnormalities. A matched ventilation/perfusion defect is identified in the right lung base (arrows, upper image) and corresponds to an abnormality seen on the chest X-ray (circle, left image). In light of this triple match, this lung scan is associated with an intermediate probability for pulmonary embolism. (Also seen is central airway deposition of the radioaerosol.)

◼ AORTIC DISSECTION (AD) – INTRODUCTION

💻 55

Aortic dissection (AD)

Risk factors
- Hypertension
- Connective tissue disorders (Marfan, Ehlers–Danlos)
- Vasculitis
- Trauma (deceleration trauma, MVA)
- In females: pregnancy risk factor

If ruptured: 80% mortality rate; 50% of patients die before they even reach the hospital.

Stanford classification system divides AD into two groups:
- A = originates in ascending aorta
- B = originates in the descending aorta

Type A is an emergency and usually has to be treated surgically because of risk:
1. Extension into aortic valve → aortic insufficiency, arrhythmia
2. Rupture into pericardium → pericardial tamponade
3. Occlusion of coronary arteries

Type B can be usually managed medically.

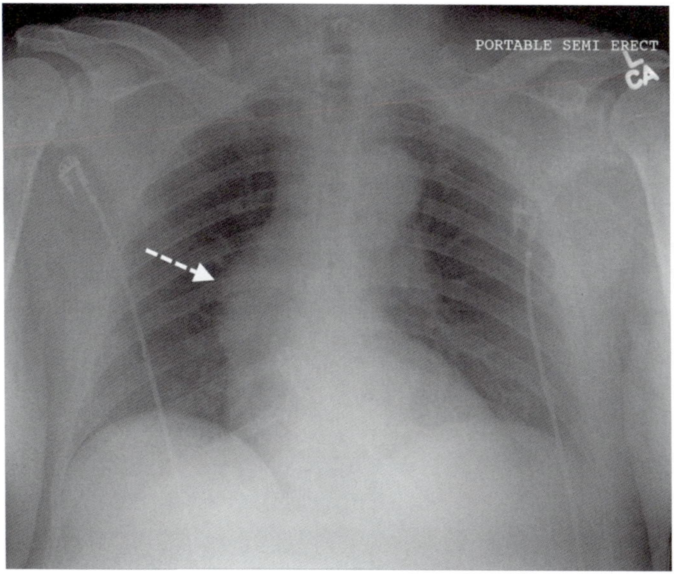

I-88

TYPE A AORTIC DISSECTION   56

There is abnormal contour of the ascending aorta with widening of the right mediastinum on this radiograph.

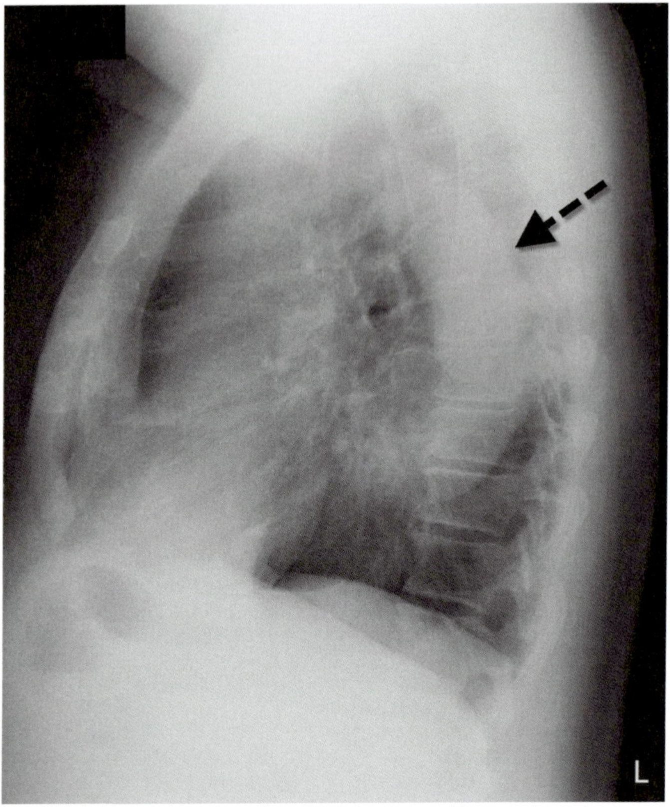

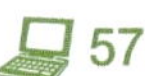

I-89

■ AORTIC ANEURYSM 57

- Thoracic aortic aneurysm.
- Prominence of aortic arch and/or descending aorta.
- Can often not be distinguished from dissection – clinical history and symptoms important (trauma, acute chest pain).
- CT confirms in this case a partially thrombosed aortic aneurysm (right bottom: axial oblique reformatted CT).

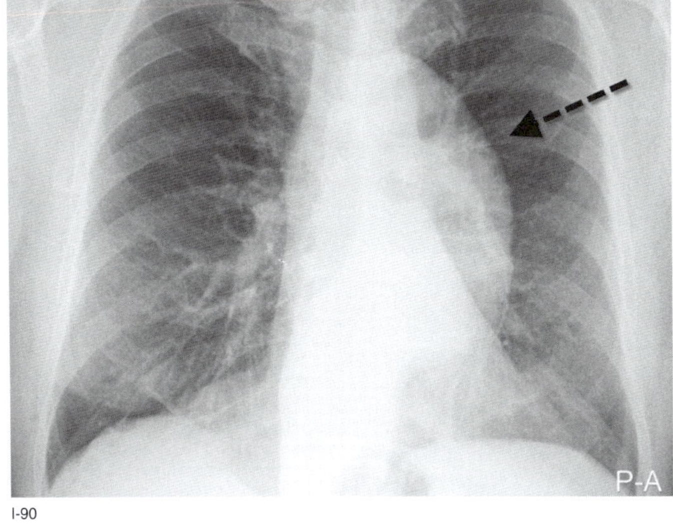

I-90

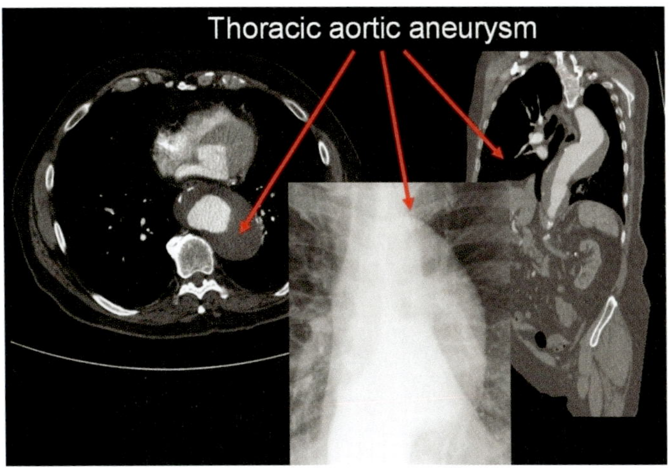

I-91

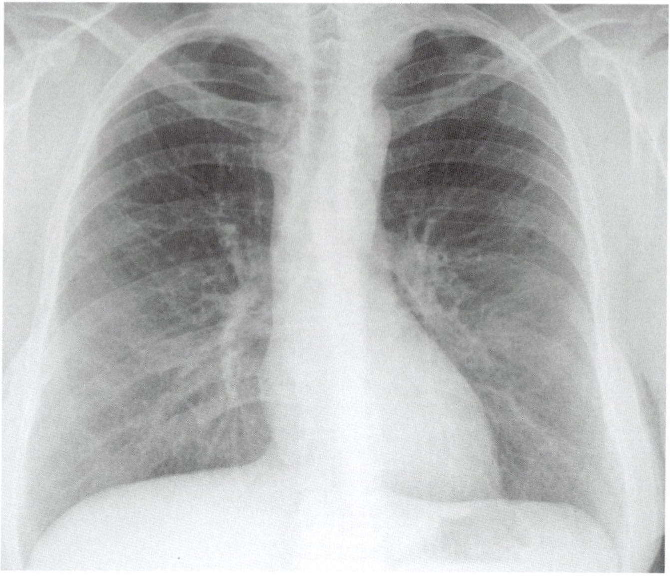

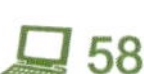

I-92

AORTIC COARCTATION   58

- Figure 3 Sign (right middle and bottom image)
- Rib notching – most often 4th–8th ribs (arrows right middle image)
- Rib notching because 4th–8th intercostal arteries anastomose with internal mammary artery to form collaterals for descending aorta

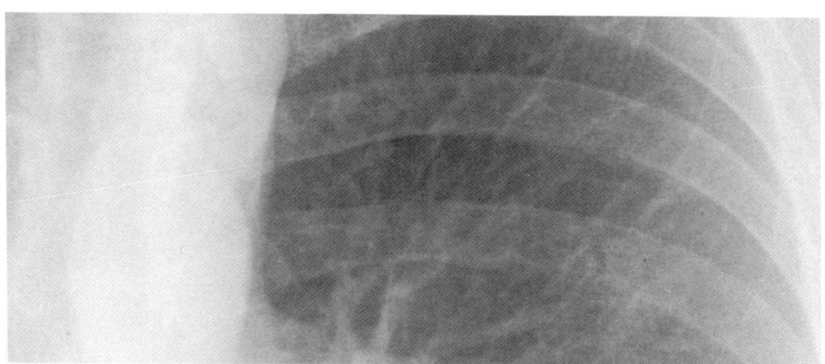

I-93

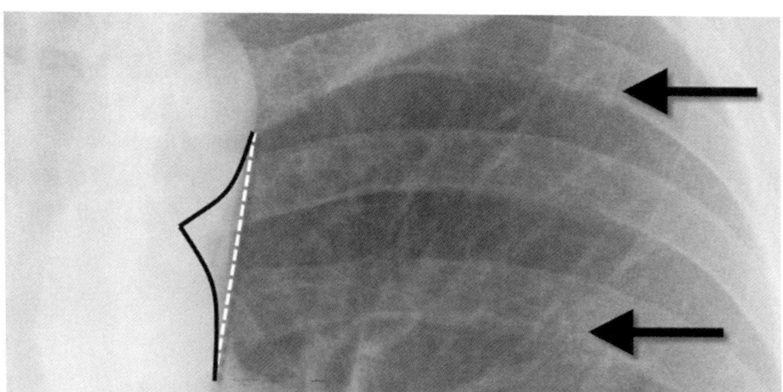

I-94

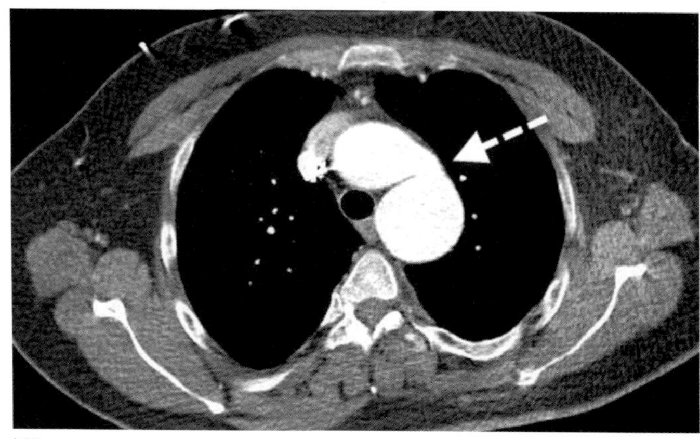

I-95

■ PNEUMOMEDIASTINUM/ PNEUMOPERICARDIUM – INTRODUCTION 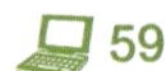 59

Pneumomediastinum/Pneumopericardium

Etiology is multifactorial:
- Blunt force or penetrating chest trauma
- Endobronchial or esophageal procedures
- Neonatal lung disease
- Mechanical (hyperbaric) ventilation
- Chest surgery or other invasive procedures

Findings
- Air within the mediastinal space.
- Radiolucent streaks (free air) along margins of heart, within the retrosternal space, or surrounding trachea.
- Ring around the artery (tubular artery) sign: radiolucent area surrounding the right pulmonary artery (on lateral chest radiograph).
- Thymic sail sign: in infants with pneumomediastinum, the thymic lobes are shifted upward resembling a full sail.
- Continuous diaphragm sign: free air between the pericardium and diaphragm, causing the central parts of the diaphragm to become apparent.
- Pneumopericardium: in the pericardial cavity.

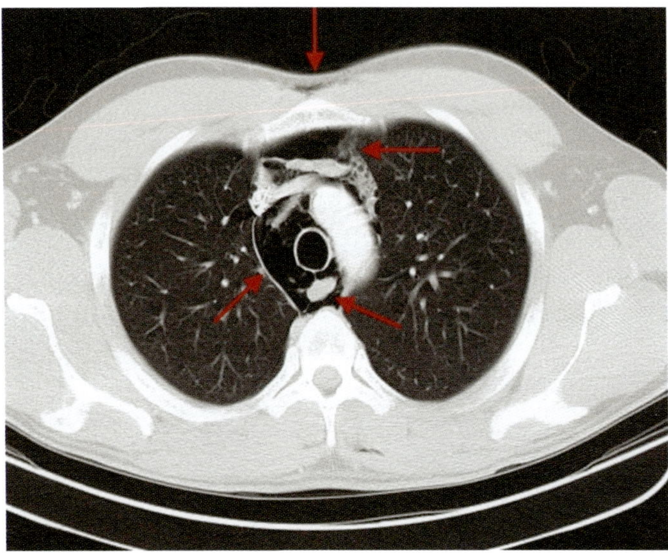

I-96

▪ PNEUMOMEDIASTINUM 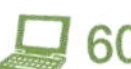 60

Air is seen within the mediastinum – separating mediastinal structures, such as trachea, esophagus and aorta.

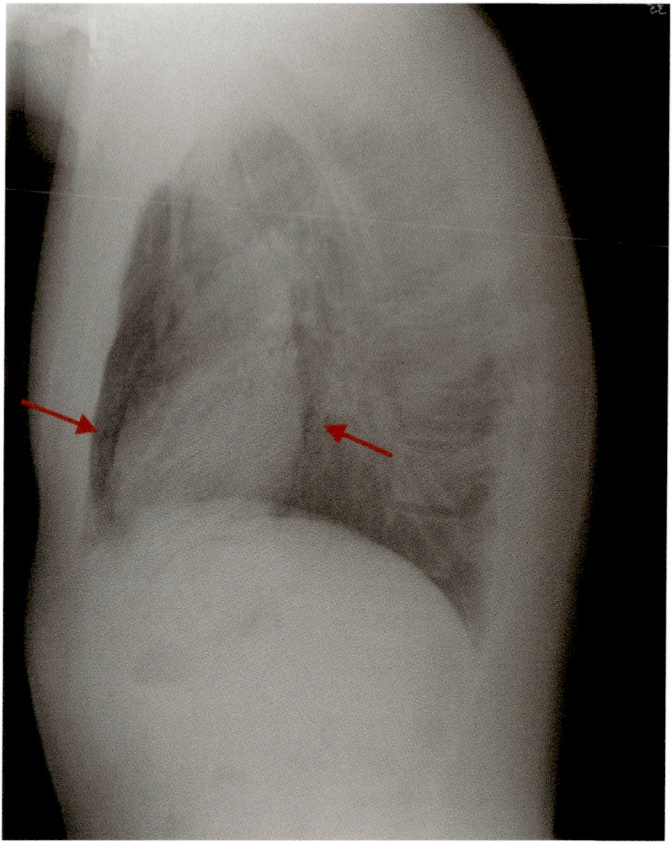

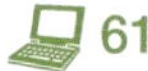

I-97

■ PNEUMOPERICARDIUM   61

Linear lucencies (air) are seen anterior and posterior to the heart border, outlining the pericardium.

6. Chest Wall & Diaphragm

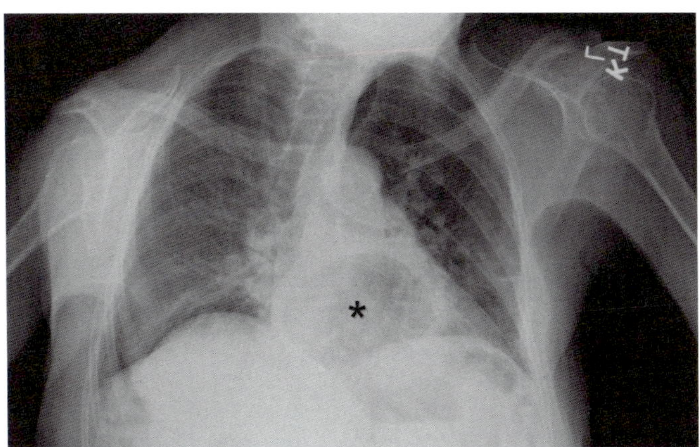

I-98

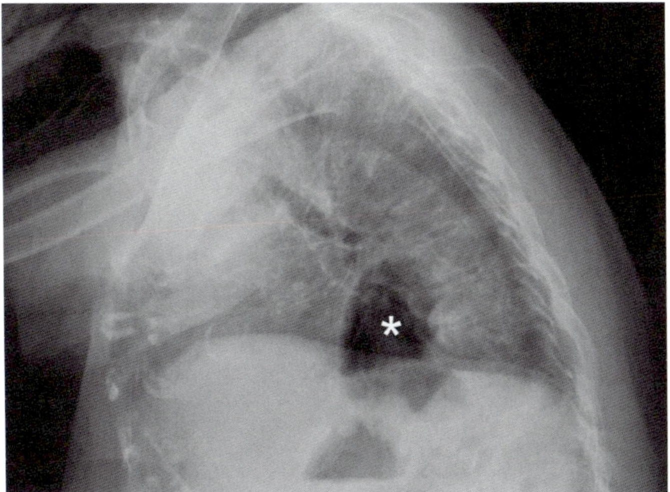

I-99

■ DIAPHRAGMATIC HERNIA 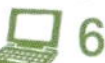 62

Large area of air lucency projecting over the medial inferior mediastinum (asterisk) consistent with a hiatal hernia.

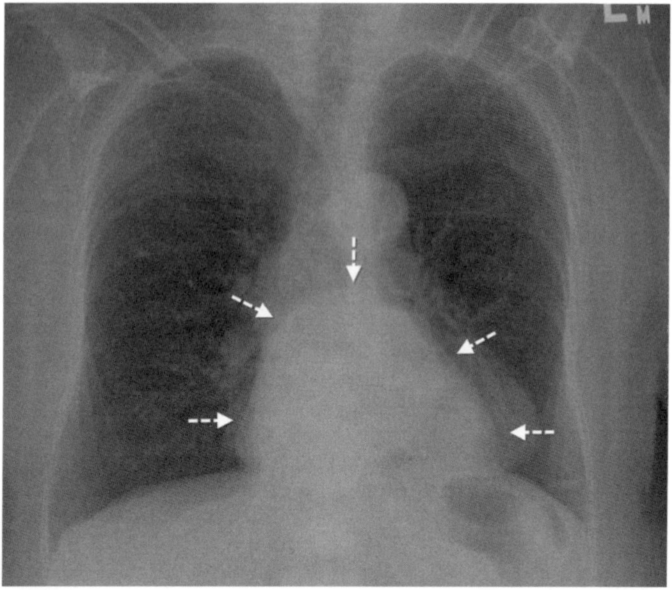

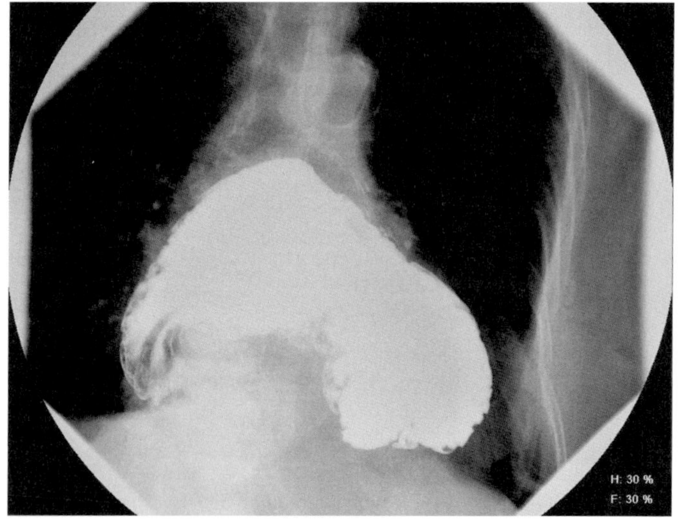

I-100

I-101

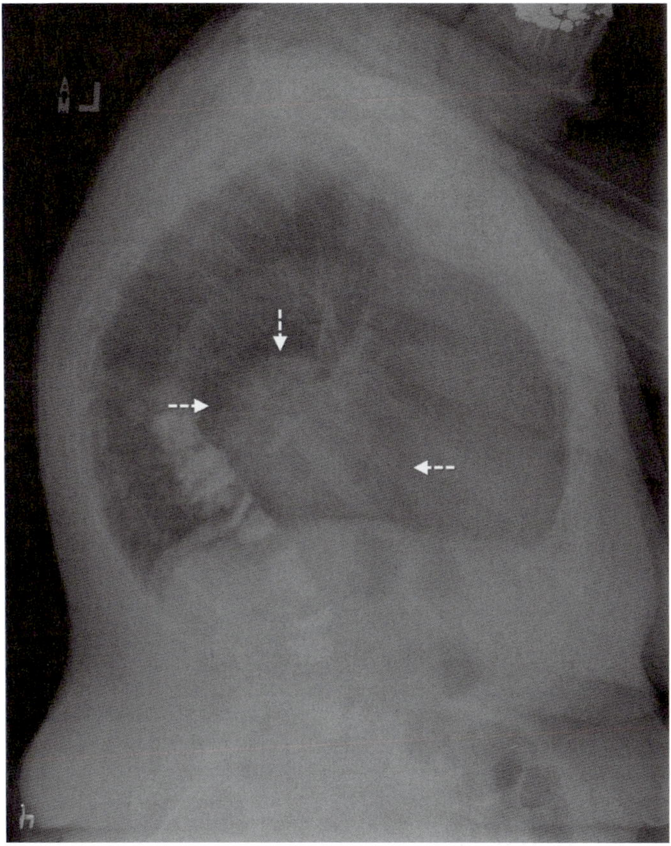

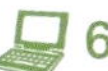

I-102

HIATAL HERNIA WITH ORGANOAXIAL ROTATION

63

Frontal chest radiograph (left top image) shows a large mass projecting over the medial inferior mediastinum (arrows), consistent with a hiatal hernia. However, an upper GI study confirms an organoaxial rotation of the stomach (left bottom image).

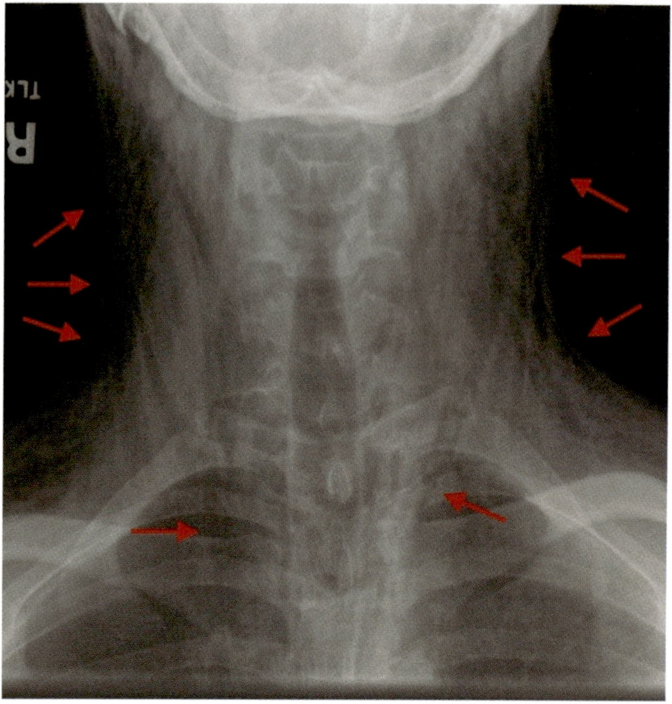

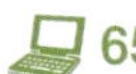

I-103

■ SUBCUTANEOUS EMPHYSEMA   65

Air is seen on these frontal and lateral radiographs of the neck within the subcutaneous soft tissues of the neck and chest.

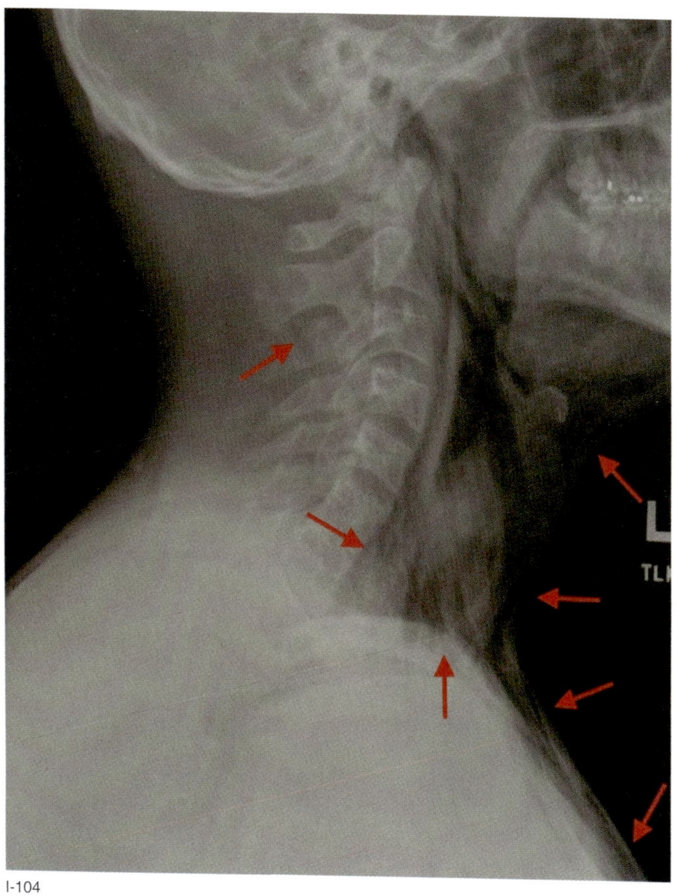

I-104

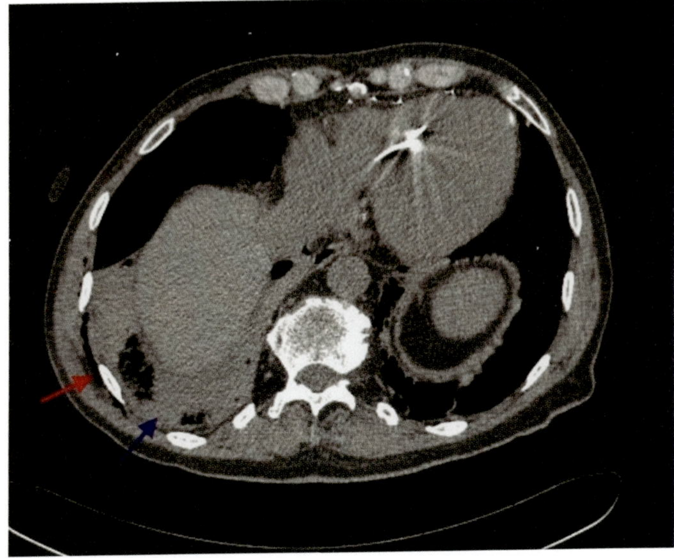

I-105

SERIAL RIB FRACTURES WITH HEMOPNEUMOTHORAX

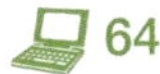 64

CT in soft tissue (top image), bone (right top image), and lung (right bottom image) windows demonstrate acute fractures of the right sixth through ninth ribs laterally and posterolaterally (red arrows) and a tiny right hemopneumothorax (blue arrows in lung window). Also seen is a pleural effusion/hemorrhage and parenchymal contusion/hemorrhage (blue arrows in soft tissue and bone windows).

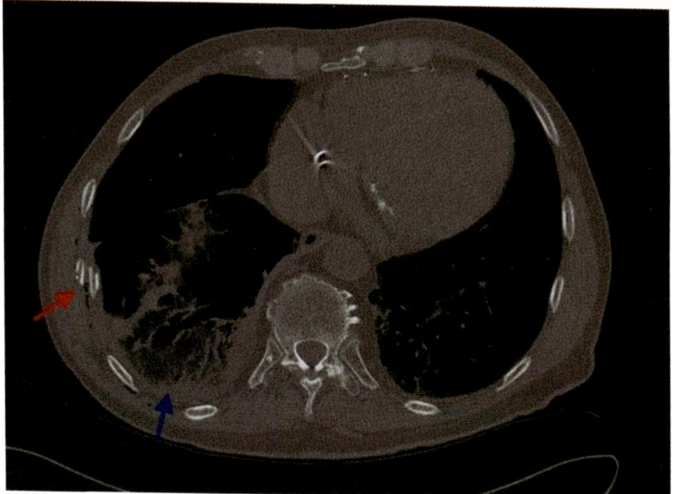

I-106

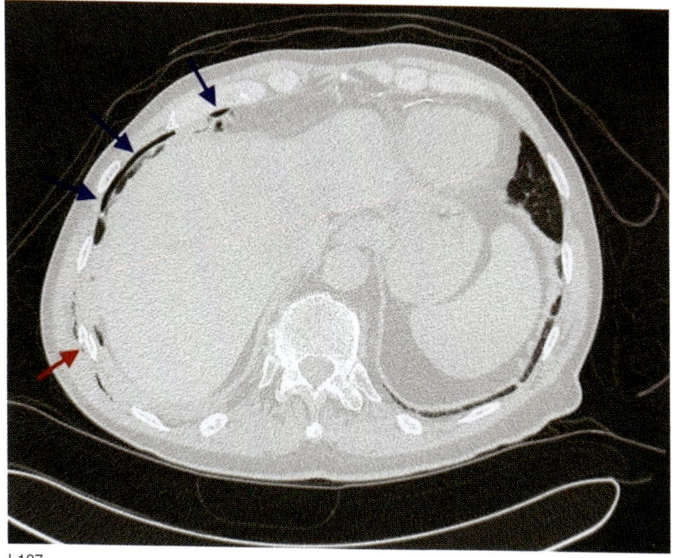

I-107

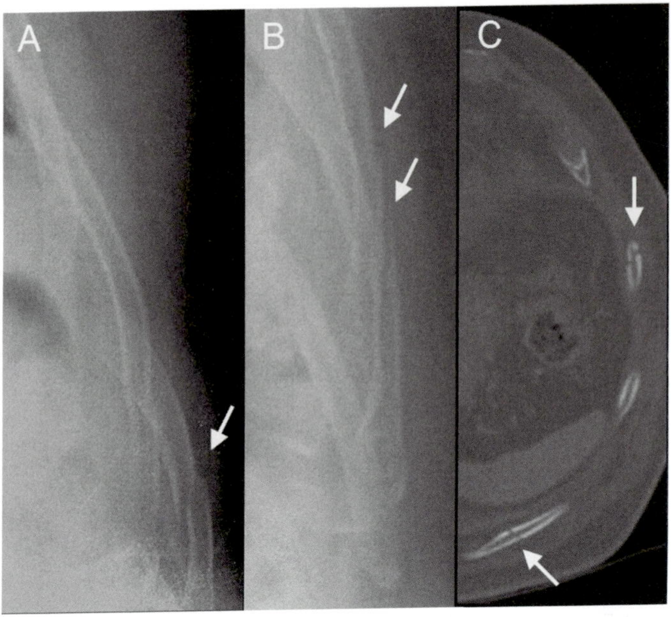

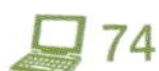

I-108

■ SERIAL RIB FRACTURES   74

PA radiograph of the chest (A) and dedicated rib view (B) demonstrate acute nondisplaced fractures of the left eighth and ninth lateral ribs. CT of the chest in bone window (C) confirms fractures of the left eigth and ninth ribs but detects additional fractures of the posterior left 10th, 11th, and 12th ribs as well as the lateral aspect of the left 9th, 10th, and 11th ribs (arrows).

7. Devices

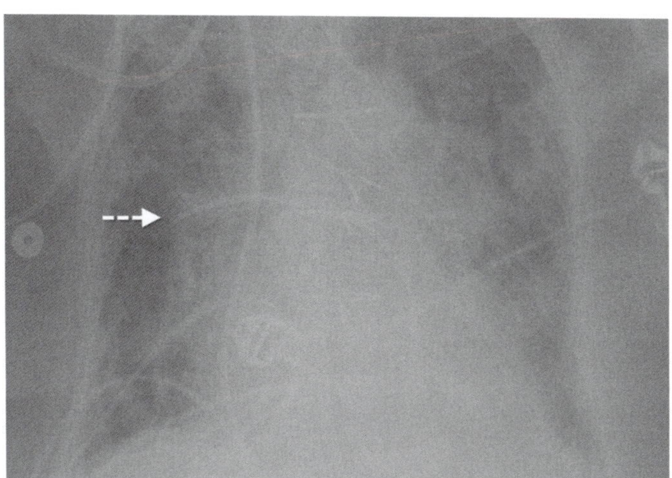

I-109

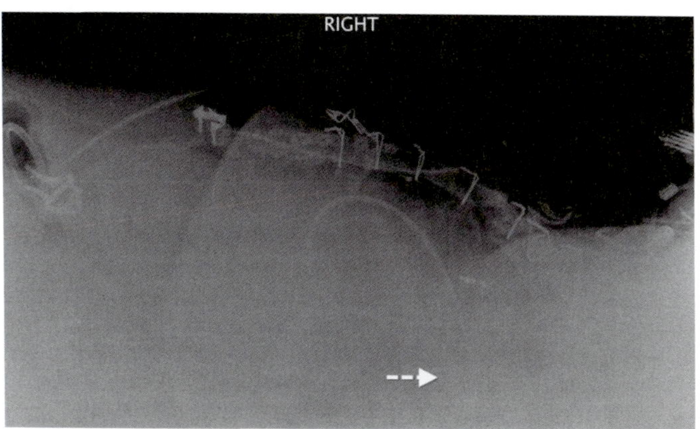

I-110

CORRECT SWAN–GANZ CATHETER PLACEMENT

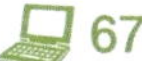 67

Correct Swan–Ganz catheter placement in the right pulmonary artery
First image = frontal view; second image = lateral view

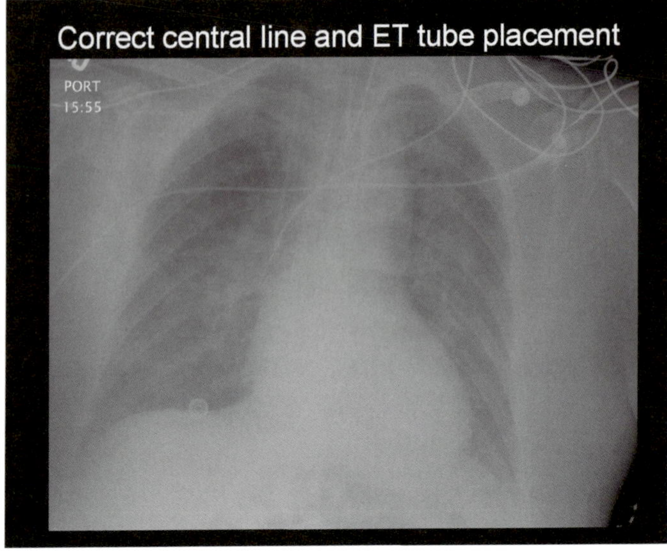

I-111

CORRECT ENDOTRACHEAL TUBE AND CENTRAL-LINE PLACEMENT 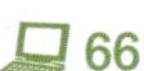 66

- ET tube tip between sternoclavicular joint and carina (right arrow)
- Central-line tip between proximal and distal SVC (left arrow)

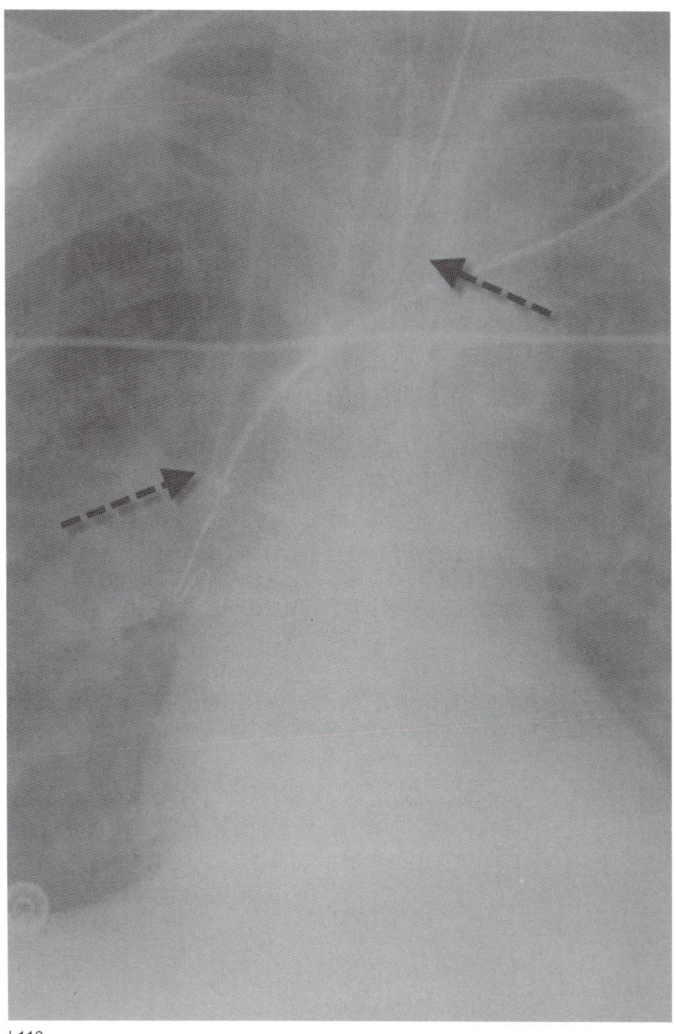

I-112

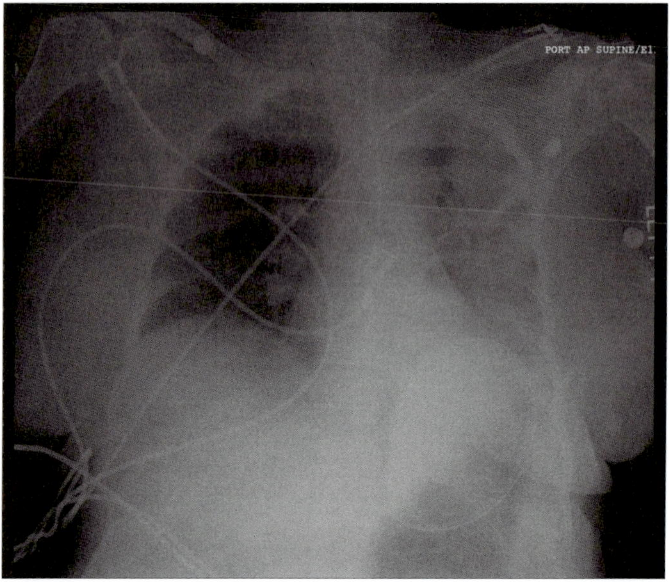

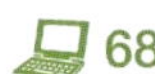

I-113

ENDOTRACHEAL (ET) TUBE MISPLACEMENT

68

- ET tube in right main stem bronchus (white arrow)
- Opacification and low volume of left lung secondary to hypoventilation (black arrow)

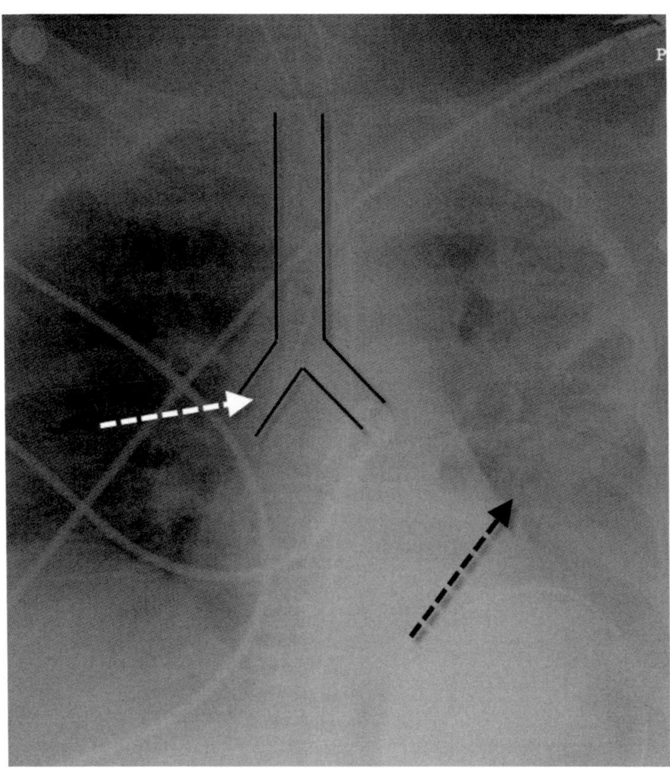

I-114

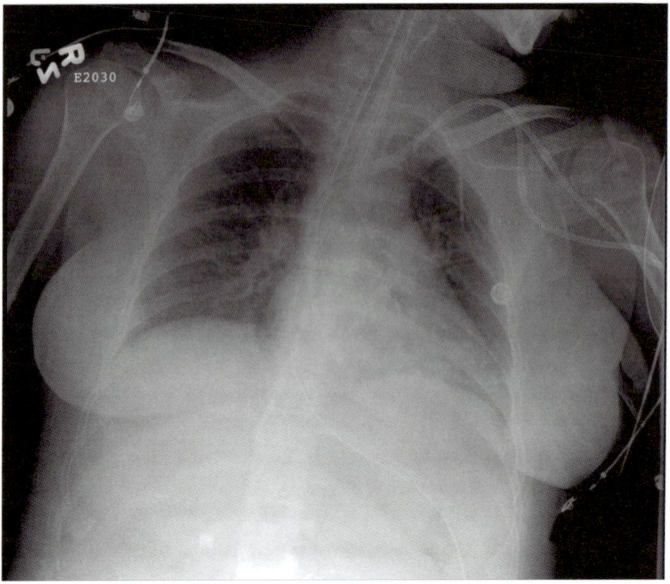

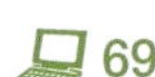

I-115

ET TUBE AND CENTRAL-LINE MISPLACEMENT

69

- ET tube in right main stem bronchus (white arrow)
- Central line in right atrium (right black arrow)
- Central line in IVC (left black arrow)

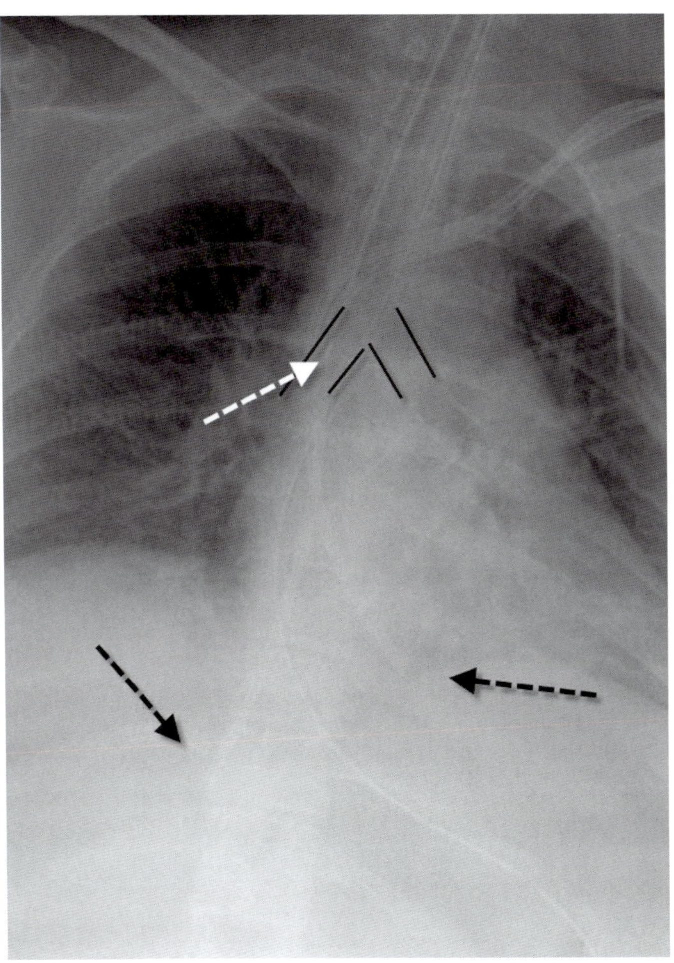

I-116

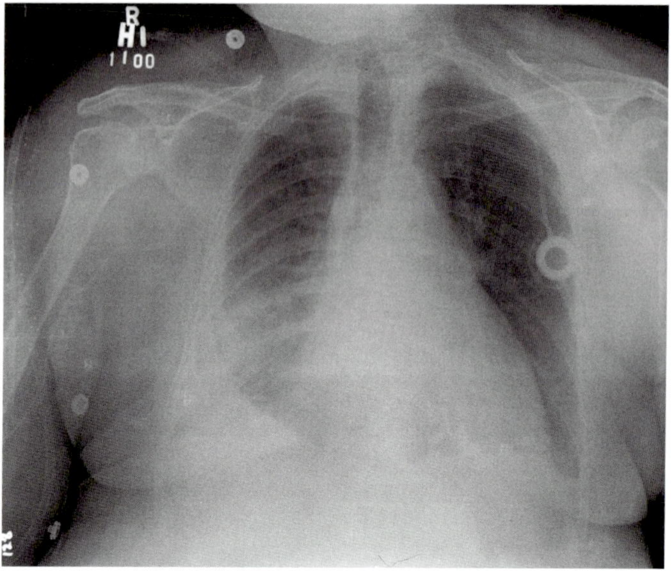

I-117

■ MISPLACED PICC 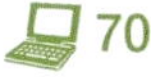 70

Misplaced peripherally inserted central catheter (PICC)

A right PICC has a somewhat serpiginous course with the tip projecting over the right lower neck (magnified view, right image). Also noted is a moderate right pleural effusion.

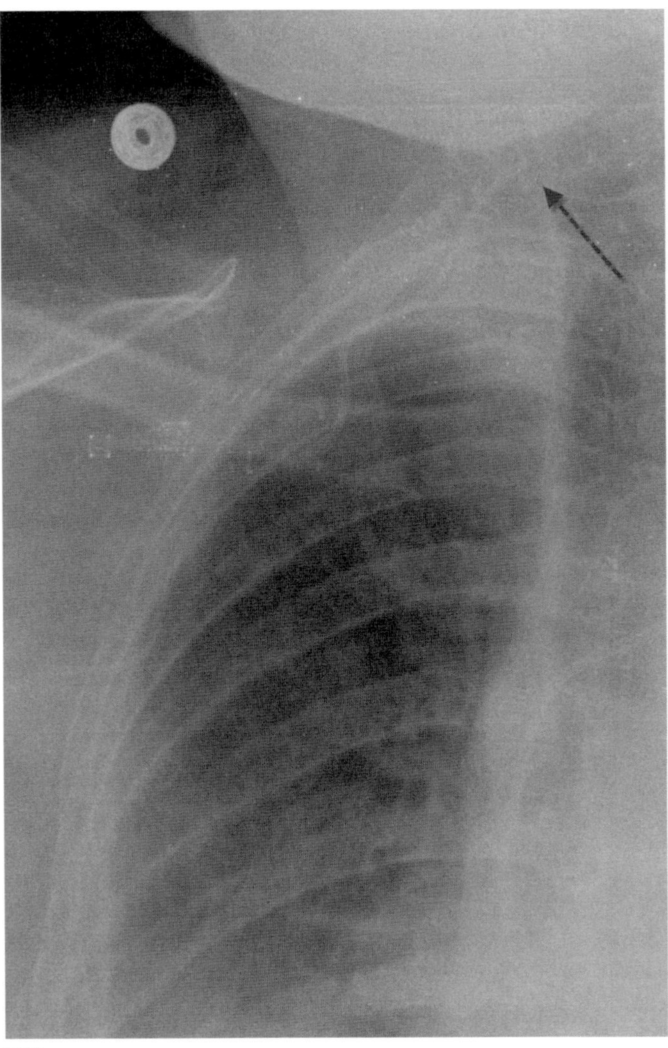

I-118

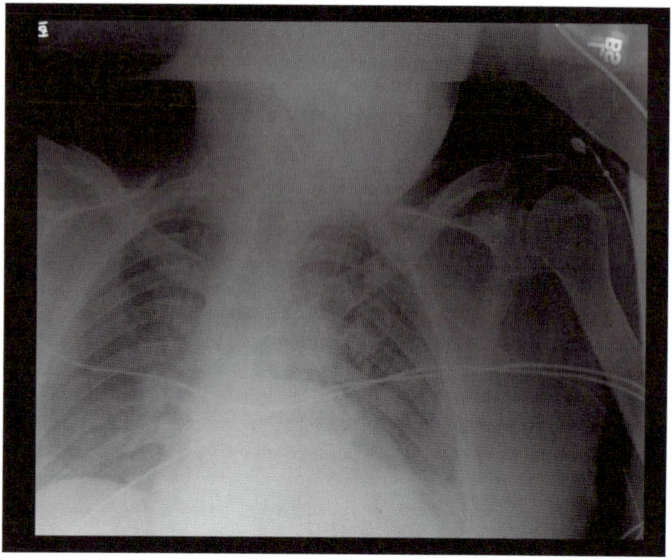

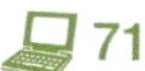

I-119

CENTRAL-LINE MISPLACEMENT   71

Tip of left IJ (bottom arrow) and PICC line (top arrow) in left brachiocephalic vein

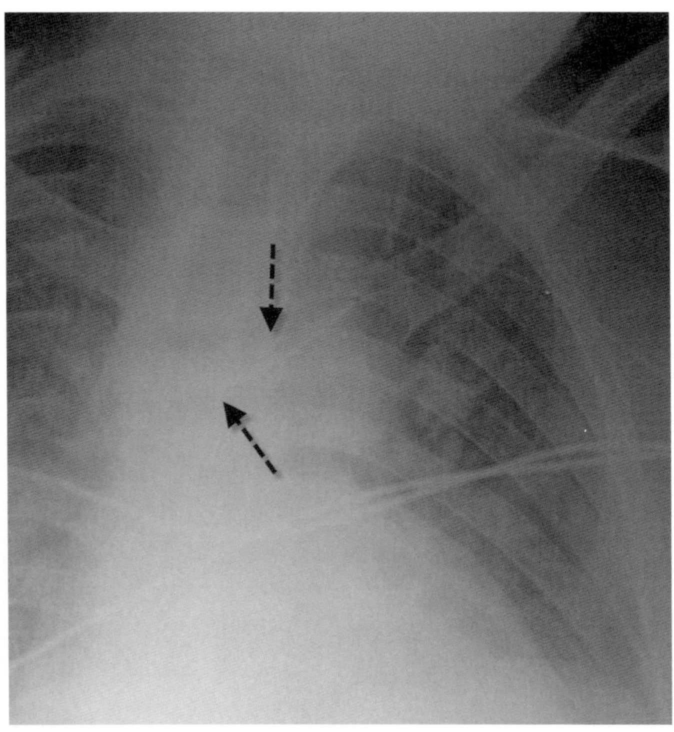

I-120

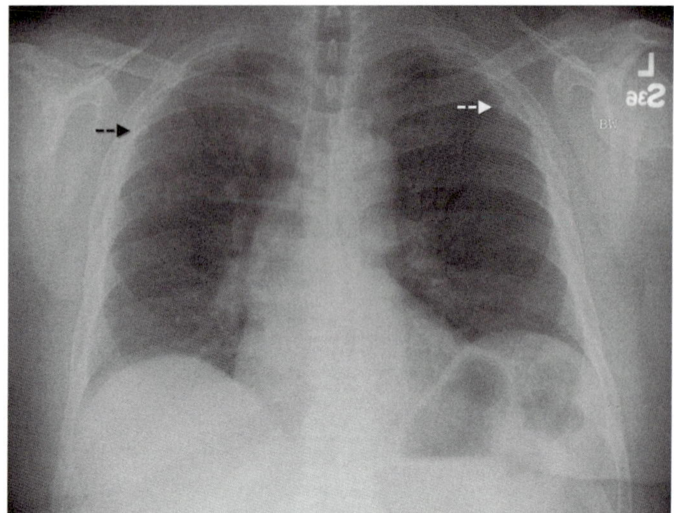

I-121

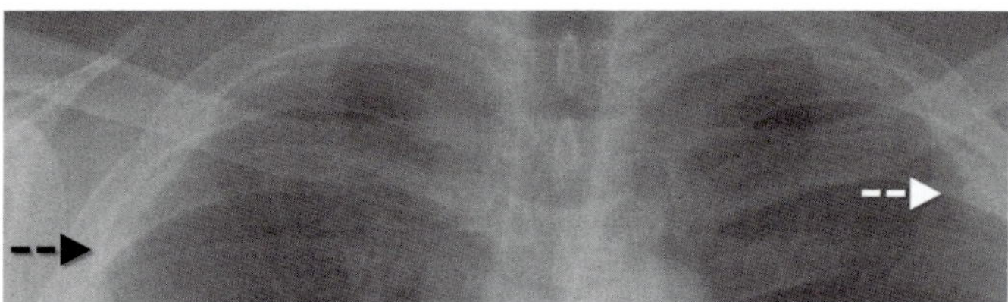

I-122

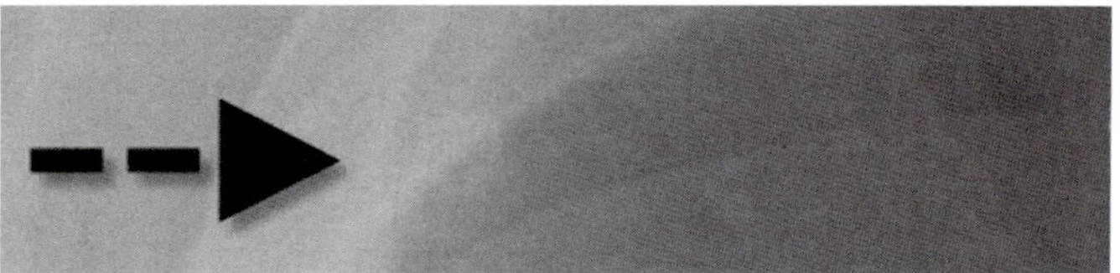

I-123

BUTTONS MIMICKING LUNG LESIONS 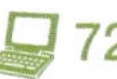 72

The buttons from the patient's gown are projecting over the lung apices (arrows) and can be potentially mistaken for lung lesions.

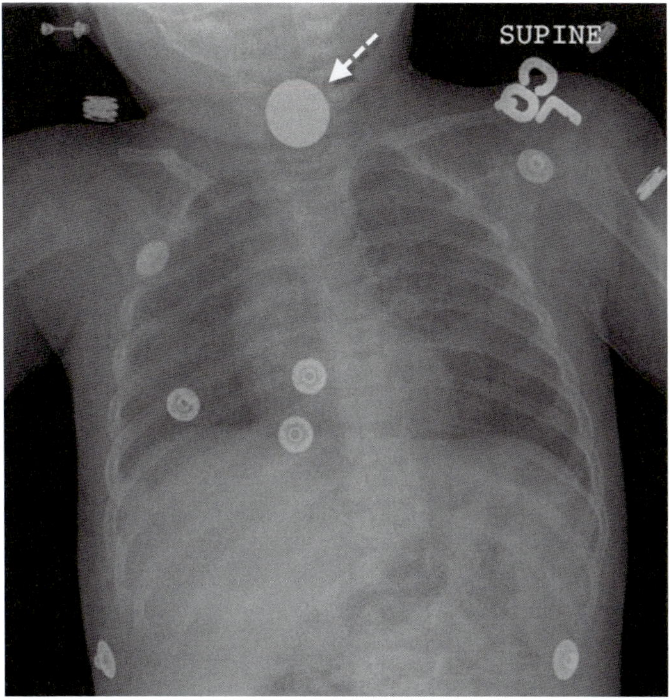

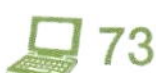

I-124

■ FOREIGN BODY: COIN IN ESOPHAGUS   73

Don't be confused by all the other lead buttons! There is a coin-shaped foreign body projecting over the lower neck (first image, white arrow). On the lateral view it projects over the esophagus/trachea (second image, black arrow). However, it has to be in the esophagus, because it is en face on the PA view. If it would be in the trachea, it would be en face on the lateral view. The reason is that the posterior wall of the trachea is membranous and has the least resistance, allowing the esophagus to orient in an AP position.

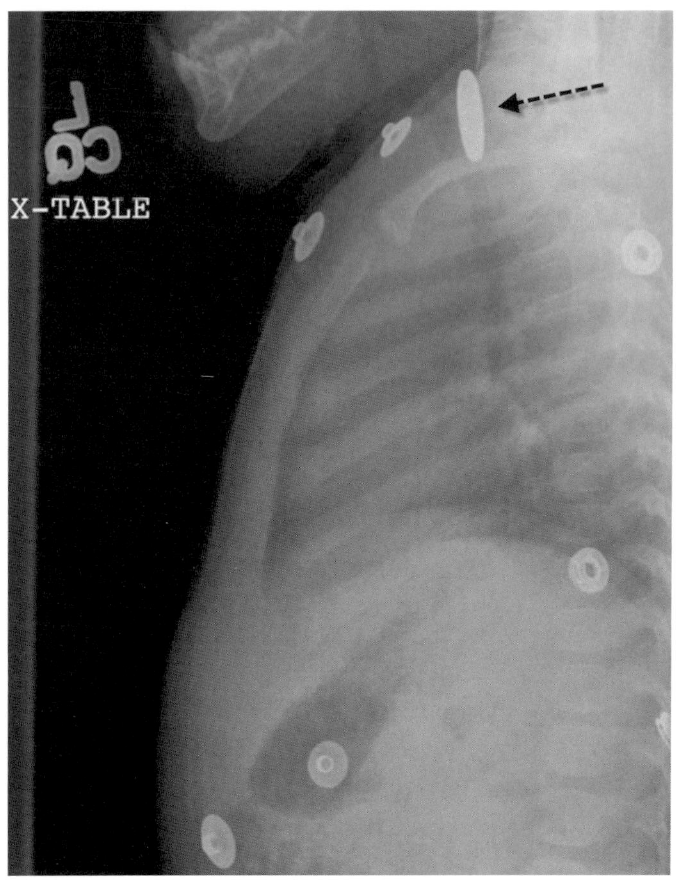

I-125

Once again: en face on the PA view: in the esophagus; en face on the lateral view: in the trachea!

References

There are many freely available high-quality review articles about specific topics discussed in this book. These selections of references are only references to high-quality journal articles that are freely and directly available.

How to get access to these articles?
Each reference has a so-called "PMID" at the end. Please use that number and go on the following hyperlink by exchanging "PMID" with that respective number: *http://www.ncbi.nlm.nih.gov/pubmed/PMID*

That hyperlink provides the abstract and also further links to direct access to these full text articles.

1. Ho ML, Gutierrez FR. Chest radiography in thoracic polytrauma. AJR Am J Roentgenol. 2009 Mar;192(3):599–612. PMID: 19234253

2. Kaewlai R, Avery LL, Asrani AV, Novelline RA. Multidetector CT of blunt thoracic trauma. Radiographics. 2008 Oct;28(6):1555–1570. PMID: 18936021

3. Kuhlman JE, Pozniak MA, Collins J, Knisely BL. Radiographic and CT findings of blunt chest trauma: aortic injuries and looking beyond them. Radiographics. 1998 Sep–Oct; 18(5):1085–1106. PMID: 9747609

4. Van Hise ML, Primack SL, Israel RS, Müller NL. CT in blunt chest trauma: indications and limitations. Radiographics. 1998 Sep–Oct;18(5):1071–1084. PMID: 9747608

5. Creasy JD, Chiles C, Routh WD, Dyer RB. Overview of traumatic injury of the thoracic aorta. Radiographics. 1997 Jan–Feb;17(1):27–45. PMID: 9017797

6. Restrepo CS, Lemos DF, Lemos JA, Velasquez E, Diethelm L, Ovella TA, Martinez S, Carrillo J, Moncada R, Klein JS. Imaging findings in cardiac tamponade with emphasis on CT. Radiographics. 2007 Nov–Dec;27(6):1595–1610. PMID: 18025505

7. Alkadhi H, Wildermuth S, Desbiolles L, Schertler T, Crook D, Marincek B, Boehm T. Vascular emergencies of the thorax after blunt and iatrogenic trauma: multi-detector row CT and three-dimensional imaging. Radiographics. 2004 Sep–Oct;24(5):1239–1255. PMID: 15371605

8. O'Conor CE. Diagnosing traumatic rupture of the thoracic aorta in the emergency department. Emerg Med J. 2004 Jul;21(4):414–419. PMID: 15208221

9. Han D, Lee KS, Franquet T, Müller NL, Kim TS, Kim H, Kwon OJ, Byun HS. Thrombotic and nonthrombotic pulmonary arterial embolism: spectrum of imaging findings. Radiographics. 2003 Nov–Dec;23(6):1521–1539. PMID: 14615562

10. Sybrandy KC, Cramer MJ, Burgersdijk C. Diagnosing cardiac contusion: old wisdom and new insights. Heart. 2003 May;89(5):485–489. PMID: 12695446

11. Iochum S, Ludig T, Walter F, Sebbag H, Grosdidier G, Blum AG. Imaging of diaphragmatic injury: a diagnostic challenge? Radiographics. 2002 Oct; 22 Spec No:S103-16. PMID: 12376604

1. Anatomy

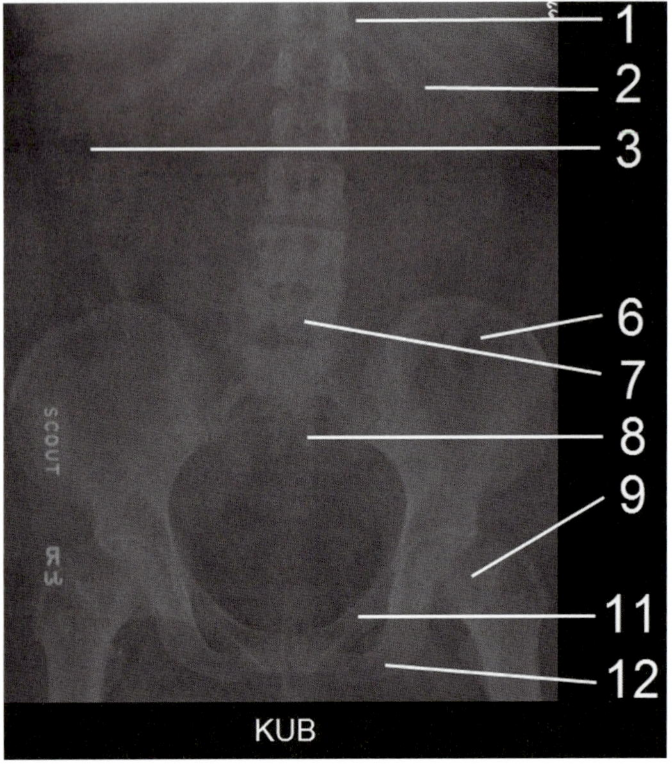

II-1

■ **NORMAL ABDOMINAL AP RADIOGRAPH**   75

1. T12 (12th thoracic) vertebral body
2. 12th rib
3. Liver
4. Right and left kidney (opacified with contrast material)
5. Right and left ureter (opacified with contrast material)
6. Bowel gas
7. L5 (5th lumbar) vertebral body

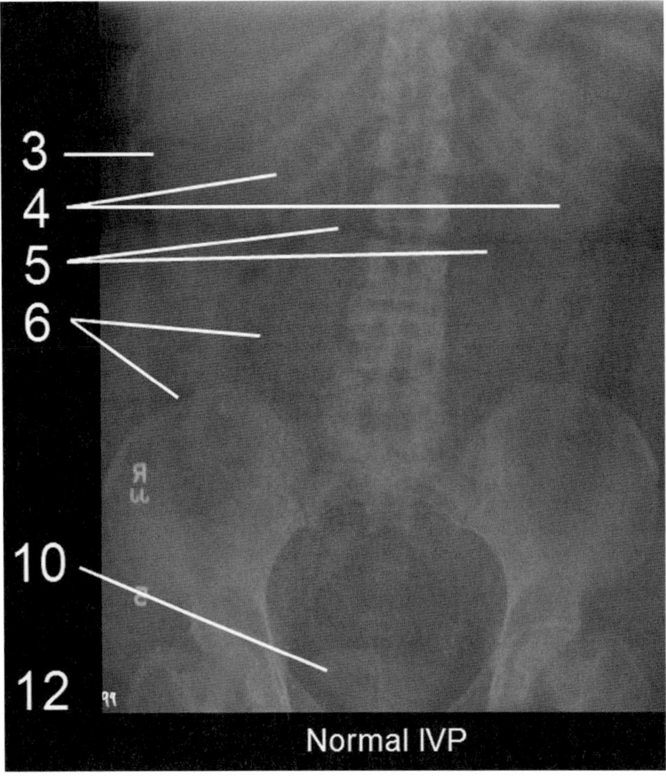

II-2

8. Sacrum
9. Left femoral neck
10. Urinary bladder (filled with contrast material)
11. Superior pubic ramus
12. Ischium

2. Technique

■ TECHNIQUES   ⌨ 76

Techniques:
- KUB (supine)
- KUB (upright)
- Lateral decubitus view
- Computed tomography (with or without oral/intravenous contrast)
- Ultrasonography

KUB: ideally upright, can detect air fluid levels (eg, in small bowel obstruction or paralytic ileus) and small amounts of free air, radiopaque structures (stones, foreign bodies)

Left lateral decubitus for questionable free air or if patient cannot be positioned upright.

Advantage: quick, low radiation exposure; disadvantage: limited evaluation of problem.

Ultrasonography: searching for (nonradiopaque) stones, biliary/urinary obstruction, ovarian, uterine, and testicular pathologies.

Advantage: quick, cheap, no radiation; disadvantage: operator dependent, difficult to interpret

Computed tomography: ideal for evaluation of masses, further localization (eg, point of obstruction), source of infection, details otherwise not appreciable on ultrasonography and plain radiographs.

Advantage: quick, complete "internal" overview, easier to interpret; disadvantage: high radiation exposure.

On optimal radiograph outlining seen of:
- Liver
- Spleen
- Kidneys
- Bladder

Evaluate for:
- Presence
- Size
- Position
- Configuration

Evaluate for:
- Obstruction (small bowel normally <3 cm, large bowel normally <5 cm)
- Masses (abnormal organ outlines)
- Calcifications (renal stones, gallstones, appendicolith)
- Abnormal air collections (pneumoperitoneum, portal venous gas, biliary air, infection/abscess)
- Fractures
- Device localization (tubes etc.)
- Do not forget the lung bases! (infection, neoplasm)

Limitations: soft tissue injuries -> better contrast enhanced CT or ultrasound

3. Liver & Gallbladder   🖥 79

▧ LIVER & GALLBLADDER

Cholelithiasis – Introduction

- Most gallstones are not radiopaque
- Can show radiolucent center with calcified rim
- Solitary or in clusters
- In expected location of gallbladder or common bile duct
- Sludge = thickened gall juice (can form stones)

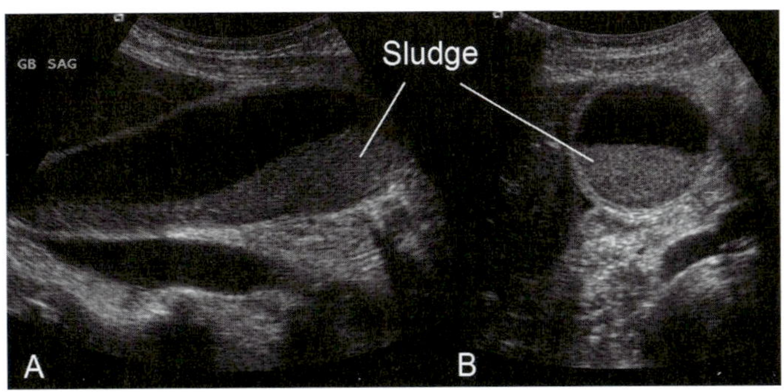

II-3

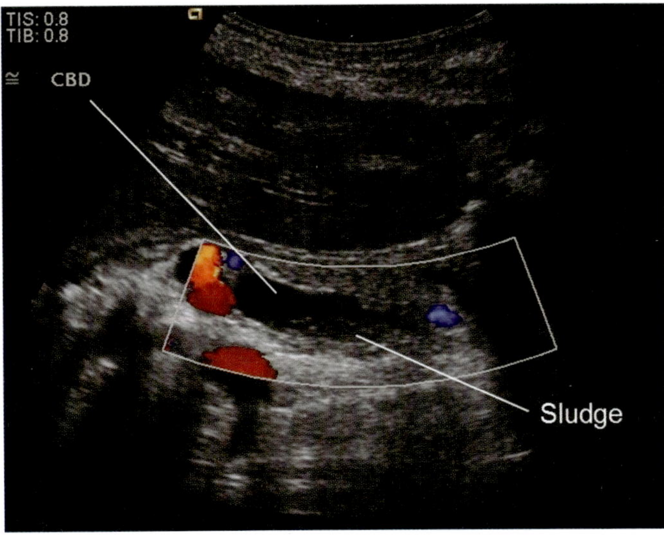

II-4

Gallbladder sludge 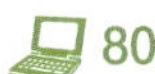 80

Upper image demonstrates sludge in the gallbladder

Lower image shows sludge in the common bile duct

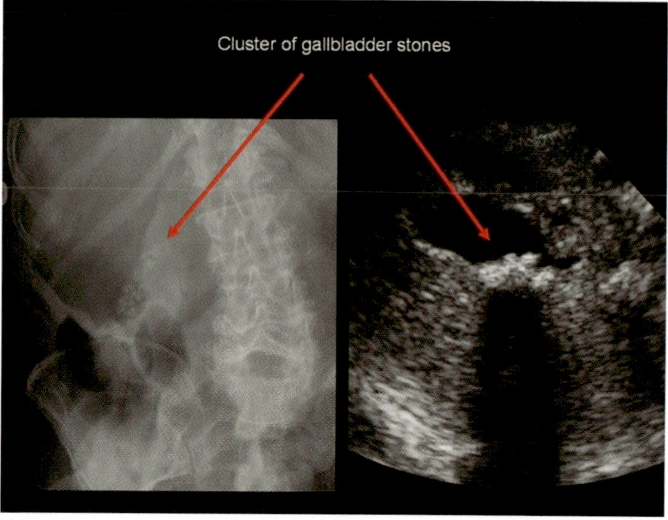

II-5

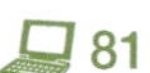 CHOLELITHIASIS   81

In this case, we can see a nice cluster of gallbladder stones on plain film and ultrasound.

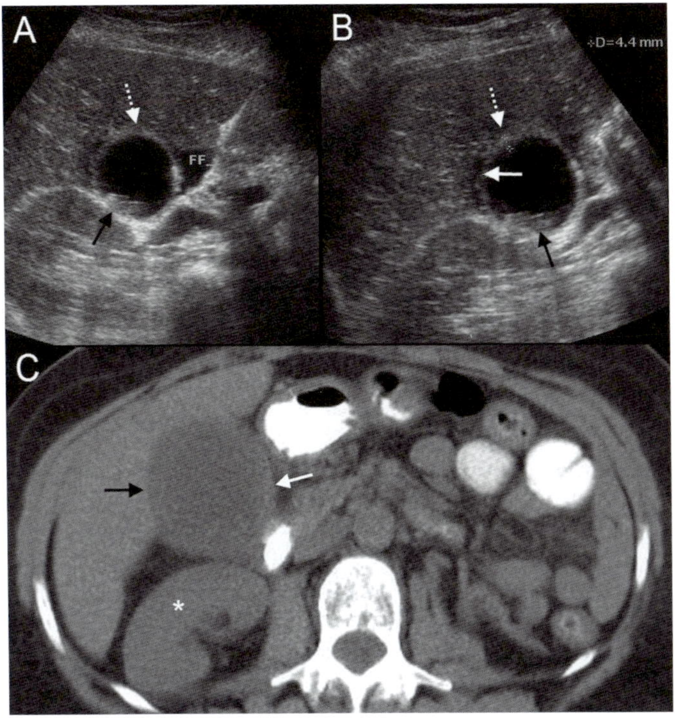

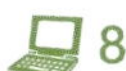

II-6

ACUTE CHOLECYSTITIS – US/CT/CORRELATION

83

Grayscale ultrasound images (A, B) of the right upper abdomen demonstrate stones within the gallbladder lumen (black arrows), gallbladder wall thickening (4.4 mm, dotted arrows) and free pericholecystic fluid (FF and full white arrow). These findings (in addition to positive Murphy's sign and distended common bile duct beyond 7 mm) are consistent with acute cholecystitis. Contrast enhanced CT of the abdomen (C) in the same patient demonstrates again pericholecystic fluid (black arrow), gallbladder wall thickening and a distended gallbladder, the shadowing stones on ultrasound are not radiopaque and barely identified in the gallbladder lumen. Incidental note is made of a malrotated right kidney (asterisk).

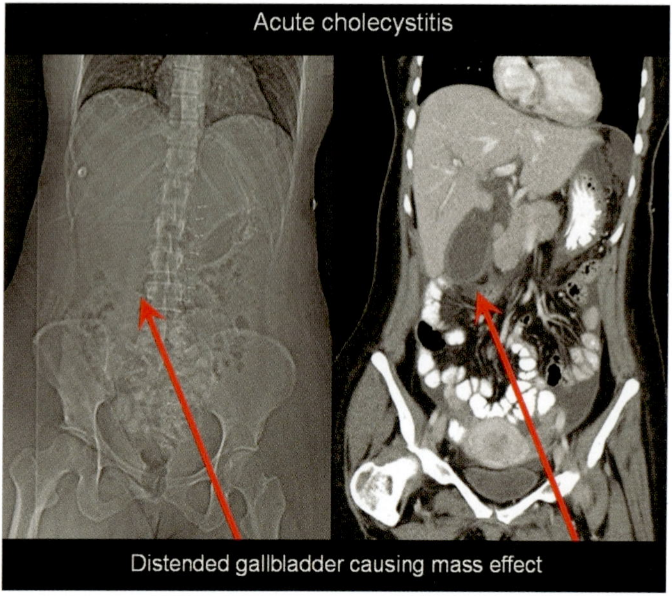

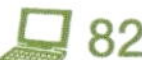

II-7

ACUTE CHOLECYSTITIS 82

The distended and inflamed/edematous gallbladder causes mass effect, also seen on the KUB (here topogram).

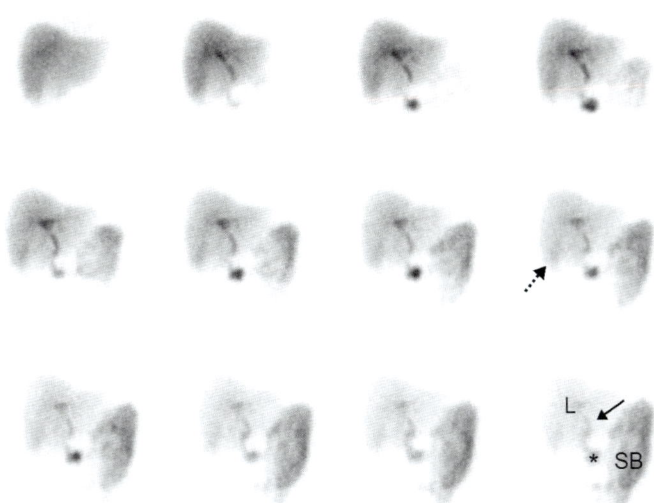

II-8

ACUTE CHOLECYSTITIS – HIDA SCAN    84

HIDA scan images obtained over 60 min after injection of 99 mTc Mebrofenin (top left image obtained at time zero, bottom right image obtained after 60 min). Prompt and homogeneous tracer uptake is noticed throughout the liver (L), followed by tracer uptake in the small bowel (SB). The gallbladder cannot be identified after 60 min and even after Morphine injection (to increase the intrabiliary pressure to help open the gallbladder). Please notice an area of increased hepatic activity in the expected area of the gallbladder fossa (dotted arrow), which is referred to as the rim sign and suggestive of acute cholecystitis due to the increased blood flow to the inflamed neighboring liver parenchyma. Asterisk is at the level of the papilla Vateri.

Patient needs to be at least 4 hours and a maximum of 24 hours NPO to exclude false positive findings!

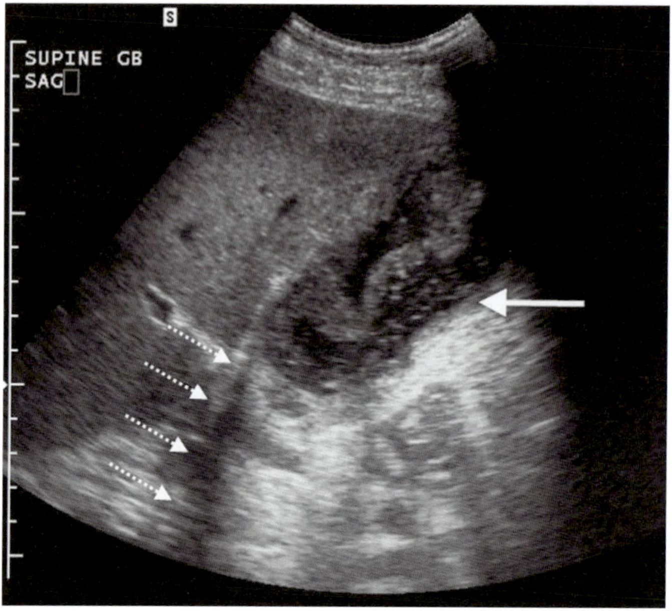

II-9

GANGRENOUS CHOLECYSTITIS – ULTRASOUND

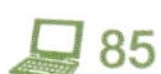

Echogenic and shadowing (dotted arrows) areas within the edematous gallbladder wall (full arrow) represent air within the gangrenous gallbladder.

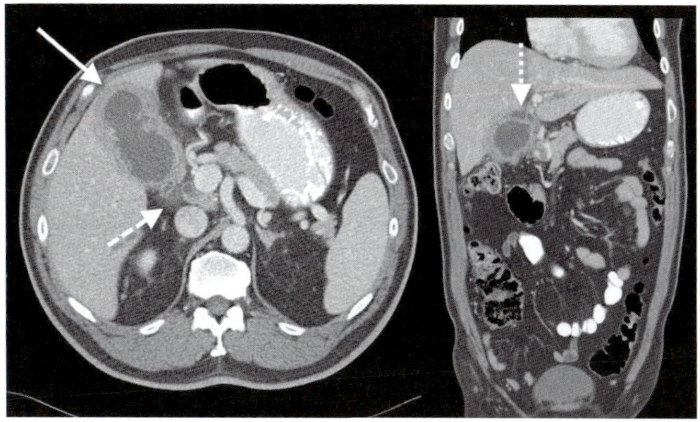

II-10

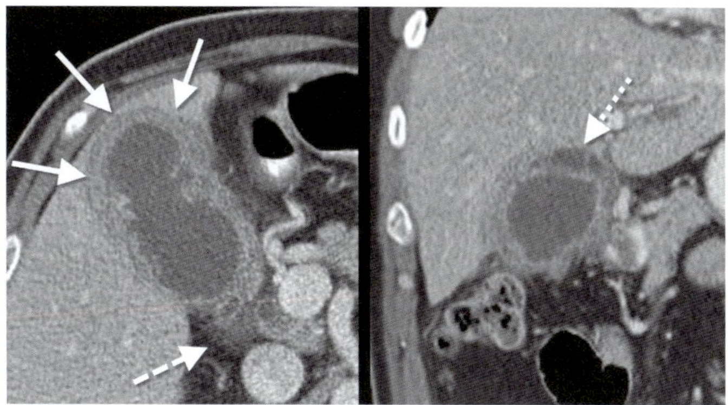

II-11

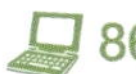 GANGRENOUS CHOLECYSTITIS – CT   86

Distended gallbladder with wall thickening (full arrows), pericholecystic fluid (dotted arrow) and surrounding fat stranding (dashed arrows) are signs of an acute inflammatory process.

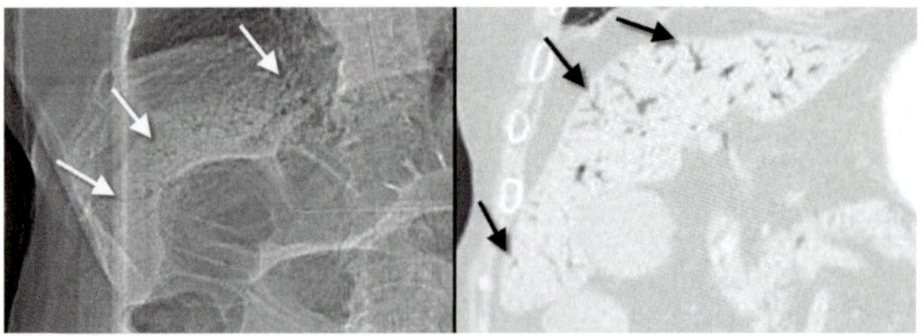

II-12

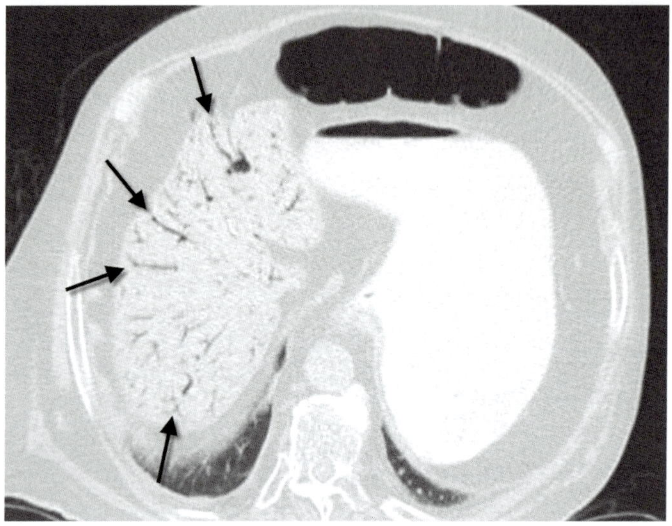

II-13

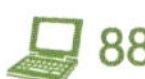 PORTAL VENOUS GAS 88

Upper left image: supine abdominal radiograph, upper right image: coronal CT of the abdomen in lung window. Lower image: axial CT of the abdomen in lung window at the level of the liver. Note is made of air in the intrahepatic portal venous system (arrows). Portal venous gas comes usually from pneumatosis — the air is transported (usually via superior mesentery vein) into the portal system. It might be confused by pneumobilia; however, portal venous gas is more peripherally located in the liver, since it is pushed away in the direction of the portal venous flow.

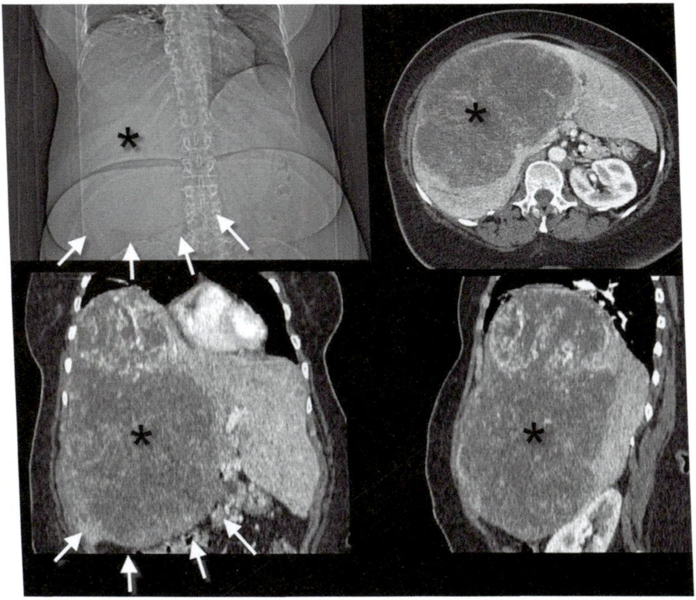

II-14

LIVER MASSES 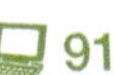 91

This liver mass "(Leiomyosarcoma, asterisk) occupies almost the entire right upper abdomen. On the abdominal radiograph, one can anticipate the large mass effect by the tumor (arrows) because of the lack of bowel gas in the right upper quadrant and the increased opacity of the mass.

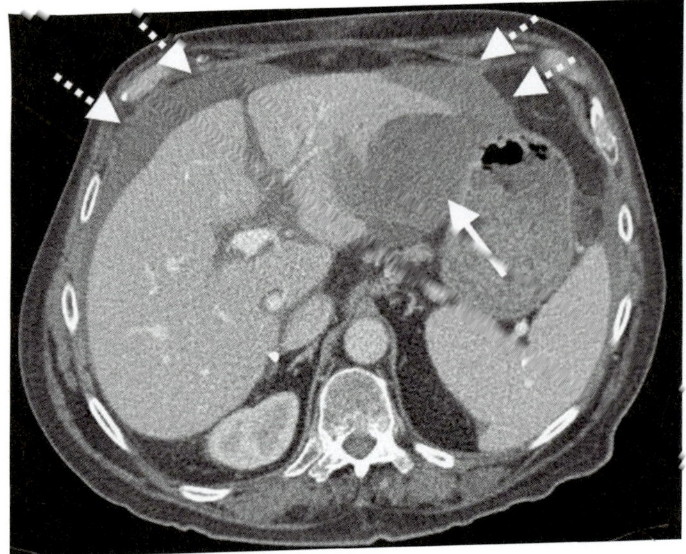

II-15

■ SUBCAPSULAR HEMATOMA (AFTER BIOPSY) 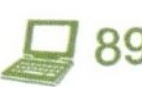 89

In the lateral segment of the left hepatic lobe there is a subcapsular hematoma (measuring 5.7 × 6.7 cm in axial dimensions, solid arrow). There is also a small amount of acute blood products in the perihepatic space anterior to the left and right hepatic lobes (dotted arrows).

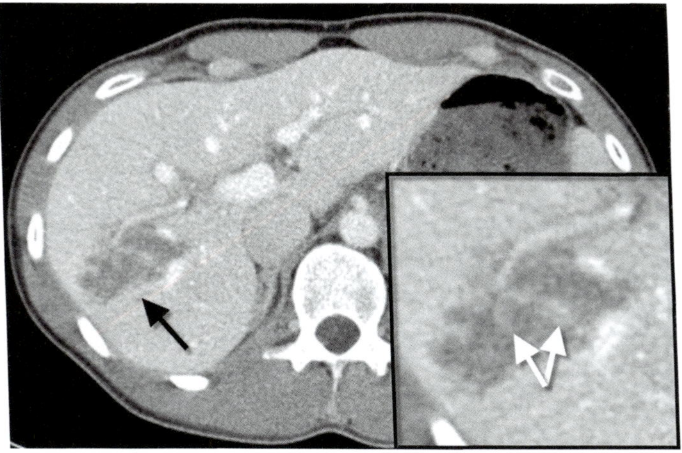

II-16

■ LIVER LACERATION 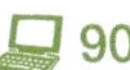 90

Contrast enhanced CT of the abdomen shows a lobulated low attenuation area in the lateral aspect of the right lobe of the liver (black arrow). Magnification (right lower corner) demonstrates higher density material (white arrows) compatible with active extravasation of contrast.

4. Pancreas

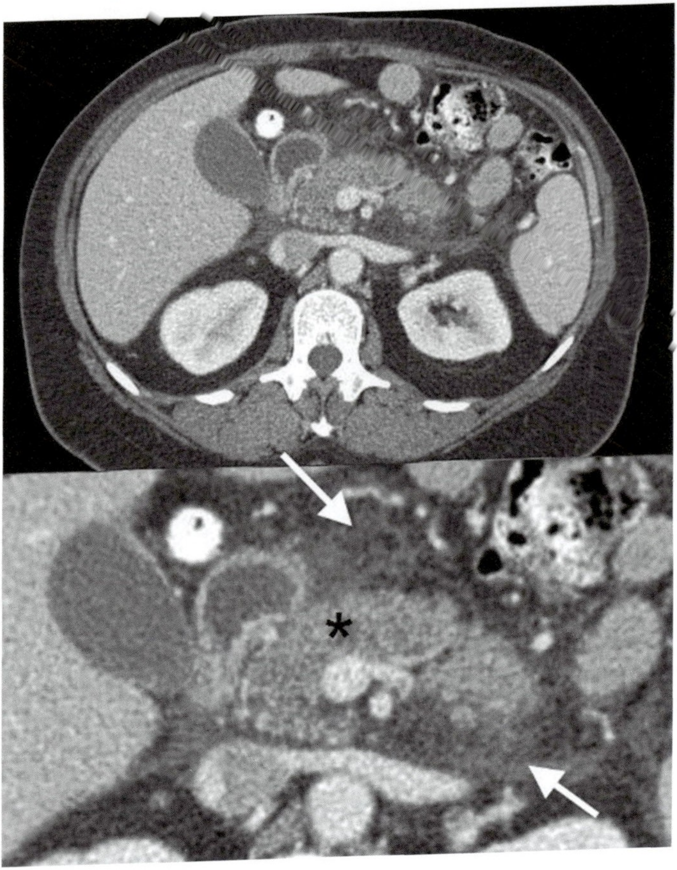

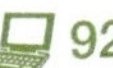

II-17

ACUTE PANCREATITIS   92

Contrast enhanced CT of the abdomen shows a thickened pancreas (asterisk) and peripancreatic fat stranding (arrows). Important to look for sequel of acute pancreatitis such as bleeding, portal vein, splenic and superior mesenteric vein/artery thrombosis, aneurysm, and pseudocyst formation.

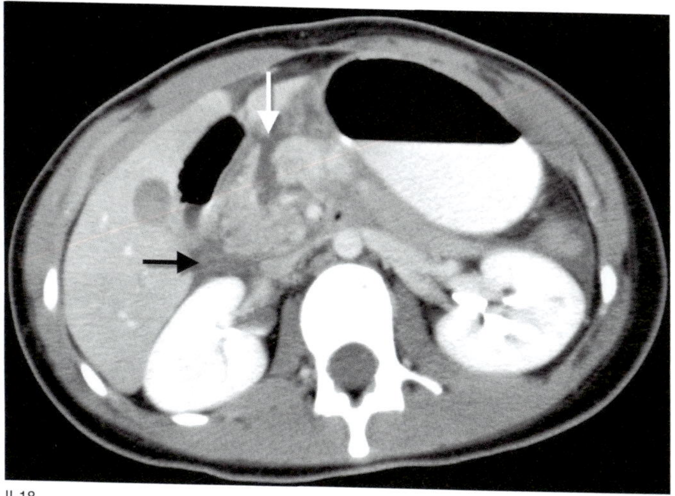

II-18

■ PANCREATIC LACERATION 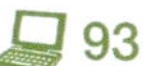 93

Contrast enhanced CT of the abdomen shows a linear nonenhancing area involving the head/neck of the pancreas (white arrow). There is also a small amount of peripancreatic fluid (black arrow), containing some higher density material, suggestive of hemorrhage.

Pancreatic lacerations are graded on CT as following:
- Grade A: pancreatitis or superficial laceration (<50% pancreatic thickness)
- Grade B1: deep laceration (>50% pancreatic thickness) of the pancreatic tail
- Grade B2: transection of the pancreatic tail
- Grade C1: deep laceration (>50% pancreatic thickness of the pancreatic head
- Grade C2: transection of the pancreatic head

5. Spleen

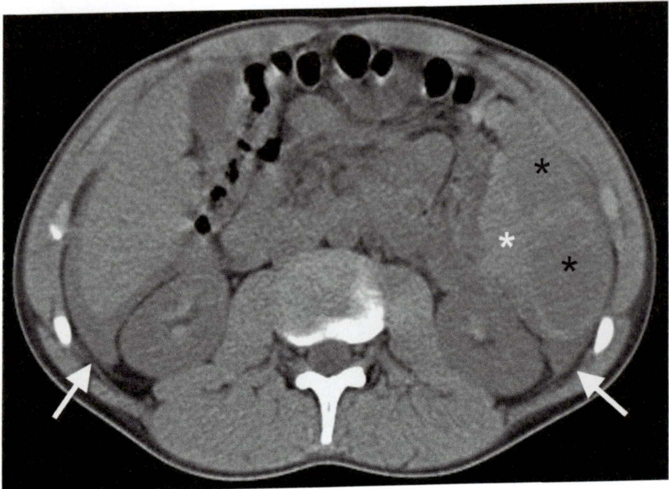

II-19

■ SPLENIC LACERATION 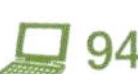 94

Noncontrast enhanced CT of the andomen shows low attenuation areas within the spleen (black asterisks), representing splenic hemorrhage. The white asterisk indicates normal (denser) splenic tissue. Also seen is a small amount of perisplenic and perihepatic fluid/hemorrhage (arrows).

■ SPLENIC LACERATION 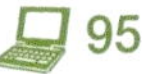 95

Right image: Contrast enhanced CT of the abdomen demonstrates a linear low-attenuation area extending through the spleen (arrow), consistent with a grade IV splenic laceration.

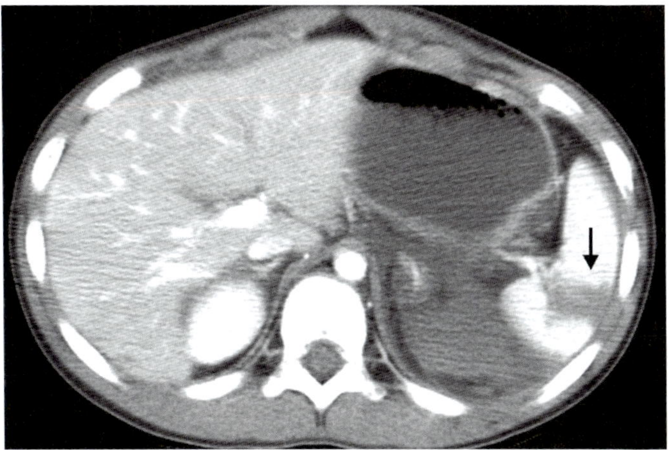

II-20

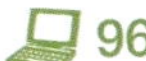 CLASSIFICATION OF SPLENIC TRAUMA 96

Classification of splenic trauma by the American Association for the Surgery of Trauma (AAST):

Grade I:

- Subcapsular hematoma involving <25%
- Capsular laceration <1 cm deep

Grade II:

- Subcapsular hematoma involving 25–50% of the surface area or intra-parenchymal <5 cm in diameter
- Capsular laceration 1–3 cm deep without involvement of a trabecular vessel

Grade III:

- Subcapsular hematoma involving >50% of the surface area or a ruptured subcapsular hematoma or a intraparenchymal hematoma 5 or more cm in size or expanding
- Laceration >3 cm or one involving trabecular vessels

Grade IV:

- Laceration involving segmental or hilar vessels with devascularization of >25%

Grade V ("Shattered" spleen):

- Avulsed spleen with total devascularization

6. Adrenal Glands

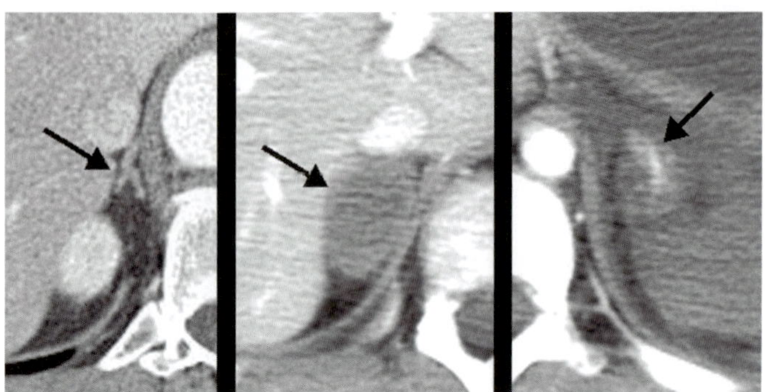

II-21

■ ADRENAL HEMORRHAGE   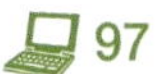 97

Contrast enhanced CT of the abdomen in three different patients: the left image demonstrates a normal right adrenal gland (arrow), the middle image shows a right adrenal gland that is smoothly enlarged by intermediate-attenuation material (arrow, middle image), consistent with a subacute hemorrhage. The third image demonstrates high attenuation material within the left adrenal gland (arrow), indicative of an acute bleed.

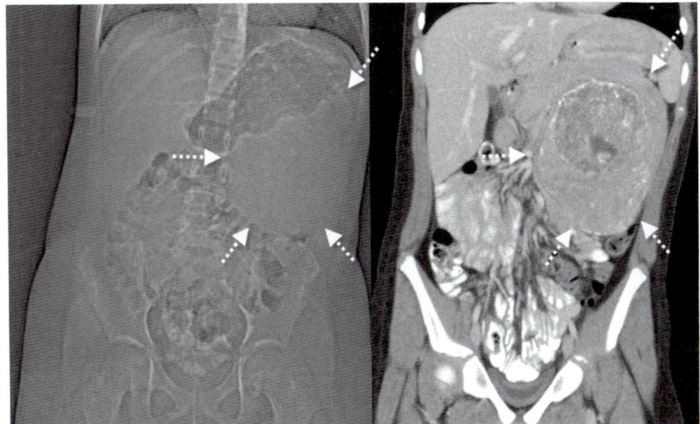

II-22

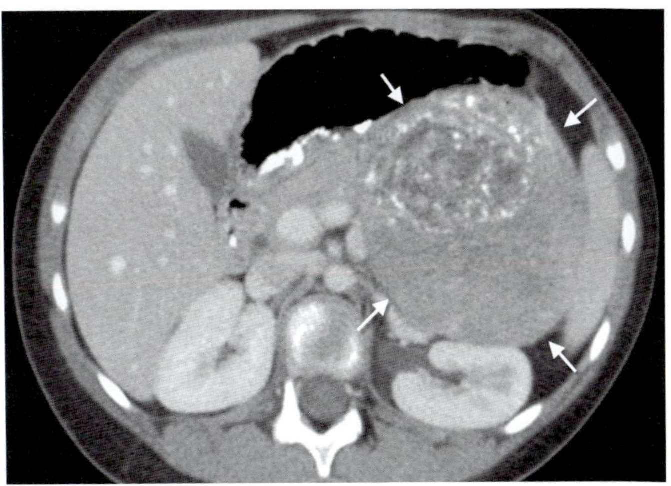

II-23

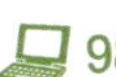 ADRENAL MASSES – NEUROBLASTOMA   98

This 7-year-old child has a large neuroblastoma (white arrows, lower image = axial CT) arising from the left adrenal gland, occupying the entire left upper abdomen (left upper image CT topogram ~ KUB; right upper image: coronal reformatted CT).

7. Kidneys & Urinary Tract

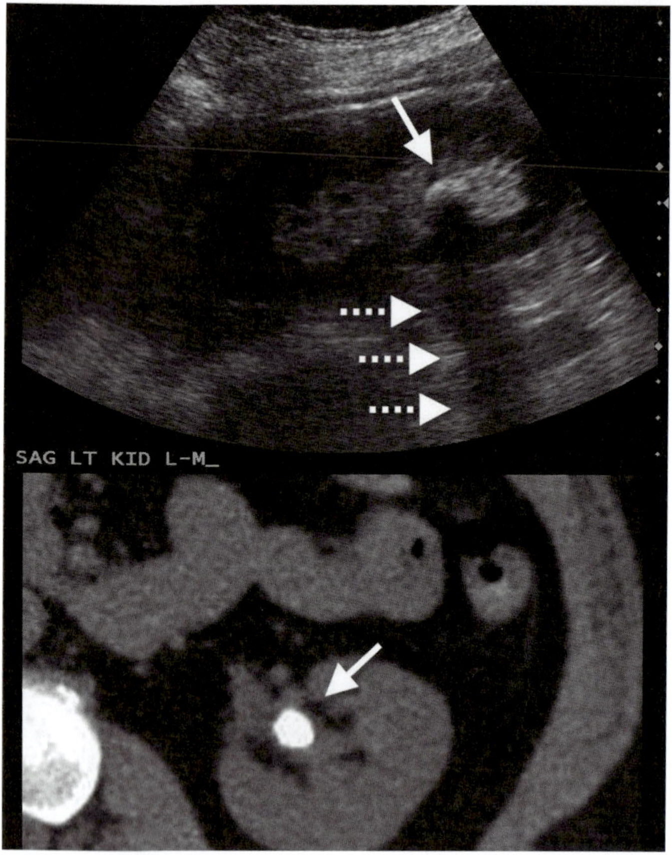

II-24

NEPHROLITHIASIS – NONOBSTRUCTING RENAL STONE

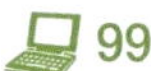 99

Ultrasound image (top) demonstrates a shadowing (dotted arrows) echogenic focus within the left lower renal pole (white arrow), consistent with a renal calculus. Noncontrast CT (stone protocol, lower image) demonstrates again the high attenuation calculus. There are no signs of obstruction in either CT or US.

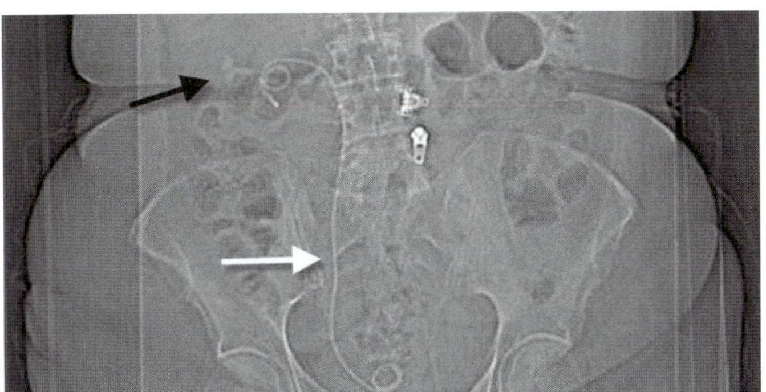

II-25

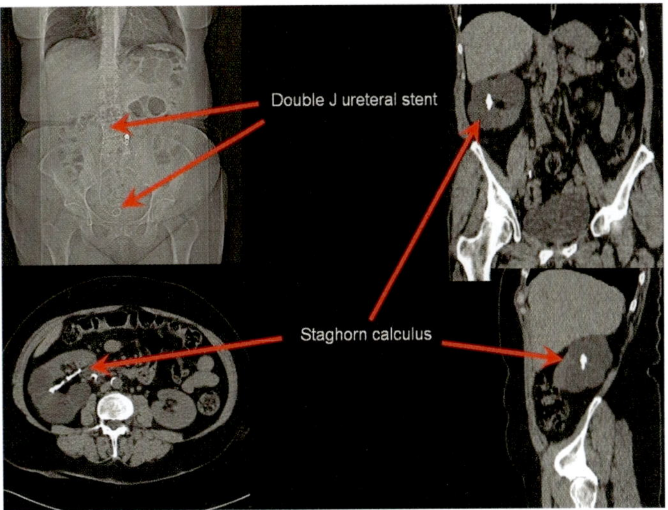

II-26

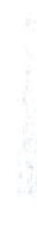

NEPHROLITHIASIS – NONOBSTRUCTING RENAL STONE (STAGHORN CALCULUS)

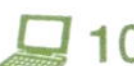 100

There is a Staghorn calculus in the right kidney (upper image, black arrow). Also noted a right double J ureteral stent (upper image, white arrow) – likely placed because of stone obstruction. Lower image shows CT in axial, coronal and sagittal reformations as well as the full KUB. Renal low densities are cysts.

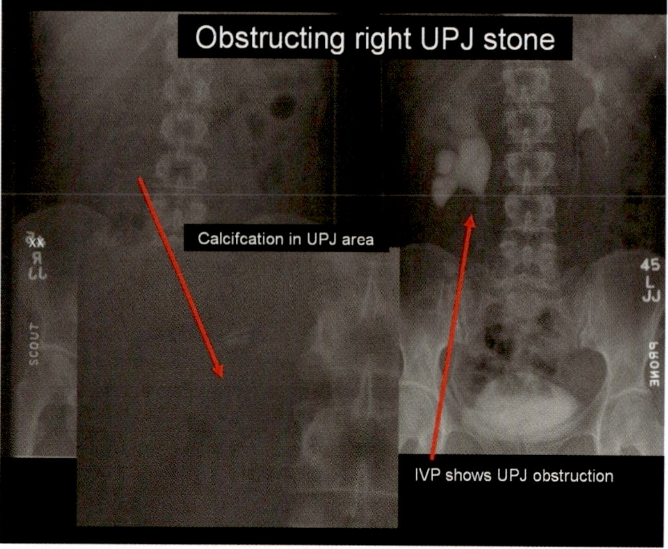

II-27

■ OBSTRUCTING RIGHT UPJ STONE   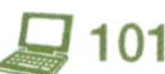 101

A calcification is noticed in the right renal area and along the right ureter on the abdominal radiograph. (Calcification in UPJ area better appreciated on the magnified area below). A subsequent intravenous pyelogram (IVP, right image) confirms a right ureteropelvic junction (UPJ) obstruction.

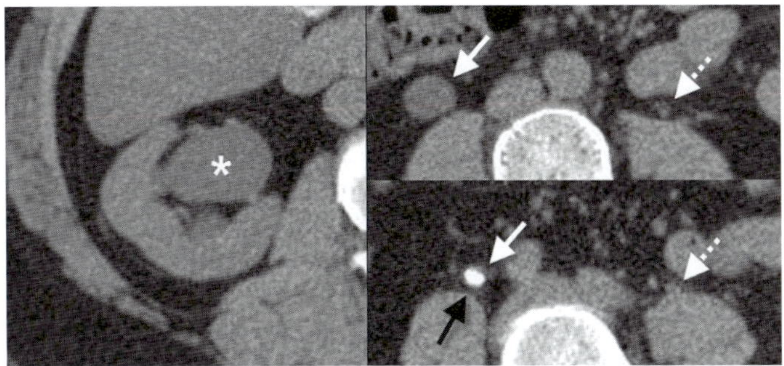

II-28

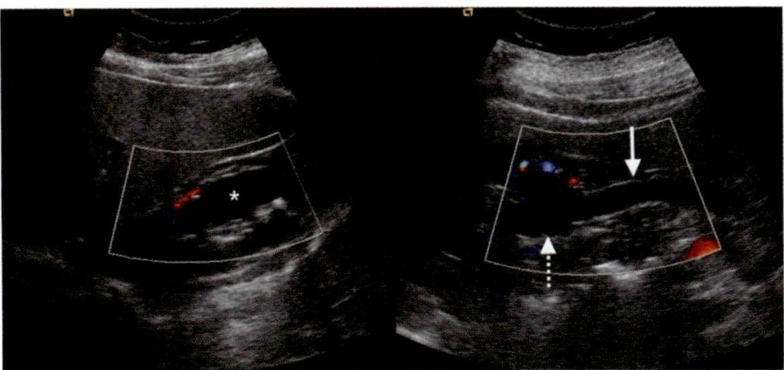

II-29

■ OBSTRUCTING MID URETER STONE 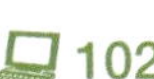 102

Noncontrast CT of the abdomen (stone protocol, upper image row) demonstrates a 7 × 6 by 12-mm calculus (black arrow) within the mid right ureter (white arrows) causing moderate hydroureteronephrosis (asterisk). Compare the size of the dilated right ureter proximal to the obstructing calculus with the collapsed left ureter (dotted arrows). An ultrasound of the kidneys in the same patient (lower image) demonstrates moderate to severe dilatation of the right renal collecting system (asterisk), ureteropelvic junction (dotted arrow), as well as the proximal ureter (full arrow).

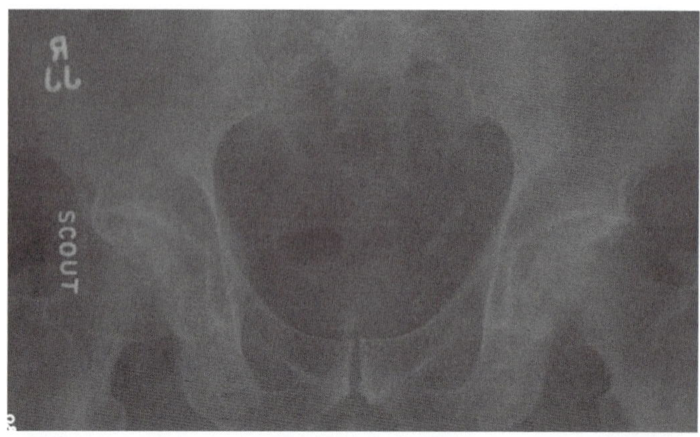

II-30

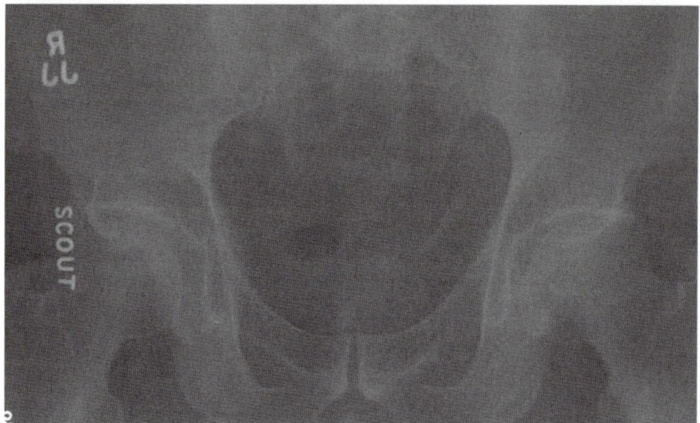

II-31

■ OBSTRUCTING URETERAL CHAIN OF STONES

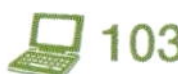 103

Chain of distal left ureteral stones (mid-size arrows, upper image = magnified view) causing left hydronephrosis (long arrow), evident on the right IVP image. Note is made of surgical clips inferior to the ureteral stones (short arrow), not to mistake for stones.

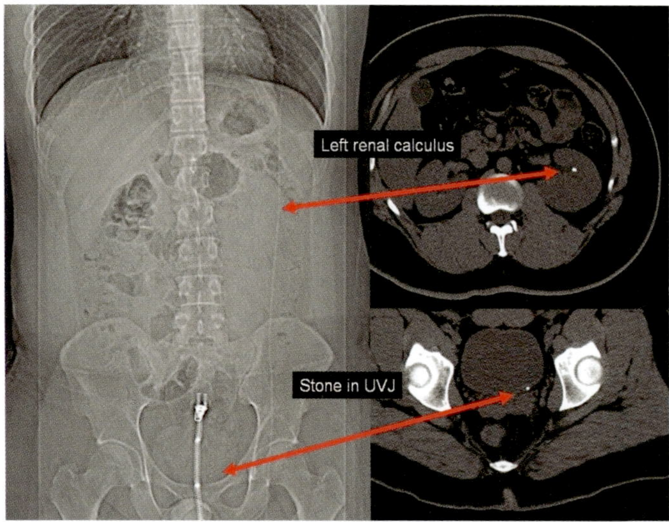

II-32

■ OBSTRUCTING LEFT UVJ STONE 💻 104

Distal left ureteral stone (at the UVJ) causing hydronephrosis (seen as edematous swollen left kidney – compared to the right kidney). Also noted a nonobstructing left renal stone.

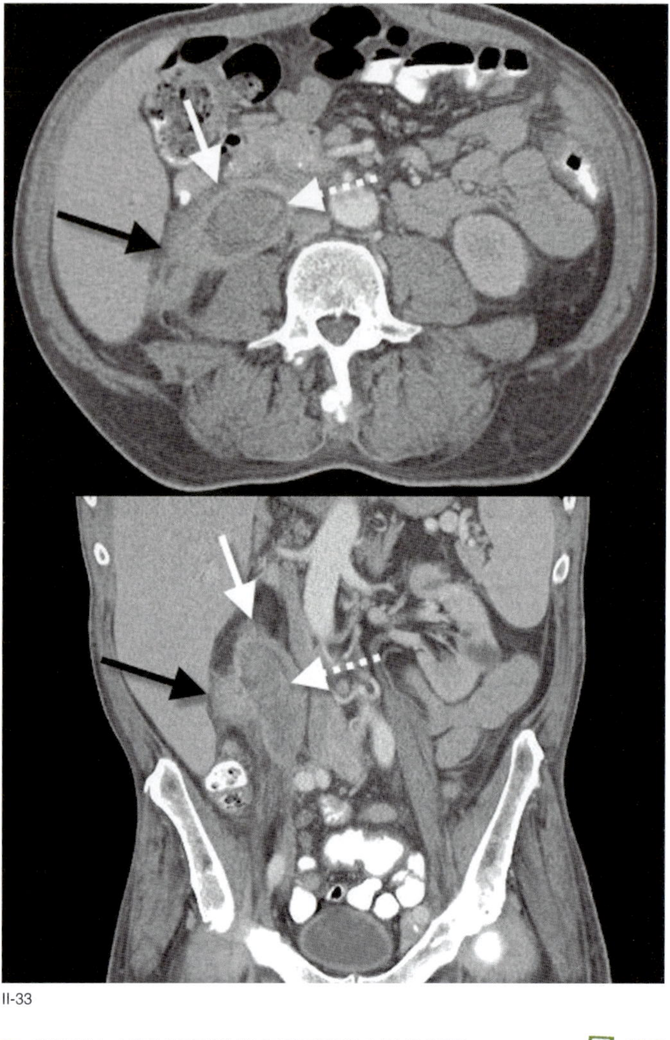

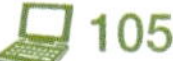

II-33

■ RENAL HEMORRHAGE FROM TUMOR 💻 105

There is a perinephric hematoma (white arrows). Additional smaller areas of stranding (black arrows) and denser components (white dotted arrow) represent new bleed. A right renal cancer was the source of bleed.

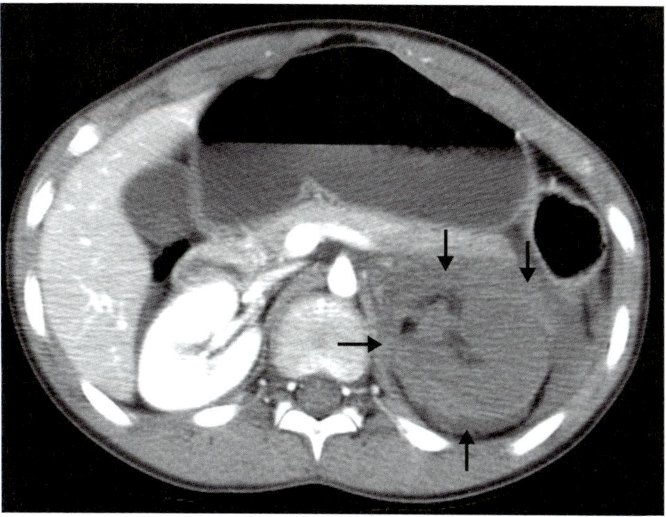

II-34

■ RENAL HILUM AVULSION

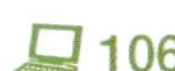 106

Contrast enhanced CT of the abdomen shows an edematous and non-enhancing left kidney. Also seen is perirenal hemorrhage (black arrows). The kidney is completely avulsed from its hilum (grade V injury).

■ CLASSIFICATION OF RENAL TRAUMA 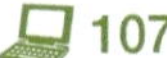 107

Classification of renal trauma by the American Association for the Surgery of Trauma (AAST):

Grade I:

- Hematuria with normal imaging studies
- Parenchymal contusions
- Nonexpanding subcapsular hematomas

Grade II:

- Nonexpanding perinephric hematomas confined to the retroperitoneum
- Superficial cortical lacerations less than 1 cm in depth without collecting system injury

Grade III:

- Renal lacerations greater than 1 cm in depth that do not involve the collecting system

Grade IV:

- Renal lacerations extending through the kidney into the collecting system
- Injuries involving the main renal artery or vein with contained hemorrhage
- Segmental infarctions without associated lacerations
- Expanding subcapsular hematomas compressing the kidney

Grade V ("Shattered" kidney):

- Ureteropelvic avulsions
- Complete laceration or thrombus of the main renal artery or vein

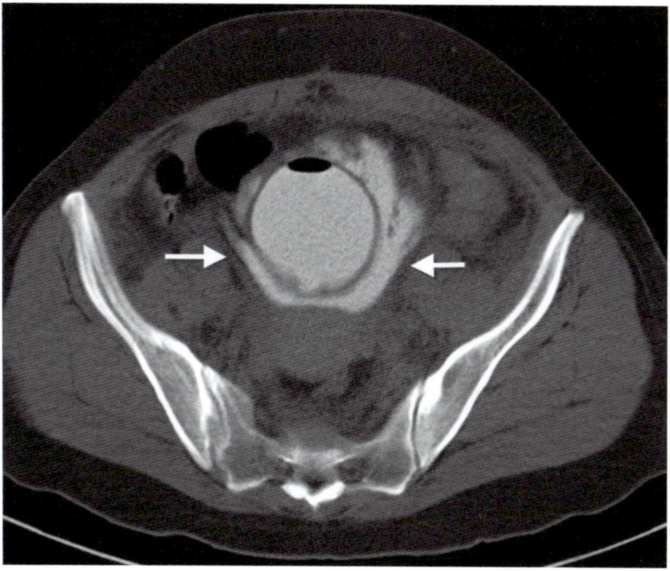

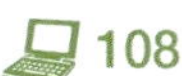

II-35

▮ EXTRAPERITONEAL BLADDER PERFORATION 💻 108

CT of the pelvis after retrograde instillation of water soluble contrast material through a foley catheter demonstrates extravasation of contrast into the perivesicular space. The leak is extraperitoneal since extravasated contrast is limited to the lateral paravesicular fascial planes of the pelvis.

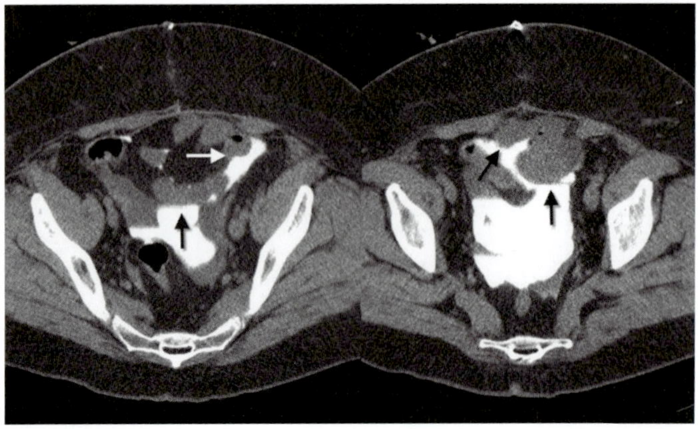

II-36

■ INTRAPERITONEAL BLADDER PERFORATION 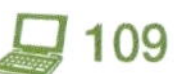 109

CT of the pelvis after retrograde instillation of water soluble contrast material through a foley catheter demonstrates contrast material surrounding adjacent small bowel loops (arrows), consistent with intraperitoneal extravasation.

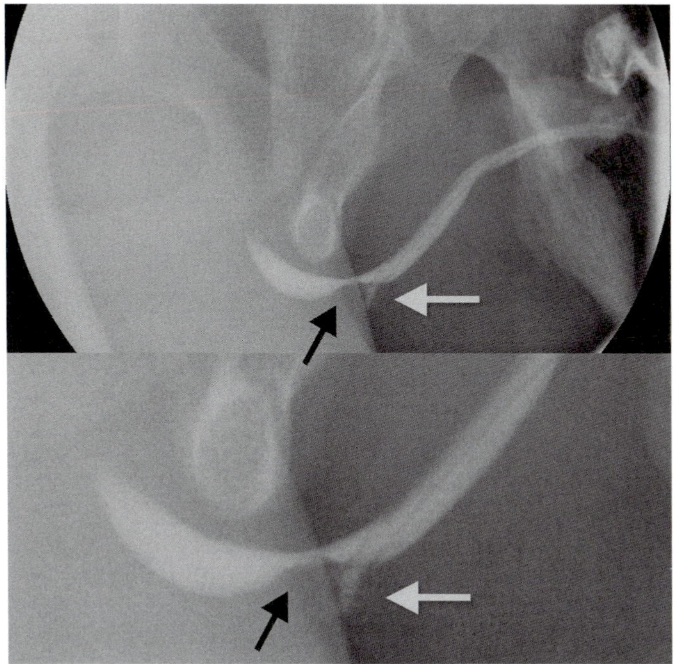

II-37

■ URETHRAL INJURY WITH SMALL BULBAR URETHRAL TEAR

💻 110

Retrograde urethrogram shows a narrowed segment of the bulbar urethra with a subtle irregularity of the contour of the posterior wall of the bulbar urethra (black arrow, lower image = magnified view). The catheter has been advanced and the tip is now projecting outside the lumen of the bulbar urethra (white arrow). Also noticed is a small amount of contrast extravasation adjacent to the catheter tip.

8. Gastrointestinal Tract

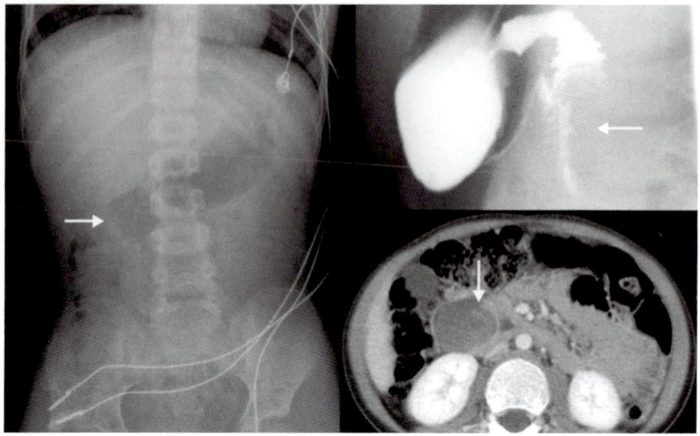

II-38

◼ DUODENAL HEMATOMA 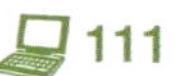 111

Abdominal radiograph demonstrates an air-filled stomach and dilated air-filled first portion of the duodenum (arrow, left image). Upper GI examination demonstrates a large mural filling defect involving the second portion of the duodenum which nearly completely obstructs the entire lumen (arrow, right upper image). Contrast enhanced CT of the abdomen demonstrates a large hemorrhage involving the duodenal wall, with some higher attenuation components, indicative of active bleed (arrow, right lower image).

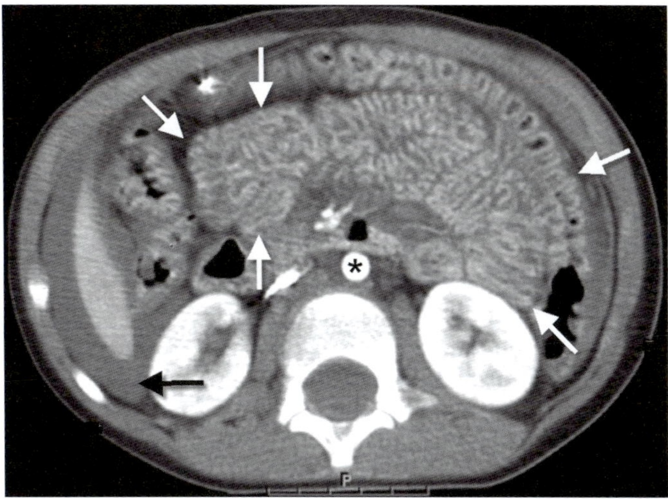

II-39

■ SHOCK BOWEL WITH HEMOPERITONEUM 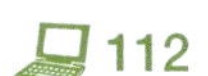 112

Contrast enhanced CT of the abdomen demonstrates a persistent bowel wall enhancement pattern in this shock hypotonic patient after MVA. There is intermediate density perihepatic fluid (black arrow), consistent with hemoperitoneum. Small caliber aorta (asterisk) is indicative of a hypotonic status/shock.

PNEUMOPERITONEUM – INTRODUCTION    113

- Pneumoperitoneum = Free intraabdominal air
- Radiographs can detect up to 1 cc of free air
- Best view: upright or left lateral decubitus
- Upright: air crescent under left hemidiaphragm, along diaphragmatic crux or between liver and right hemdiaphragm
- Decubitus: Air between abdominal wall and bowel/right liver lobe
- Supine view unreliable, may show Rigler's sign (air on both sides of bowel wall)
- Highest sensitivity for detection of free air: CT in lung windows

Pneumoperitoneum 2nd to:
- Perforated viscus (peptic ulcer, diverticulitis, appendicitis, toxic mega-colon, intestinal infarction)
- Neoplasm
- Abscess
- Iatrogenic (recent surgery/laparoscopy)

Caveat!
Mimicker: Colon interposition, hiatal hernia

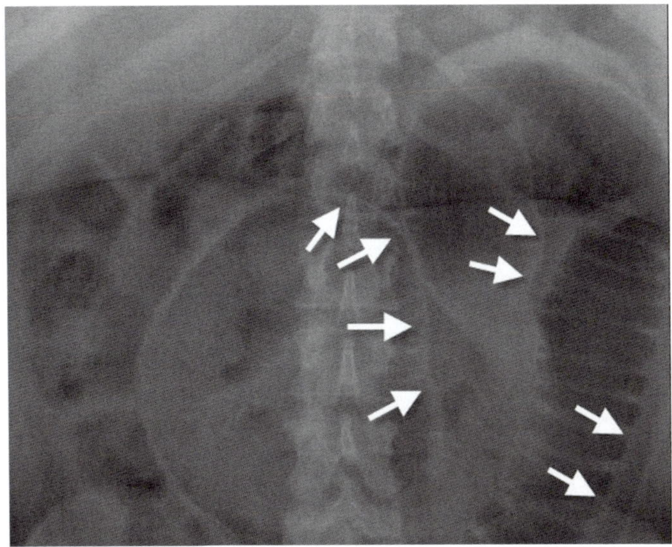

II-40

■ PNEUMOPERITONEUM WITH RIGLER'S SIGN 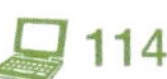 114

Free intraabdominal air with Rigler's sign. Rigler's sign: Bowel wall visualized due to bilateral (intra- and extraluminal) air contrast (arrows).

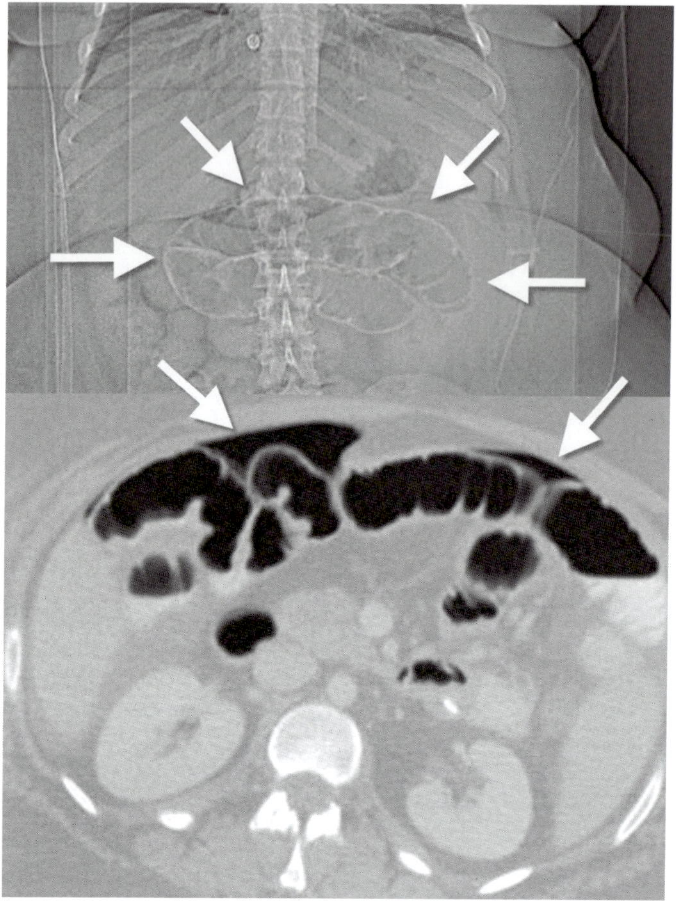

II-41

◼ PNEUMOPERITONEUM WITH RIGLER'S SIGN – CT CORRELATION

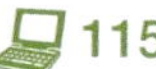 115

CT topogram (Upper image) demonstrates a typical Rigler's sign from free intraperitoneal air (arrows), which is confrmed by the subsequent CT (bottom image).

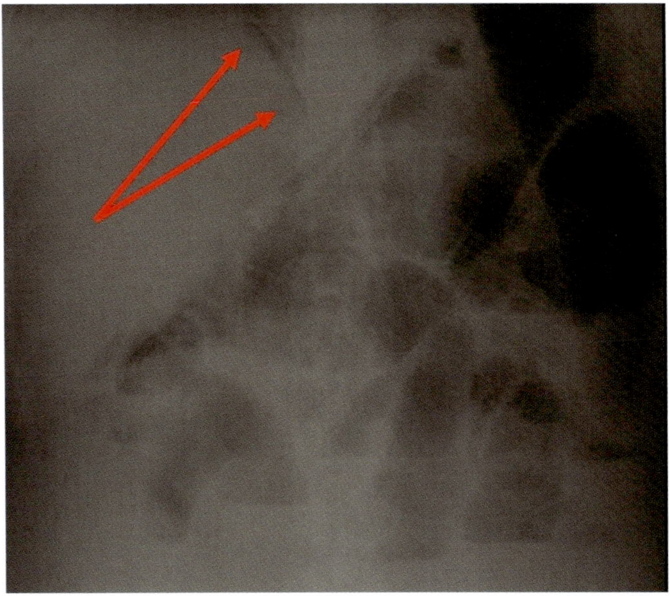

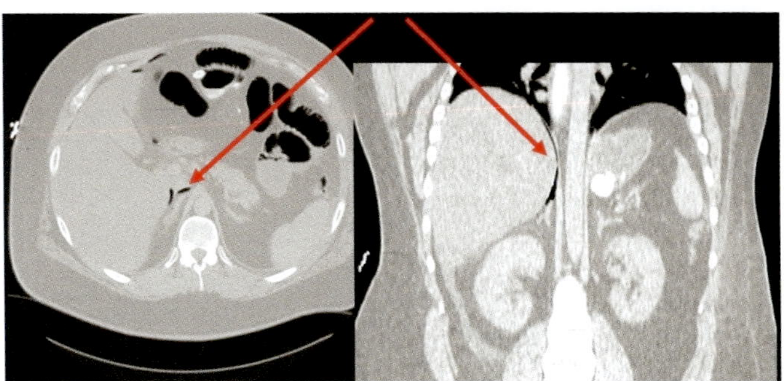

II-42

II-43

■ PNEUMOPERITONEUM 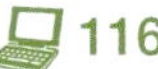 116

Free intraabdominal air is seen along diaphragmatic crux (arrows) on this upright abdominal radiograph.CT in lung windows confirms the free intra-peritoneal location of air.

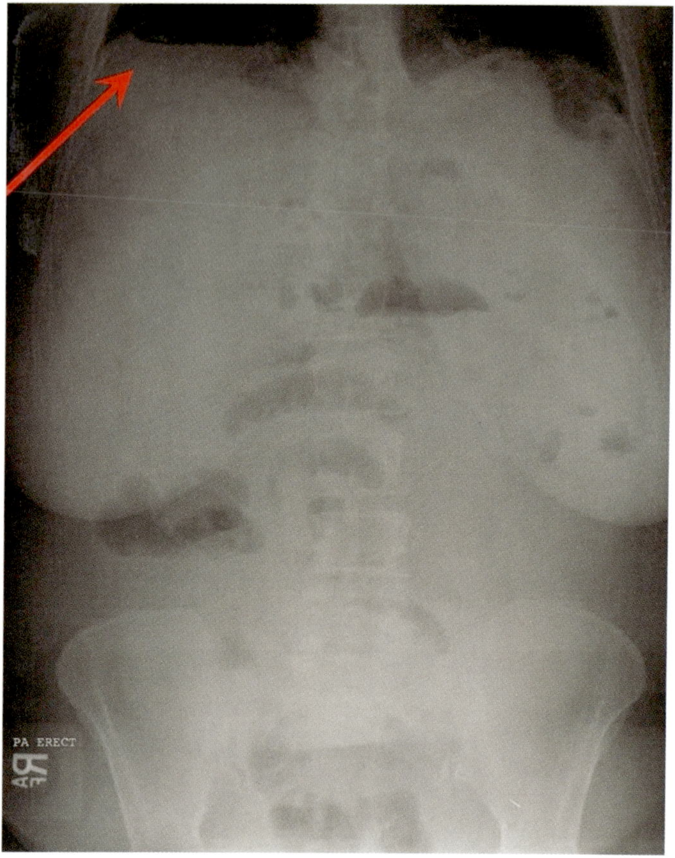

II-44

■ FREE INTRAABDOMINAL AIR
(AFTER IATROGENIC PERFORATION)
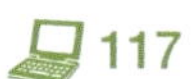 117

Upright KUB shows a crescent shaped air-fluid level below the right hemi-diaphragm (arrow). This patient underwent recent colonoscopy which was likely the culprit of perforation.

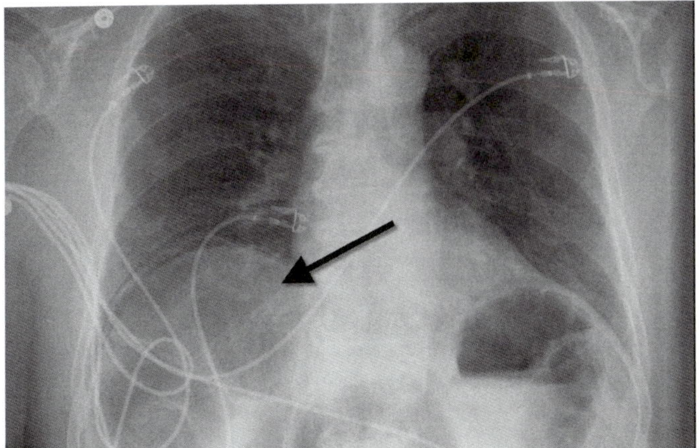

II-45

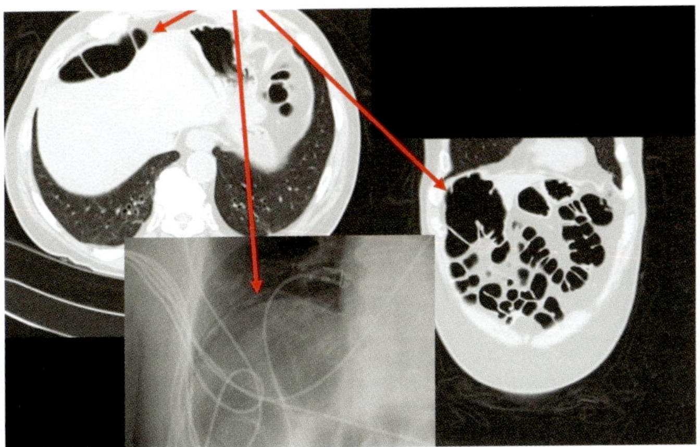

II-46

■ PNEUMOPERITONEUM MIMICKER: COLONIC INTERPOSITION

🖥 118

Patient complained about abdominal pain after colonoscopy. The lucent area over the right upper quadrant (upright KUB, upper image, black arrow) however has a haustral pattern and represents colon interposed between liver and diaphragm (as seen on CT).

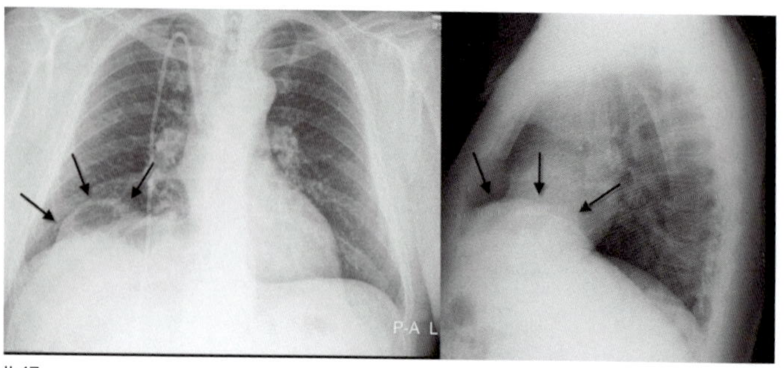

II-47

PNEUMOPERITONEUM MIMICKER: DIAPHRAGMATIC EVENTRATION

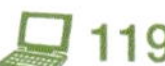 119

Eventration of right hemidiaphragm (arrows) with colon interposition. Eventration is usually due to local weakness of the diaphragm. The dense line (left image, arrows) represents the hemidiaphragm. Below you notice an air lucency, which is from bowel gas – and which might mimick free air on the first look.

■ PNEUMATOSIS – INTRODUCTION 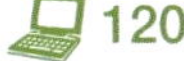 120

Pneumatosis in small bowel loops: air is seen within the bowel wall. You can differentiate intraluminal air from bowel wall air, if you see air within the dependent portions of the bowel wall. Air rises – if it is within the bowel wall it can not! On supine plain films air in the bowel wall might also appear as speckled air lucencies. One etiology is bowel obstruction – as in the following case.

Portal venous gas comes usually from pneumatosis – the air is transported (usually via SMV) into the portal system. It might be confused by pneumo-bilia; however, portal venous gas is more peripherally located in the liver, since it is pushed away in the direction of the portal venous flow.

- Speckled air seen in association with bowel loops on radiograph
- Air seen in bowel wall (on CT)
- Air seen in portal venous system

Caveat:
Pneumobilia can mimick pneumatosis in liver -> History important (previous ERCP, biliary surgery)

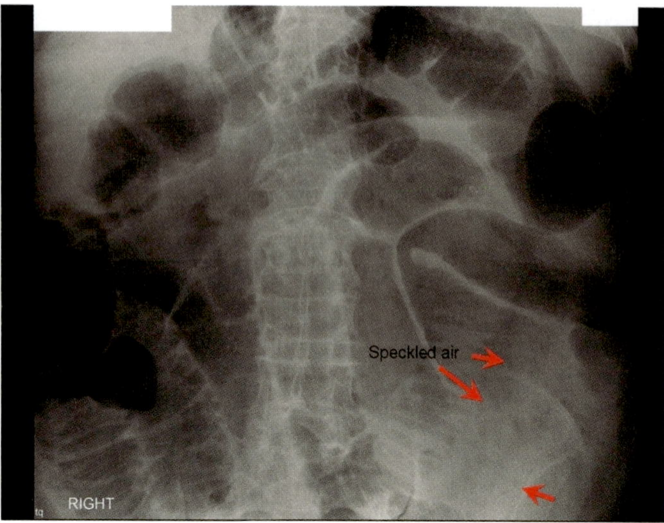

II-48

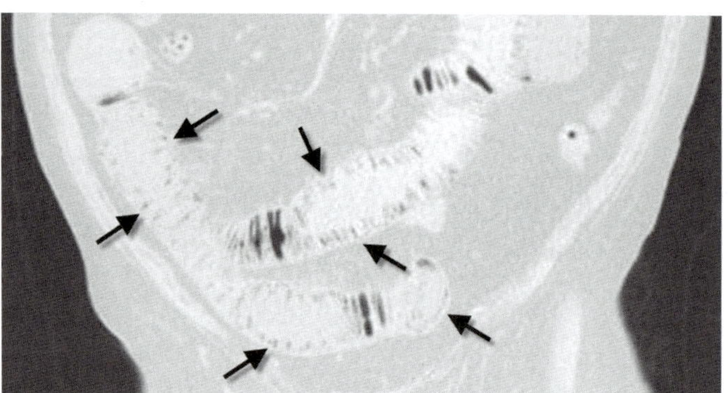

II-49

PNEUMATOSIS 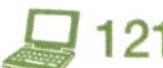 121

Speckled air lucencies are noted in association with several bowel loops (arrows, abdominal radiograph at the top). These lucencies correlate with air in several bowel loops (arrows, coronal reformatted CT in lung window, lower image). This patient has a small bowel obstruction which is a common etiology for pneumatosis.

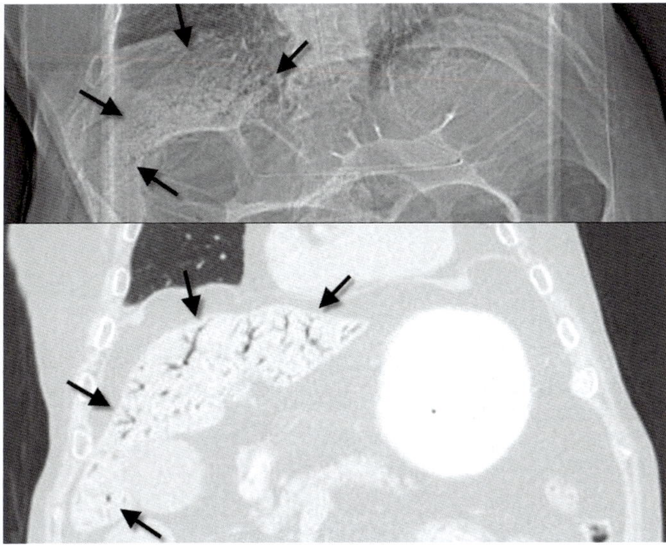

II-50

PNEUMATOSIS – PORTAL VENOUS GAS   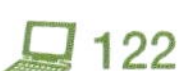 122

Linear, radiating air lucencies are noted projecting over the liver (arrows, CT topogram at the top). These lucencies correlate within the intrahepatic portal venous tree (arrows, coronal reformatted CT in lung window, lower image). The air is transported via SMV secondary to pneumatosis, caused by the patient's small bowel obstruction (see dilated bowel loops in the upper image).

■ BOWEL OBSTRUCTION – INTRODUCTION 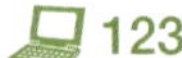 123

- Dilated small bowel (> 3cm)
- Dilated large bowel (> 5 cm)
- Air fluid levels on upright view
- On supine view small bowel loops may have a circular configuration
- No air in distal colon/rectum (if prolonged, however can still be seen in early phase)
- Look for free intraabdominal air (perforation)!

Etiologies for small bowel obstruction
- Volvulus
- Intususception
- Adhesions (postoperative)
- Hernia
- Obstructing neoplasm
- Stricture (eg, Crohn's stricture)
- Foreign bodies
- Infection/abscess

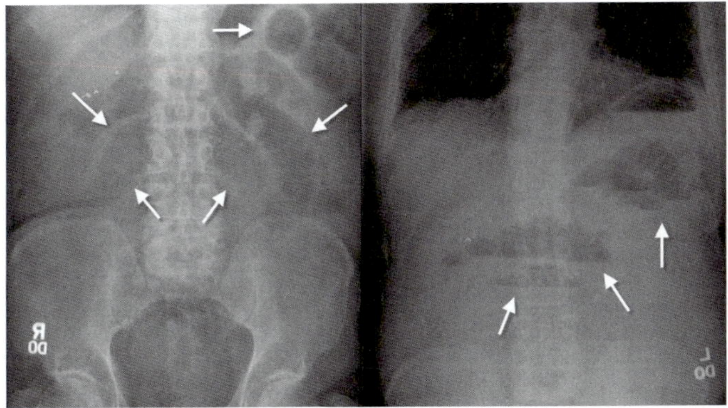

II-51

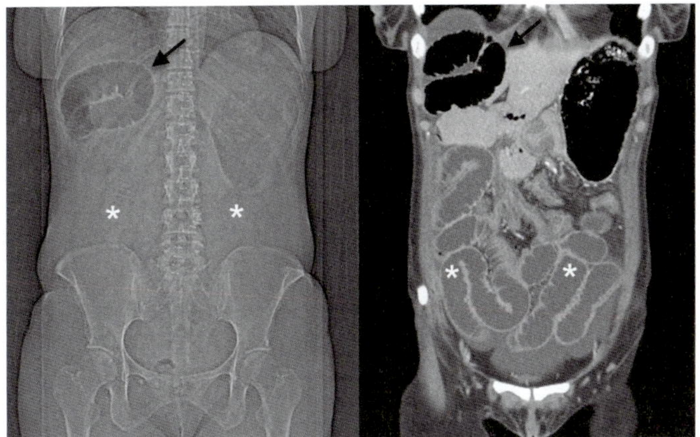

II-52

■ SMALL BOWEL OBSTRUCTION 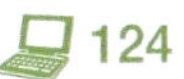 124

Upper row: Supine view (left image) demonstrates dilated air-filled small bowel loops (arrows) in a circular arrangement. The upright abdominal radiograph (right image) demonstrates air-fluid levels (arrows) within these dilated bowel loops.

Lower row: CT topogram (supine) and coronal reformatted CT demonstrate proximal air-filled dilated loop (arrow) and dilated completely fluid filled distal loops of bowel (asterisk)

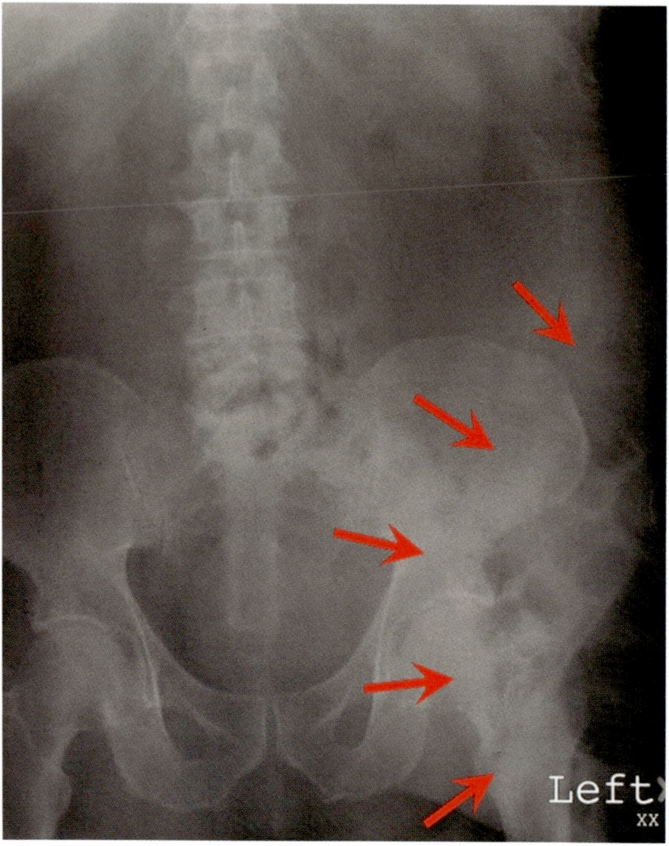

II-53

■ OBSTRUCTING ABDOMINAL WALL HERNIA ⌨ 125

This patient herniated his small bowel through an abdominal wall defect. We can appreciate the air-filled and dilated-bowel loops within the hernia (arrows), indicating obstruction. There is relative paucity of air, especially in the lower abdomen.

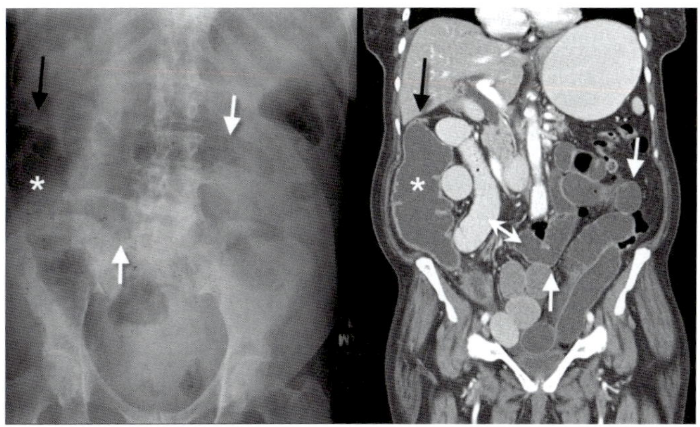

II-54

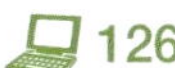 LARGE BOWEL OBSTRUCTION 126

A hepatic flexure stricture is causing large bowel obstruction proximal to this level. Note is made of a dilated, air-filled ascending colon (asterisk) with abrupt cut-off at the hepatic flexure. Coronal reformatted CT (right image) confirms a stricture at the hepatic flexure (black arrows). Also noticed are dilated air-filled small bowel loops, which subsequently also become obstructed. The reason, why some bowel loops contain contrast, some less, and some no contrast (double arrow) is, because the contrast did not have a chance to progress to the more distal loops.

By the way: both, the abdominal radiograph and CT were performed in patient supine position, therefore fluid is layering posterior and air anterior. The CT cut has been performed in a more posterior position, thus showing fluid in the bowel.

■ VOLVULUS - INTRODUCTION

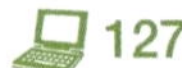 127

Volvulus
- Most common: sigmoid and cecum
- Less frequent: stomach, small bowel, transverse colon
- May lead to partial or complete obstruction

Sigmoid volvulus
- Dilated sigmoid (coffee bean shaped)
- Inverted U-shaped
- Loss of haustration
- Coffee-bean sign due to midline crease (arrow, right image)
- Rotates and points toward RUQ

Cecal volvulus
- Dilated cecum (coffee bean shaped)
- Inverted U-shaped
- Loss of haustration
- Coffee-bean sign due to midline crease
- Rotates and points toward LUQ
- Dilated cecum rests in LUQ

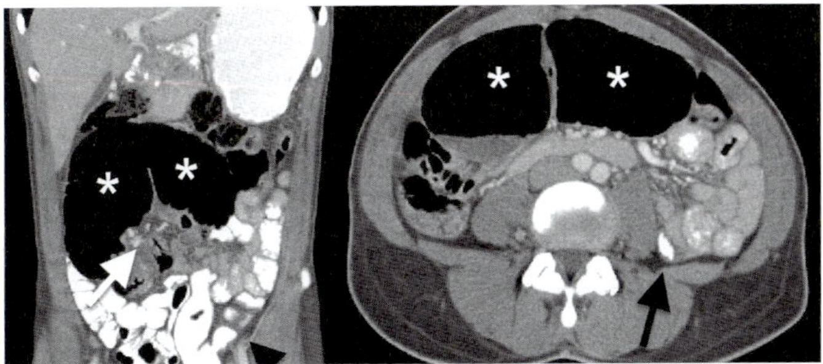

II-55

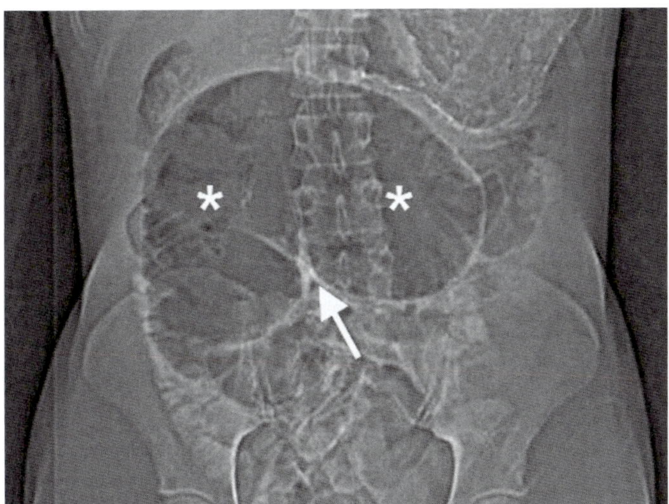

II-56

■ CECAL VOLVULUS MIMICKING
SIGMOID VOLVULUS

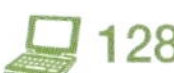 128

We see a largely dilated air-filled loop of bowel (asterisk) in the RUQ with a crease (arrow) giving it a coffee bean appearance. The crease is pointing toward the right upper quadrant which is more typical for a sigmoid volvulus. However, contrast enhanced CT (upper image) confirms that the rotated structure is indeed the cecum – rotated around the cecal mesentery (white arrow). Black arrows indicate a (rectal) contrast filled nondilated descending colon.

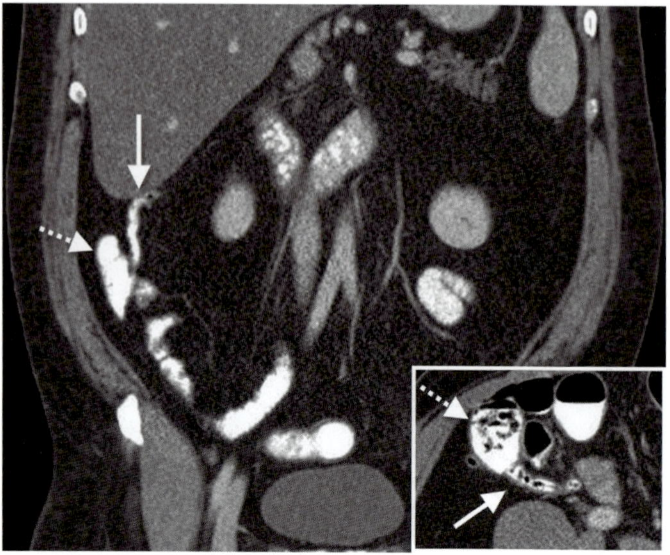

II-57

◼ NORMAL APPENDIX   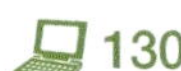 130

A normal appendix (arrow) should be patent, no more than 6 mm in diameter and contain contrast material if applied (that's why rectal contrast
useful in evaluation of appendicitis). Right lower corner demonstrates
a magnified view of a normal appendix in an axial plane. Dotted arrow
points to the cecum.

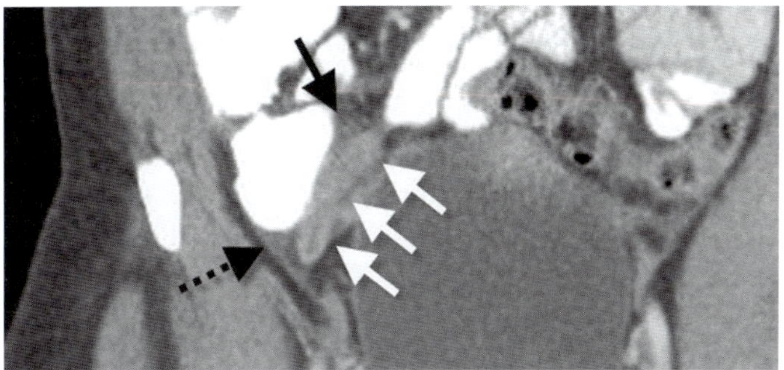

II-58

APPENDICITIS 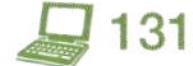 131

Coronal reformatted contrast enhanced CT of the abdomen: The appendix is thickened (arrows), contains no rectal contrast material (not patent) and demonstrates some peri-appendiceal fat stranding (black arrow) and a tiny amount of free fluid (dotted black arrow).

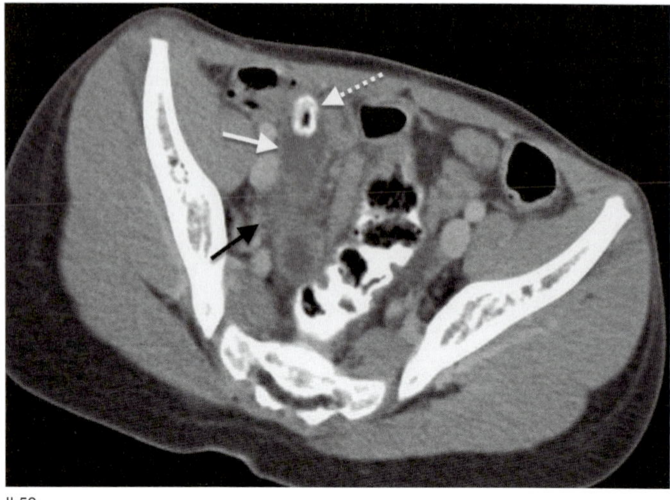

II-59

APPENDICITIS CAUSED BY AN APPENDICOLITH

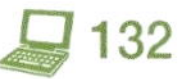 132

Axial contrast enhanced CT of the abdomen: The appendix is fluid-filled and dilated (full white arrow), up to 1.7 cm. A 1.4 × 0.9 cm appendicolith is noted in the proximal appendix (dotted white arrow). Also noted is peri-appendiceal fat stranding (black arrow), sign of an acute inflammatory process. An appendix diameter larger than 6 mm, fluid filled appendix, appendicolith, and peri-appendiceal fat stranding are indicative of acute appendicitis.

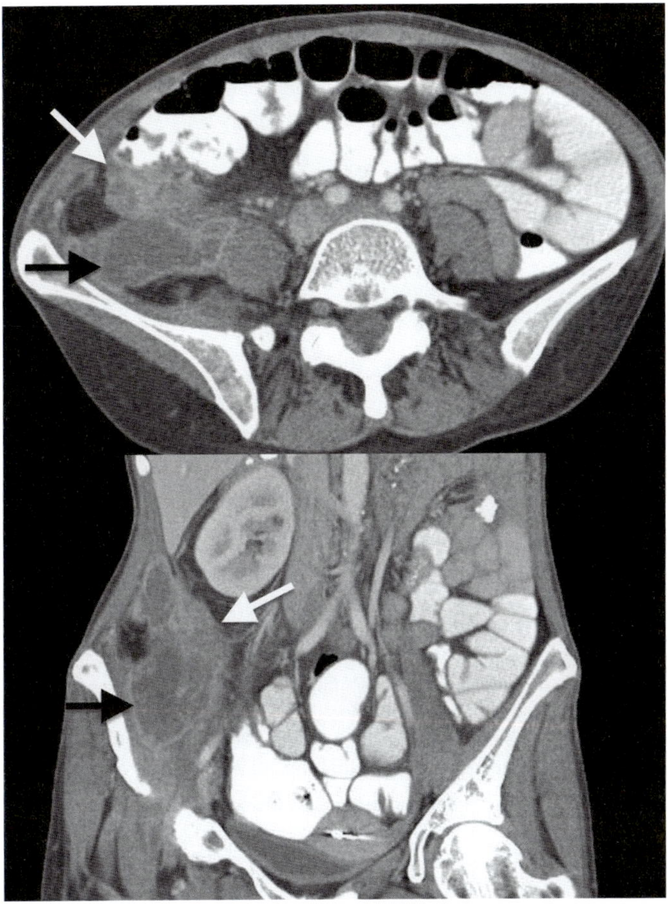

II-60

RUPTURED APPENDICITIS WITH ABSCESS FORMATION

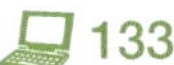 133

Contrast enhanced CT of the abdomen in axial plane (upper image) and coronal reformation (bottom image). The appendix (white arrow) is thickened and ruptured. A peri-appendiceal abscess has evolved (black arrow).

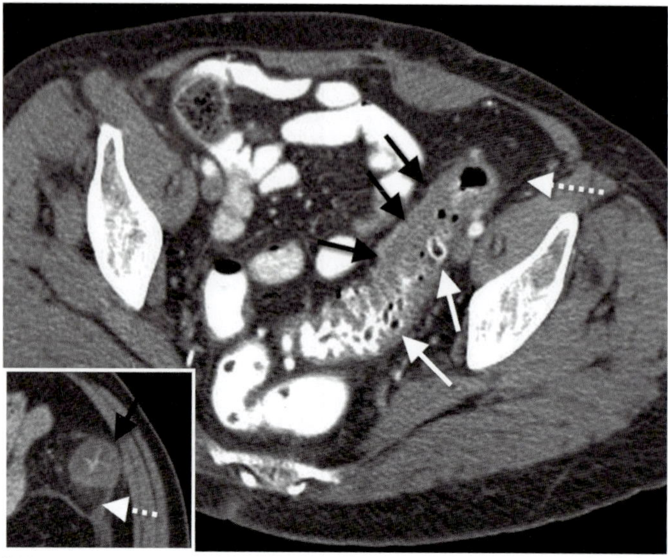

II-61

■ DIVERTICULITIS 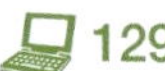 129

Contrast enhanced CT (IV, oral and rectal contrast) of the abdomen: There are scattered diverticula (white arrows) and wall thickening (black arrows) of about 8 cm of descending colon with associated fat stranding (dotted white arrow) – a classic combination for acute diverticulitis. Left lower frame magnified view of another patient with acute diverticulitis.

For distal bowel evaluation it is always advised to use rectal contrast, which allows a better evaluation of bowel wall and luminal pathologies. Otherwise collapsed bowel could mimic bowel wall thickening.

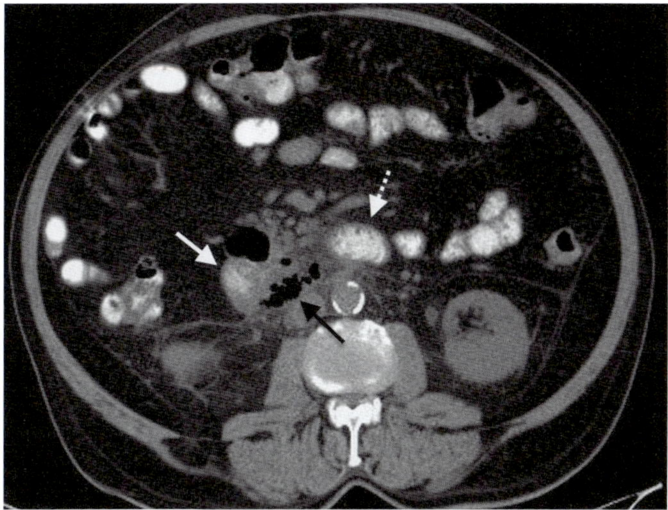

II-62

■ PERFORATED DUODENAL ULCER 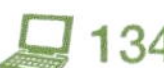 134

Axial CT of the abdomen with oral contrast demonstrates free intraabdominal air (black arrow), fat stranding and small amount of free fluid between the second portion of the duodenum (white arrow) and the proximal jejunum (dotted white arrow). This patient perforated his duodenal ulcer.

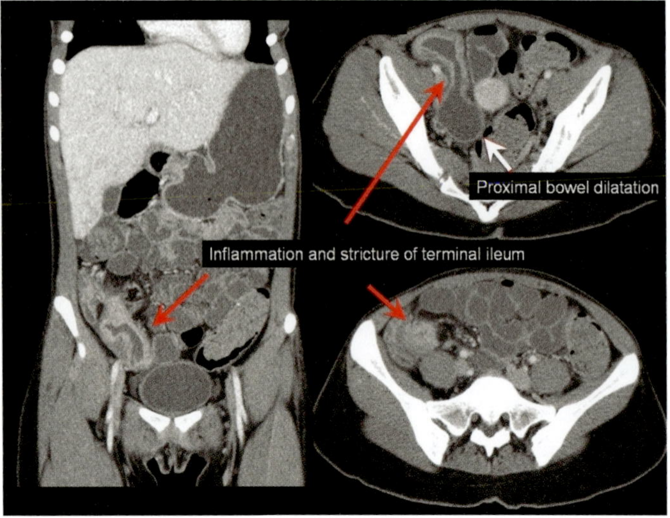

II-63

CROHN'S DISEASE CAUSING SMALL BOWEL OBSTRUCTION

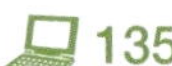 135

There is inflammation and stricture of the terminal ileum noted (red arrows) with small bowel dilatation proximal to this segment (white arrow). The terminal ileum is a typical location for a Crohn's flare.

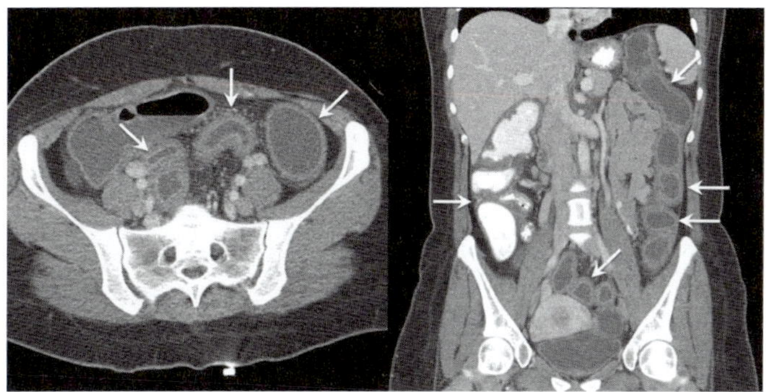

II-64

■ COLITIS 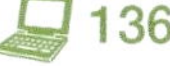 136

Axial (left image) and coronal reformatted CT of the abdomen (right image) demonstrate diffuse continuous and hyperenhancing colonic wall thickening (arrows) throughout the entire colon which is mildly distended and fluid filled. This patient suffered shigella pancolitis.

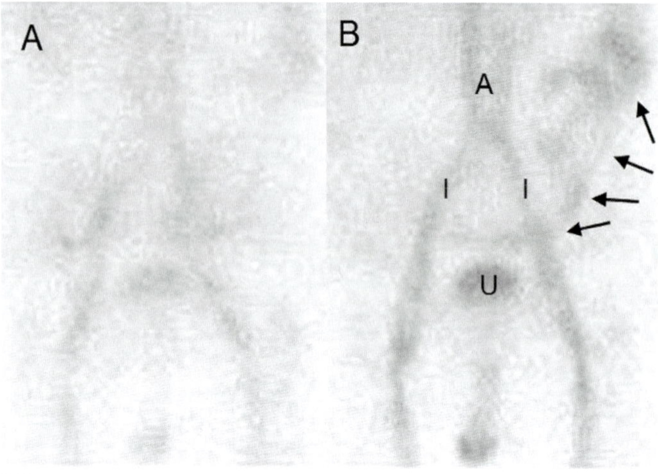

II-65

ACUTE GASTROINTESTINAL BLEED (GI BLEED) – RBC SCAN

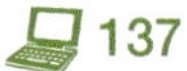 137

A tagged red blood cell (RBC) scan demonstrates initially (A) only tracer activity within the vascular system (A = aorta, I = iliac arteries) and urinary system (U = urinary bladder). Images obtained a few minutes later (B) demonstrate new tracer activity in the left abdomen (arrows) that are confined to the small bowel. This is consistent with active GI bleed. RBC scan images need to be evaluated over time where active GI bleed can be appreciated as moving tracer activity that follows the bowel pathway.

9. Female Reproductive System

■ FEMALES IN REPRODUCTIVE AGE 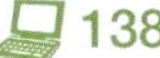 138

ANY female in reproductive age and presentation with pelvic or abdominal pain should undergo at least a qualitative (urine) beta HCG testing to rule out pregnancy!

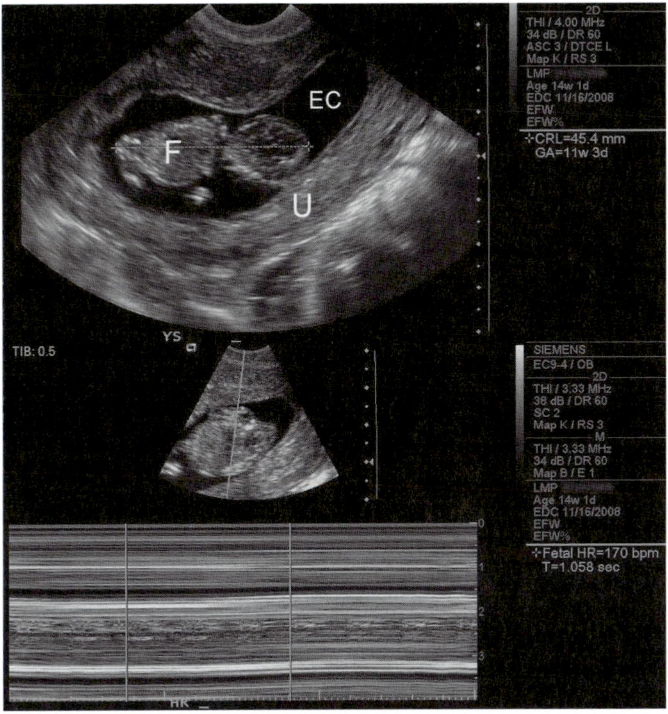

II-66

■ FIRST TRIMESTER ULTRASOUND: NORMAL INTRAUTERINE PREGNANCY 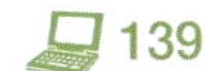 139

There is a single gestation within the endometrial cavity. F = Fetus; U = Uterus; EC = Endometrial cavity. Lower image demonstrates cardiac activity (approximately 170 bpm).

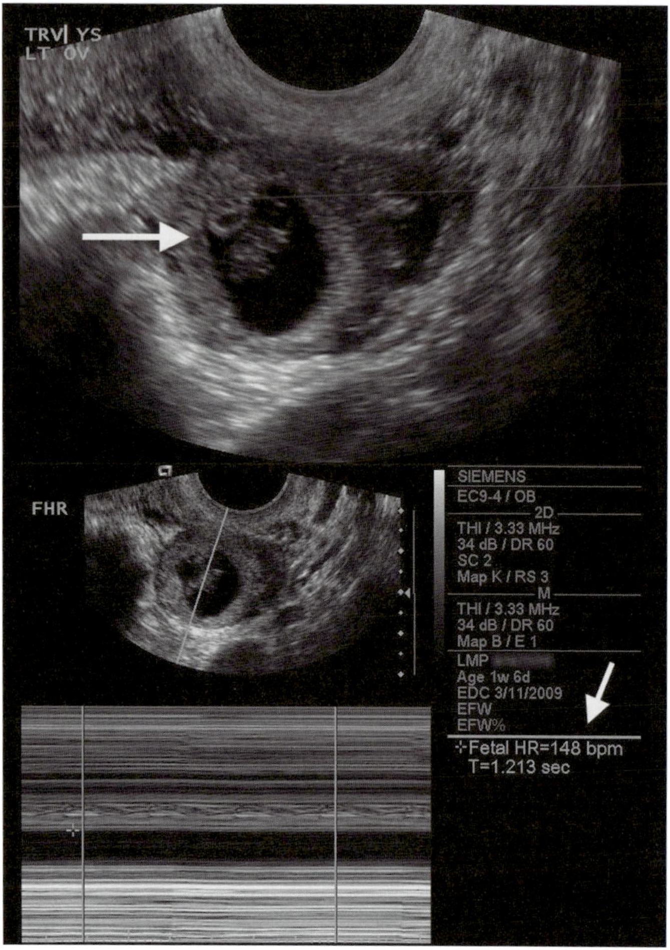

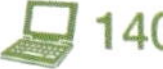

II-67

▪ ECTOPIC PREGNANCY   💻 140

Pelvic ultrasound demonstrates a gestational sac in the left ovary. Lower image shows a fetal heart rate of 148 bpm.

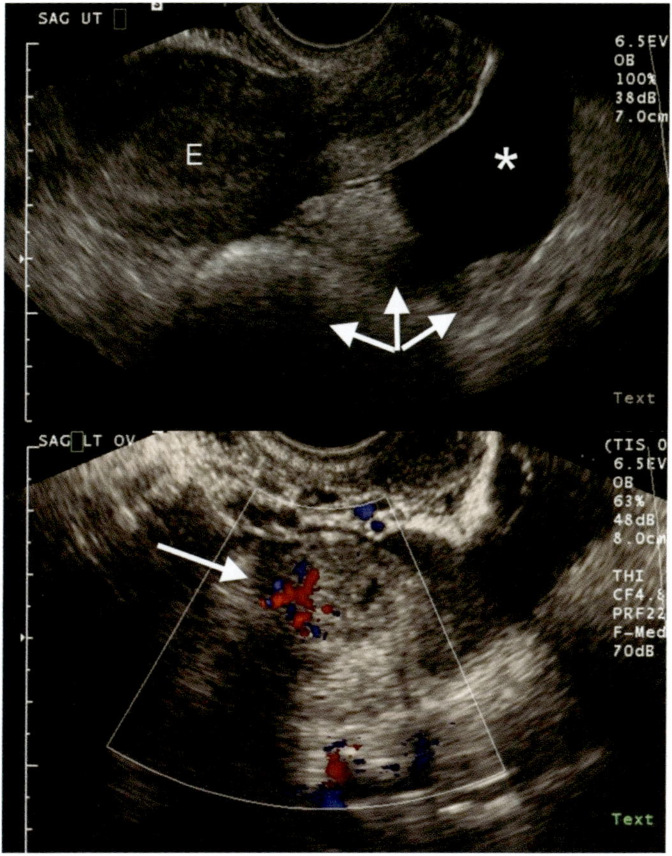

II-68

■ RUPTURED ECTOPIC PREGNANCY    141

Grayscale (top image) ultrasound demonstrates a thickened endometrial complex (E) without a gestastional sac within the uterus. There is also a moderate amount of complex fluid (arrows) in the cul-de-sac (asterisk). Color Doppler image demonstrates a complex left adnexal mass with several thickened walls and internal flow (arrow).

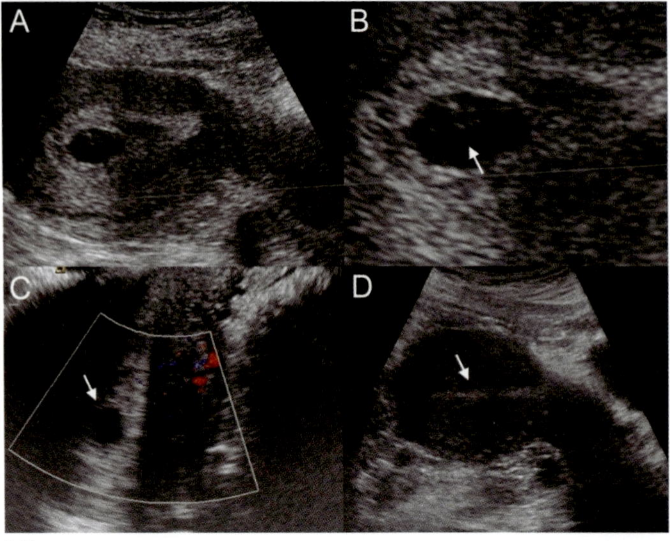

II-69

■ FETAL DEMISE 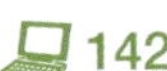 142

Sagittal pelvic ultrasound images of a 25-year-old pregnant woman demonstrate an enlarged uterus as well as a gestational sac within the uterus (A). There is a fetal pole identified within the endometrial cavity (arrow, B), however, no heart rate is identified on spectral and color Doppler images (C, arrow). This is highly concerning for fetal demise. However, this could have also represented very early pregnancy, why a follow-up ultrasound was recommended. Follow-up ultrasound one day later (D) cannot demonstrate either gestational sac or fetal pole, which have been expelled in the mean time.

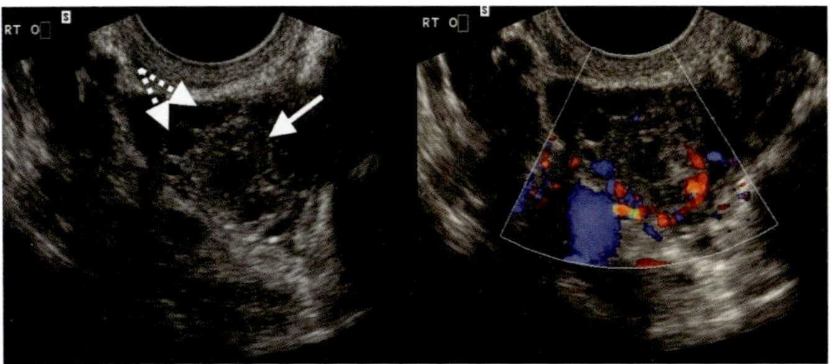

II-70

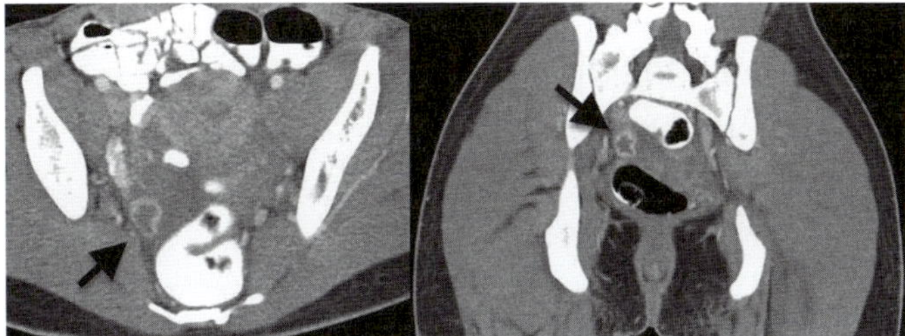

II-71

■ HEMORRHAGIC OVARIAN CYST 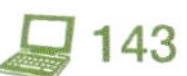 143

Upper image: Grayscale (left image) ultrasound of the pelvis demonstrates in the right ovary a 2 cm complex cyst (white arrow) with thick walls, internal debris and septations. Color Doppler image (right image) shows no flow within this lesion. This turned out to be a hemorrhagic ovarian cyst. Internal flow within this lesion would have raised suspicion for a neoplasm. However, no flow does not exclude a neoplasm and a follow-up ultrasound is warranted. A hemorrhagic cyst should have resolved or at least got smaller with time while a neoplasm does not. Dotted arrows point to physiologic ovarian follicles (should only be seen in premenopausal women).

Lower image: CT of the abdomen (performed to exclude appendicitis) demonstrates the hemorrhagic cyst as a lobulated and rim enhancing lesion in the right lower pelvis (arrows)

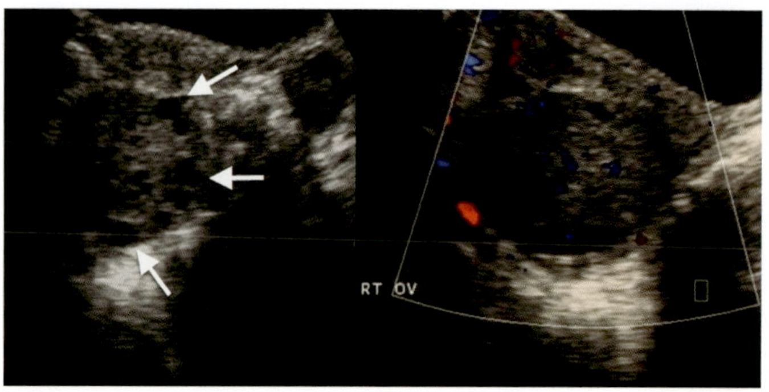

II-72

■ OVARIAN TORSION　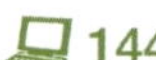 144

This woman presented with sudden onset of pelvic pain. Grayscale (left) and color Doppler images (left) demonstrate an enlarged (6 cm) and echogenic right ovary associated with multiple peripheral follicles. Color Doppler demonstrates detectable Doppler flow.

An enlarged (compare with contralateral ovary) ovary as well as peripheral located follicles are indicative of ovarian torsion.

Ovarian torsion can still be present even if flow is present. The ovary can be torsed enough to strangulate the low pressure venous outflow while still preserving the high pressure arterial inflow – causing venous congestion and subsequently infarct.

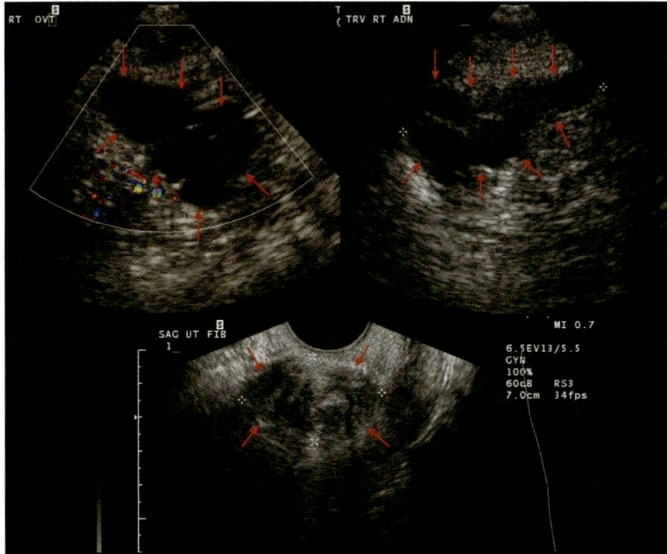

II-73

▪ HYDROSALPINX DUE TO UTERINE FIBROIDS 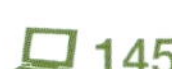 145

Sagittal color Doppler (left top) and transverse grayscale (right top) ultrasound images demonstrate a anechoic tubular structure (arrows) in the right adnexal area, compatible with a fluid filled fallopian tube – hydrosalpinx. Evaluation of the uterus (lower image) demonstrates a 7 cm heterogeneous mass (arrows) in the uterus, causing the fallopian tube obstruction.

10. Male Reproductive System

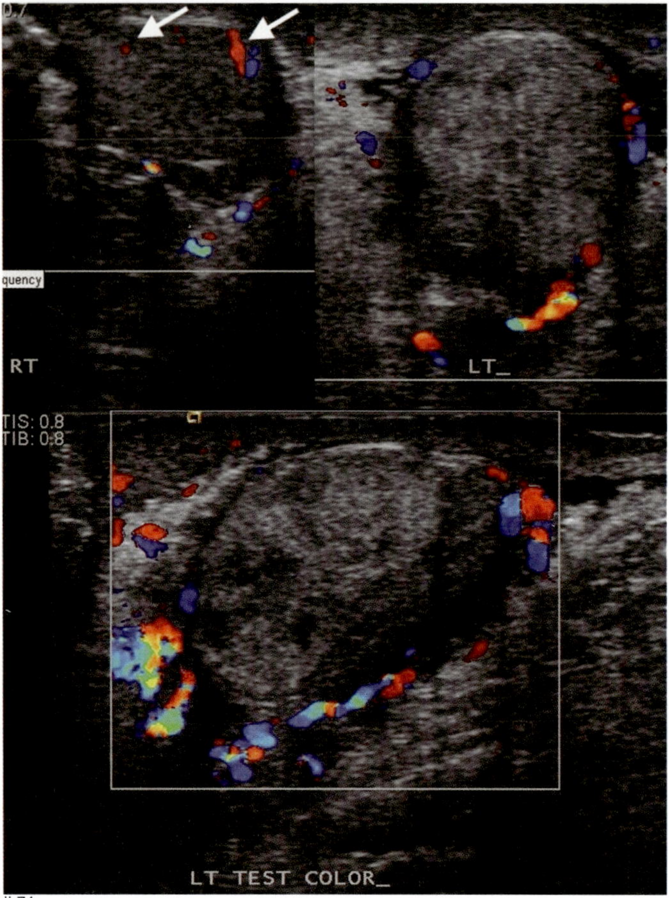

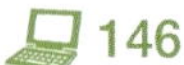

II-74

■ TESTICULAR TORSION WITH TESTICULAR INFARCT   146

Color Doppler ultrasound of the testicles demonstrates an enlarged left testicle which is heterogeneous in echotexture. There is no arterial or venous blood flow within the left testicle. (Compare to smaller right testicle showing blood flow indicated by arrows).

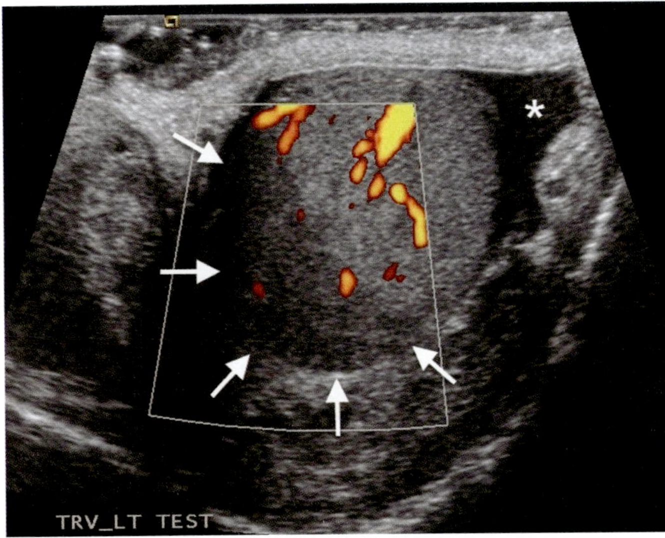

II-75

PARTIAL TESTICULAR INFARCT WITH HYDROCELE

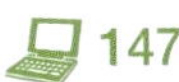 147

Power Doppler ultrasound shows a geographic area of low echogenicity in the medial mid to lower testicular area with absent blood flow (area surrounded by arrows). The speckle of color identified in the area of concern is likely artifactual. Power Doppler is more sensitive for detection of flow. However, power Doppler cannot calculate flow direction. Also noticed is a small hydrocele (asterisk).

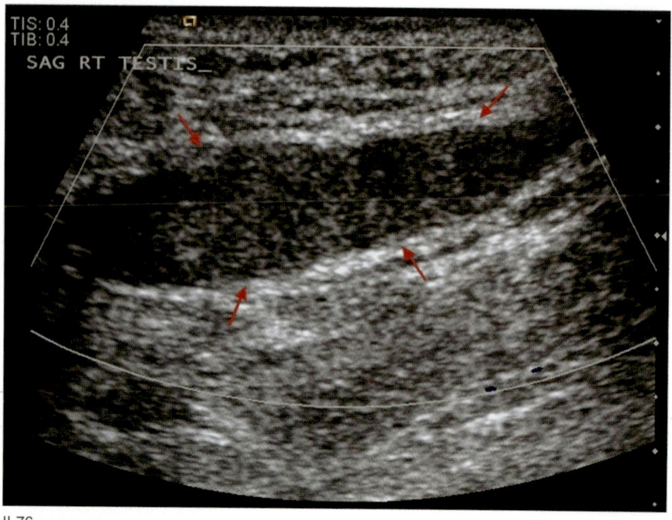

II-76

■ INFARCTED TESTIS INCARCERATED
IN INGUINAL CANAL   💻 148

The right testis (arrows) is located in the right inguinal canal. Power
Doppler ultrasound is not able to identify any intraparenchymal vascular
flow within the right testis, compatible with testicular infarct.

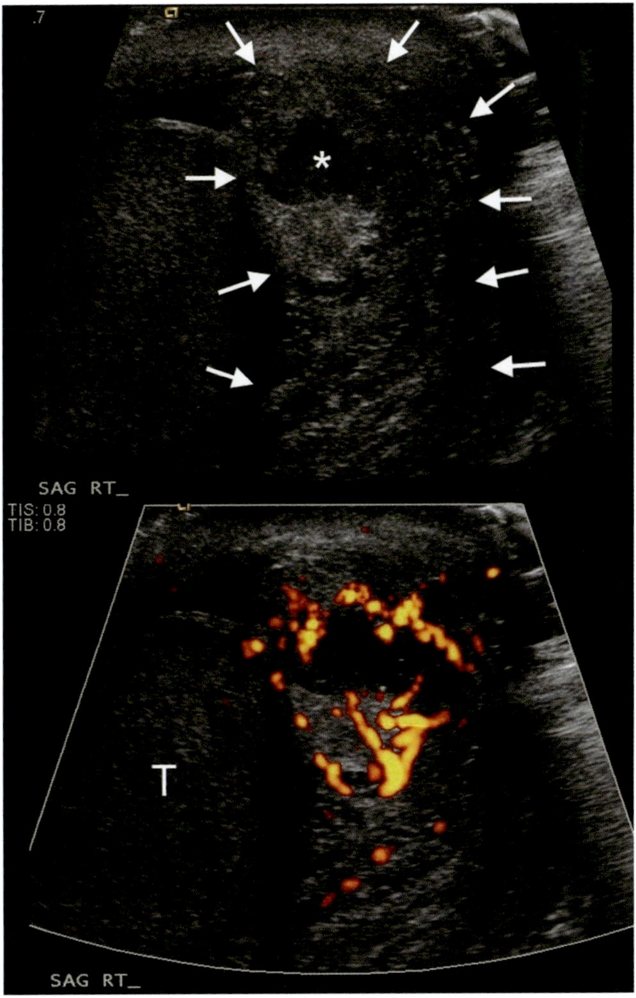

II-77

EPIDIDYMITIS WITH ABSCESS 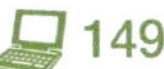 149

Grayscale ultrasound shows an enlarged right epididymal head and tail (arrows) which are heterogeneous in echotexture. There is in addition a central avascular hypoechoic area (asterisk) representing an abscess. Hyperperfusion is appreciated when compared to the neighboring testis (T).

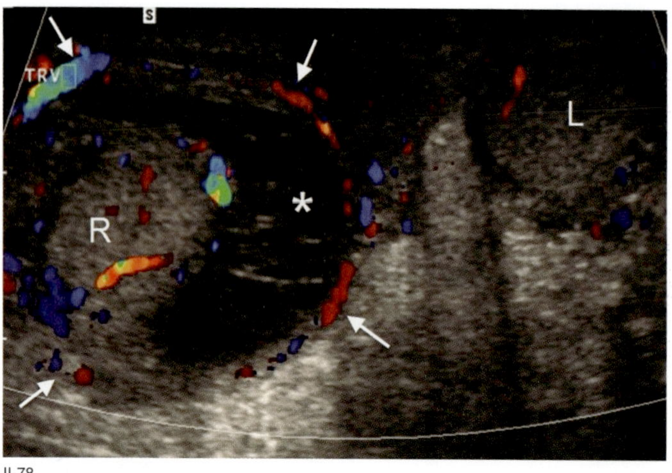

II-78

ORCHITIS AND PYOCELE 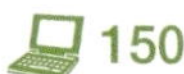 150

Color Doppler ultrasound (testicular "cleavage shot") demonstrates marked hyperemia in an enlarged right testicle (R) and scrotal wall (arrows). Compare size with left testicle (L)! There is also a right peritesticular complex fluid collection containing fine internal echoes (asterisk), consistent with a pyocele.

11. Vascular System

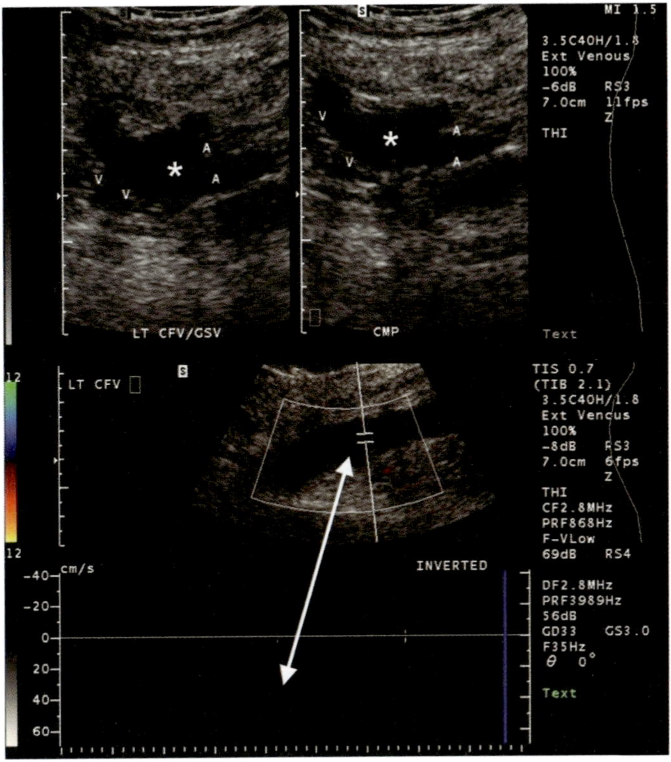

II-79

■ DEEP VEIN THROMBOSIS (DVT)

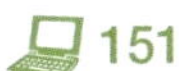 151

There is a completely occluding left common femoral vein thrombosis (asterisk, upper image). Veins (V) are not compressible (compression image to the right). Furthermore, spectral Doppler ultrasound does not reveal any flow within the vein (double arrow), confirming complete occlusion.

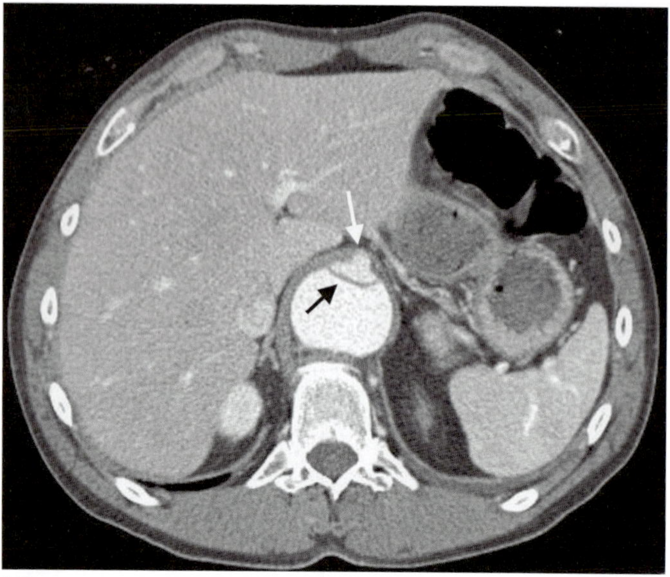

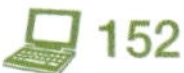

II-80

AORTIC DISSECTION

152

A dissection flap (black arrow) is noticed at the level of the celiac axis (white arrow) origin. A close look on the thoracic aorta is warranted to exclude a type A dissection (involving ascending aorta). The aorta is also aneurysmal dilated.

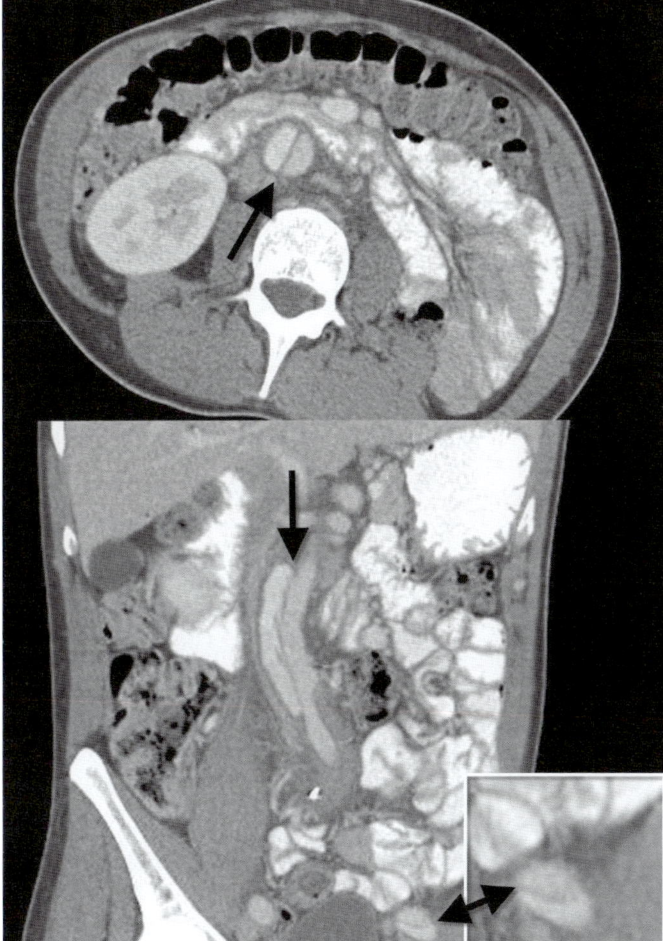

II-81

📱 153

■ AORTIC DISSECTION

Axial (top) and coronal reformatted (bottom) contrast enhanced CT of the abdomen shows a dissection flap dividing the infrarenal Aorta into two equal halves (black arrows). Magnified view (right lower corner) also shows extension of the dissection into the left external iliac artery (double arrow).

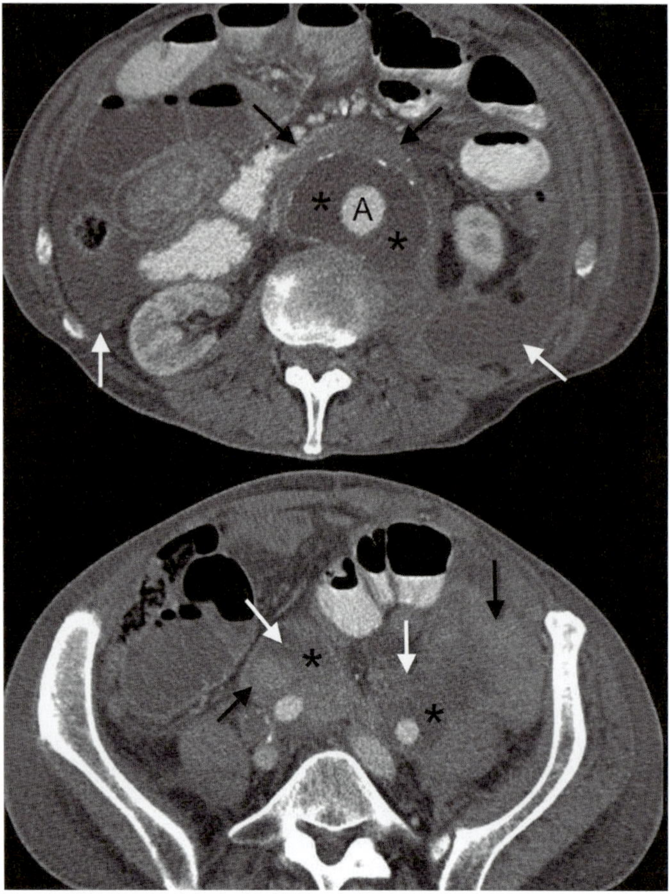

II-82

■ AORTIC ANEURYSM RUPTURE 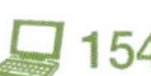 154

There is a partially thrombosed abdominal aortic aneurysm, extending into both iliac arteries (asterisk). Mixed attenuation material is surrounding the abdominal aneurysm as well as both iliac arteries and is also seen in the peritoneal space (white arrows), compatible with hemorrhage. Higher density material within the fluid (black arrows) is indicative of active hemorrhage. Note is also made of air fluid levels in several bowel loops, compatible with ileus.

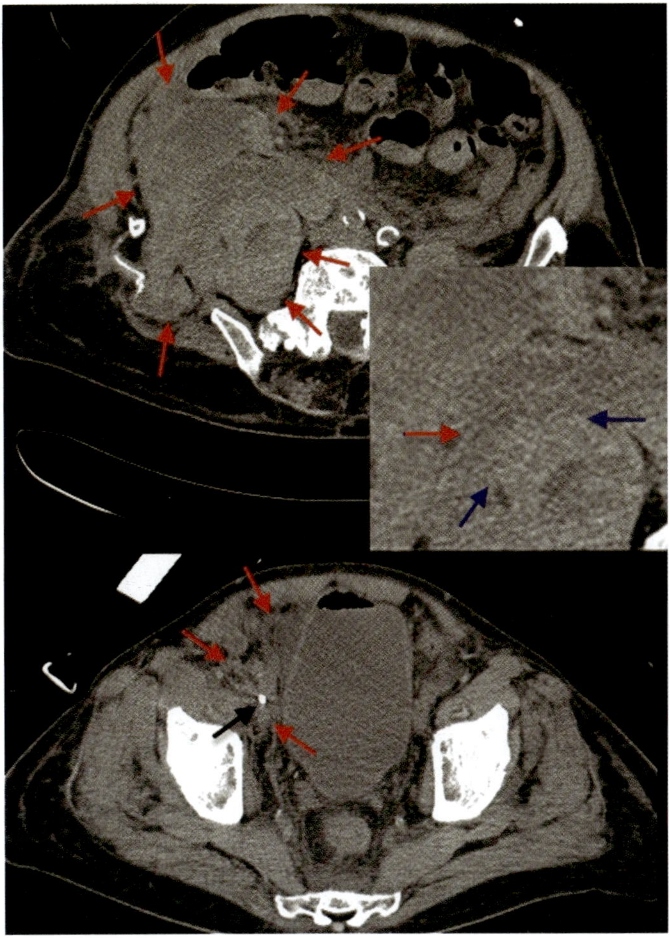

II-83

■ LARGE INTRA- AND EXTRAPERITONEAL HEMORRHAGE 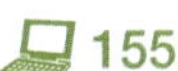 155

There is a large mixed attenuation fluid collection in the right lower abdomen and pelvis (red arrows). A right femoral line (black arrow) punctured the right external iliac artery. Higher density areas (blue arrows, magnified view) represent active bleed.

12. Devices

■ LINES AND TUBES – INTRODUCTION　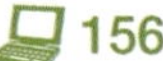 156

Make sure every tube/line/device is where it is supposed to be!
- Gastric feeding tube (terminates in stomach)
- Corpak feeding tube (terminates in jejunum)
- Nephrostomy (terminates in renal pelvis)
- Biliary drain (terminates in gallbladder or biliary system – dependent on location of obstruction)
- VP shunt (terminates in abdominal cavity)

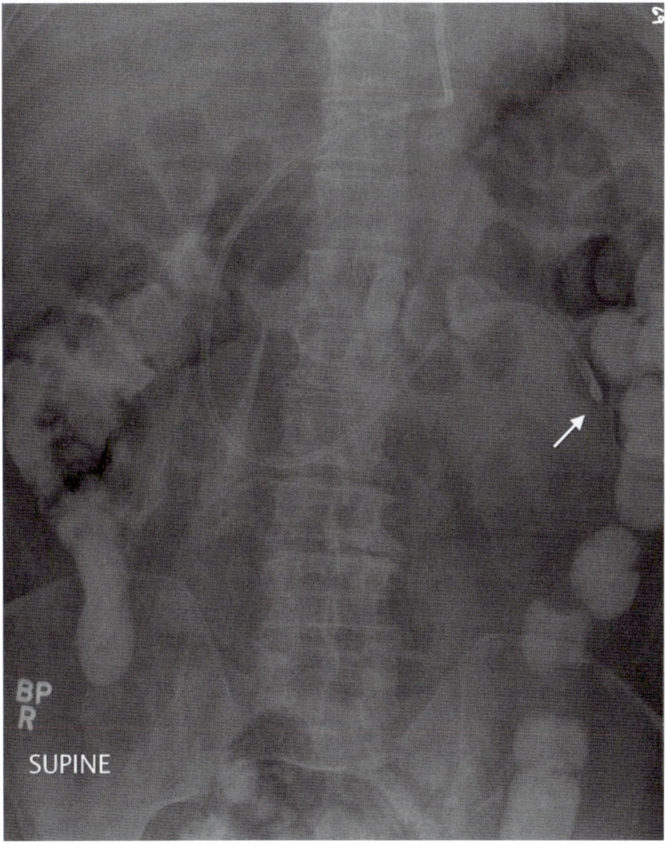

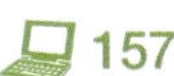

II-84

CORPAK FEEDING TUBE 157

Abdominal radiograph shows a correct position of a Corpak feeding tube with its distal tip located in jejunum (arrow). The tip should be beyond the ligament of Treitz – left to the spine.

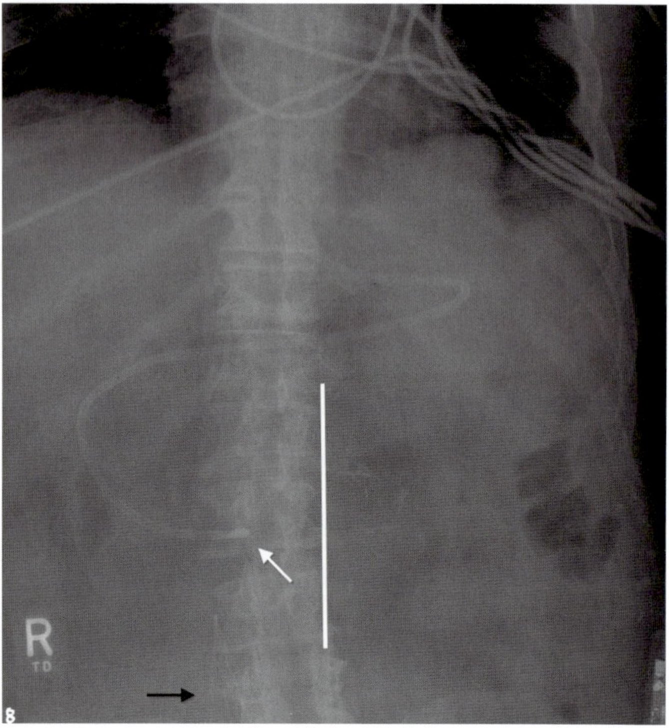

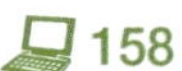

II-85

■ CORPAK FEEDING TUBE –
MISPLACEMENT IN DUODENUM   💻 158

Abdominal radiograph shows an incorrect position of a Corpak feeding tube with its distal tip located in the third portion of the duodenum (white arrow). The tip should be beyond the ligament of Treitz – left to the spine (indicated by white vertical line). Please note also an IVC filter (black arrow).

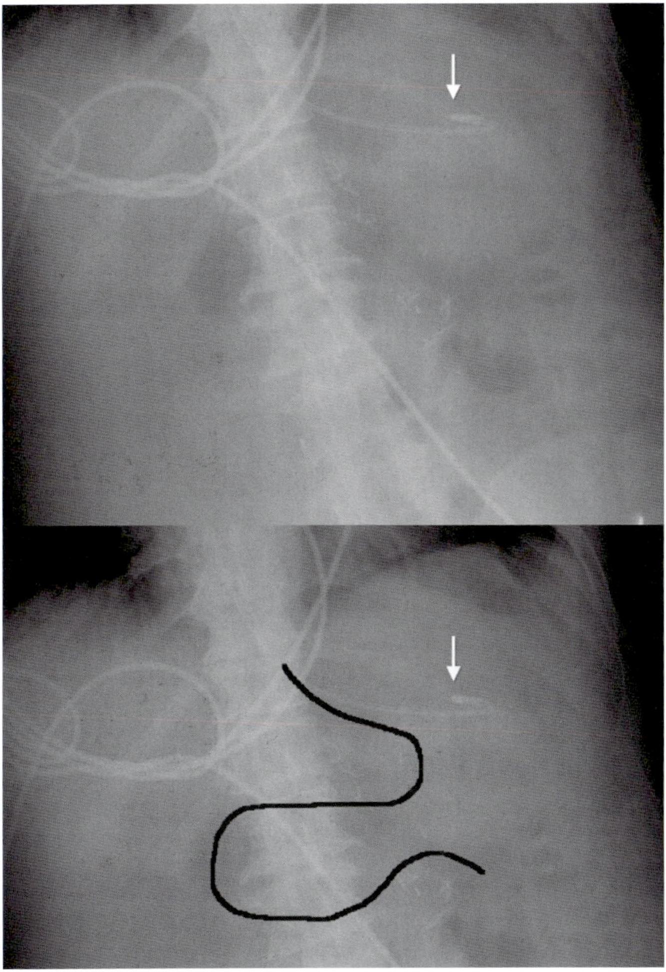

II-86

CORPAK FEEDING TUBE –
MISPLACEMENT IN STOMACH

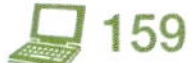 159

Abdominal radiograph shows an incorrect position of a Corpak feeding tube with its distal tip located in the stomach (white arrow). Ideal course and termination of the tube is shown in the lower image (black line).

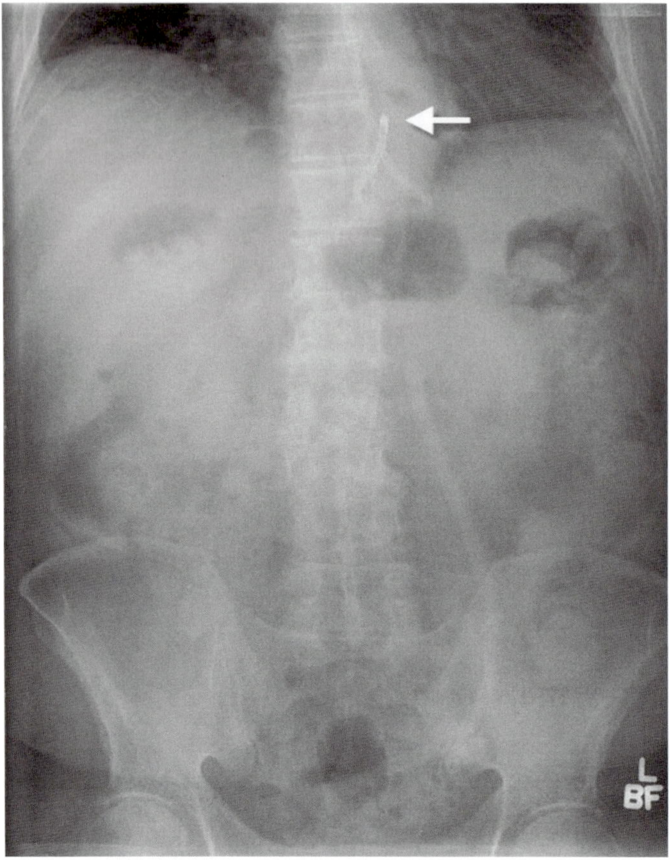

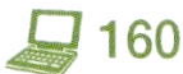

II-87

■ CORPAK FEEDING TUBE –
MISPLACEMENT IN GE JUNCTION

💻 160

Abdominal radiograph shows an incorrect position of a Corpak feeding tube curled up in the proximal stomach, coursing upward and terminating in the esophagus/GE junction (arrow).

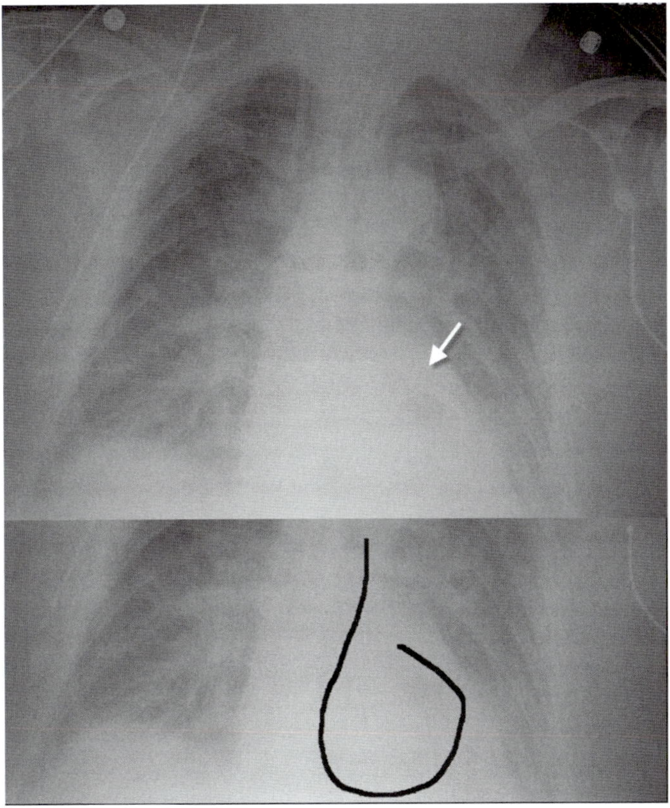

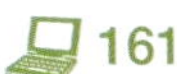

II-88

◾ CORPAK FEEDING TUBE – MISPLACEMENT
IN STOMACH/HIATAL HERNIA   161

Chest radiograph shows an incorrect position of a Corpak feeding tube, curled up within a hiatal hernia and with its distal tip located in the intrathoracic stomach (arrow). Lower image illustrates the course of the feeding tube for better conspectus.

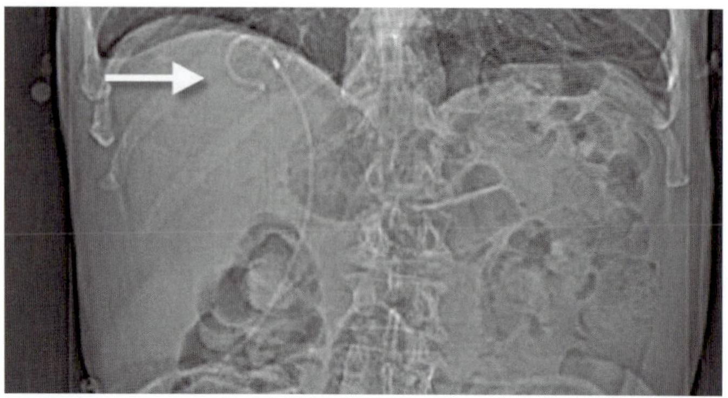

II-89

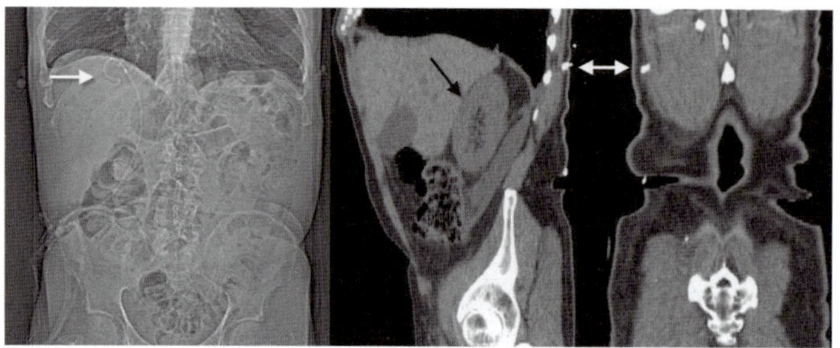

II-90

■ DISLODGED NEPHROSTOMY TUBE – IN SUBCUTANEOUS SOFT TISSUE

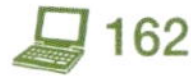 162

CT topogram (lower left and upper image) demonstrates abnormal position of a right nephrostomy tube, with its tip projecting just below the right hemidiaphragm and not in the expected location of the right kidney. Sagittal (middle image) and coronal (right image) reformatted CT images confirm that the nephrostomy tube is dislodged in the subcutaneous soft tissue of the right back (double arrow) and that the right kidney (black arrow, middle image) does not contain a tube.

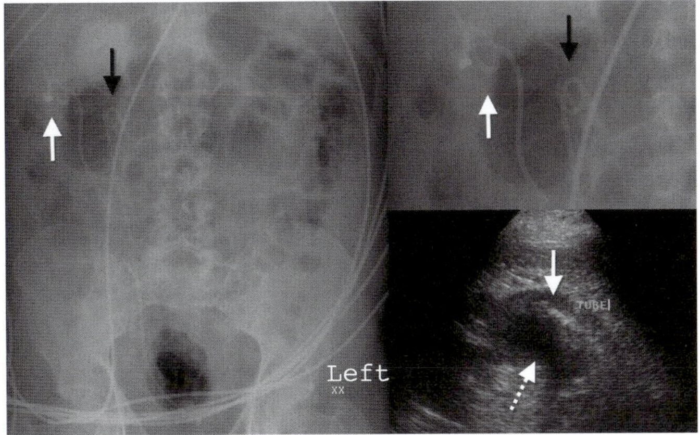

II-91

■ DISLODGED NEPHROSTOMY TUBE – IN RENAL PARENCHYMA

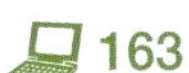 163

Abdominal radiograph shows a nephrostomy tube projecting over the right flank (white arrows), more laterally positioned than a right double J stent (black arrows) which has been also placed. The right upper image is a magnified view. Grayscale ultrasound image of the right kidney in sagittal plane (bottom right image) confirms the nephrostomy tube in an abnormal position with its tip terminating in the renal parenchyma (white full arrow). The tip should have been located in the renal pelvis (white dotted arrow) to properly drain the urine.

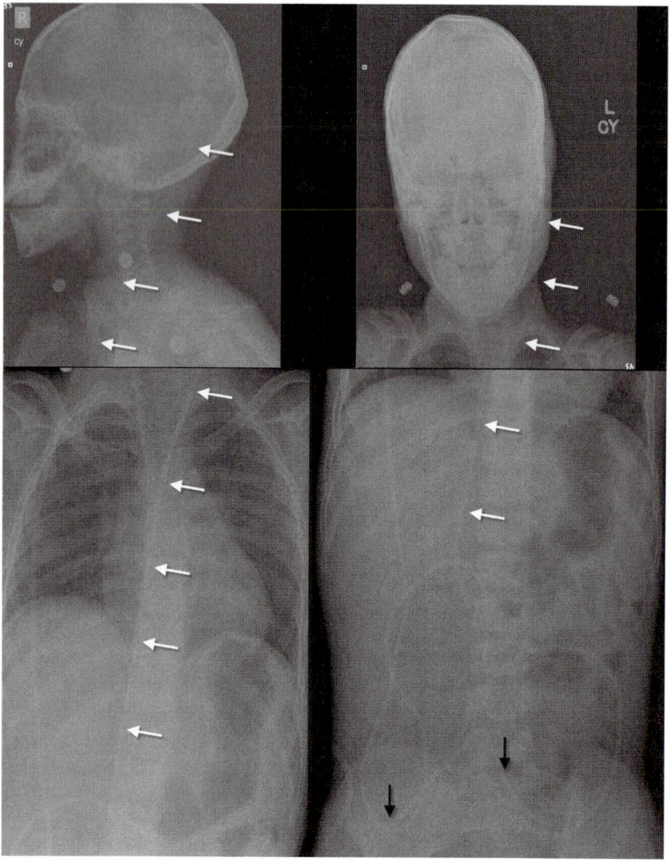

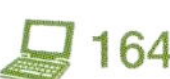

II-92

■ VENTRICULOPERITONEAL SHUNT
(VP SHUNT) – NORMAL FINDING   164

Evaluation of a VP shunt is performed by taking a frontal, lateral skull and frontal chest and abdominal radiographs to evaluate the tubing from its ventricular origin to its termination in the abdomen. A lateral radiograph of the abdomen can also be performed for confirmation of position. The course of the tubing should be continuous and without a kink. White arrows indicate the course of the left VP shunt and black arrows indicate the tip of both VP shunts.

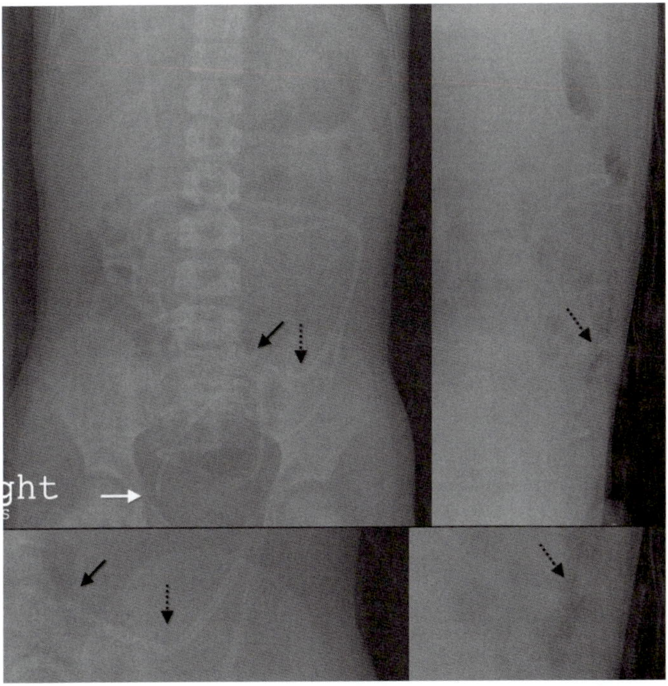

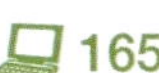

II-93

▪ MALFUNCTIONING VP SHUNT   165

Frontal (left) and lateral (right) abdominal radiographs demonstrate a left VP shunt which is coiled within the pelvis and with the tip located in the right lower quadrant (white arrow). There is no fracture or kinking in the shunt tubing. A second (nonfunctioning) shunt passes into the abdomen and is coiled in the abdomen. The distal end of the second shunt catheter is kinked (dotted black arrow, full black arrow = tip of second catheter).

Kinking of a catheter should always be confirmed with a second (perpendicular) view.

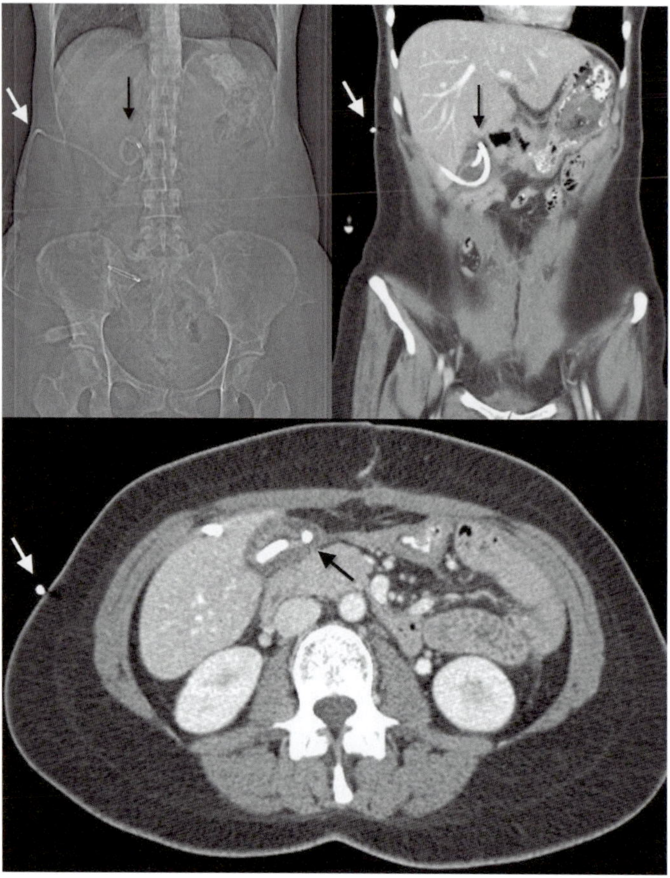

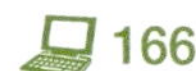

II-94

■ EXTERNAL BILIARY DRAIN – NORMAL FINDING

166

CT topogram (left upper image) and coronal reformatted (right upper image) and axial images of a contrast enhanced CT of the abdomen demonstrate an external biliary drain tubing accessing from the right lateral abdominal wall (white arrows) and terminating in a correct position within the inflamed gallbladder (black arrows).

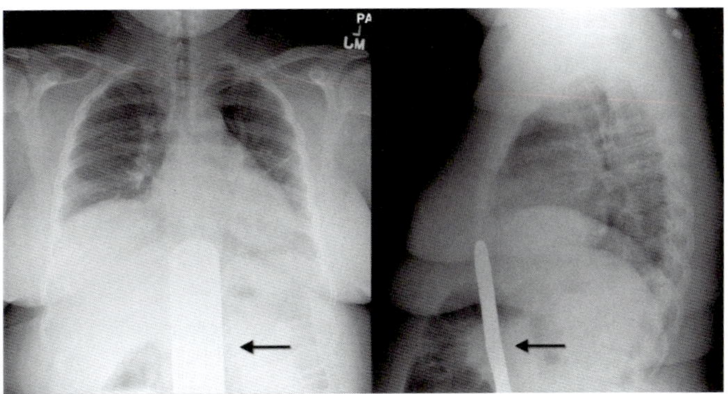

II-95

FORGOTTEN RETRACTOR 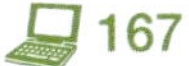 167

Radiographs in AP and lateral projection demonstrate a longitudinal metallic foreign body in the anterior upper abdomen (arrows). This surgical retractor has been forgotten after surgery. Patient was actually evaluated for pneumonia.

References

There are many freely available high quality review articles available about specific topics discussed in this book. These selections of references are only references to high quality journal articles that are freely and directly available.

How to get access to these articles?
Each reference has a so-called PMID at the end. Please use that number and go on the following hyperlink by exchanging "PMID" with that respective number: *http://www.ncbi.nlm.nih.gov/pubmed/PMID*

That hyperlink provides the abstract and also further links to direct access to these full text articles.

1. Shanbhogue AK, Fasih N, Surabhi VR, Doherty GP, Shanbhogue DK, Sethi SK. A clinical and radiologic review of uncommon types and causes of pancreatitis. Radiographics. 2009 Jul–Aug;29(4):1003–1026. PMID: 19605653

2. Sivit CJ. Imaging children with abdominal trauma. AJR Am J Roentgenol. 2009 May;192(5):1179–1189. PMID: 19380540

3. Rha SE, Ha HK, Lee SH, Kim JH, Kim JK, Kim JH, Kim PN, Lee MG, Auh YH. CT and MR imaging findings of bowel ischemia from various primary causes. Radiographics. 2000 Jan–Feb;20(1):29–42. PMID: 10682769

4. Patel SV, Spencer JA, el-Hasani S, Sheridan MB. Imaging of pancreatic trauma. Br J Radiol. 1998 Sep;71(849):985–990. PMID: 10195019

5. Freeman JL, Jafri SZ, Roberts JL, Mezwa DG, Shirkhoda A. CT of congenital and acquired abnormalities of the spleen. Radiographics. 1993 May;13(3):597–610. PMID: 8316667

6. Linsenmaier U, Wirth S, Reiser M, Körner M. Diagnosis and classification of pancreatic and duodenal injuries in emergency radiology. Radiographics. 2008 Oct;28(6):1591–1602. PMID: 18936023

7. Daly KP, Ho CP, Persson DL, Gay SB. Traumatic retroperitoneal injuries: Review of multidetector CT findings. Radiographics. 2008 Oct;28(6):1571–1590. PMID: 18936022

8. Bremnor JD, Sadovsky R. Evaluation of dysuria in adults. Am Fam Physician. 2002 Apr 15;65(8):1589–1596. PMID: 11989635

9. Létoublon C, Arvieux C. Nonoperative management of blunt hepatic trauma. Minerva Anestesiol. 2002 Apr;68(4):132–137. PMID: 12024070

10. Kawashima A, Sandler CM, Corl FM, West OC, Tamm EP, Fishman EK, Goldman SM. Imaging of renal trauma: A comprehensive review. Radiographics. 2001 May–Jun;21(3):557–574. PMID: 11353106

11. Aguirre DA, Santosa AC, Casola G, Sirlin CB. Abdominal wall hernias: Imaging features, complications, and diagnostic pitfalls at multi-detector row CT. Radiographics. 2005 Nov–Dec;25(6):1501–1520. PMID: 16284131

12. Gupta A, Stuhlfaut JW, Fleming KW, Lucey BC, Soto JA. Blunt trauma of the pancreas and biliary tract: a multimodality imaging approach to diagnosis. Radiographics. 2004 Sep–Oct;24(5):1381–1395. PMID: 15371615

13. Ramchandani P, Buckler PM. Imaging of genitourinary trauma. AJR Am J Roentgenol. 2009 Jun;192(6):1514–1523. PMID: 19457813

14. Ingram MD, Watson SG, Skippage PL, Patel U. Urethral injuries after pelvic trauma: evaluation with urethrography. Radiographics. 2008 Oct;28(6):1631–1643. PMID: 18936026

15. Titton RL, Gervais DA, Hahn PF, Harisinghani MG, Arellano RS, Mueller PR. Urine leaks and urinomas: Diagnosis and imaging-guided intervention. Radiographics. 2003 Sep–Oct;23(5):1133–1147. PMID: 12975505

16. Ali M, Safriel Y, Sclafani SJ, Schulze R. CT signs of urethral injury. Radiographics. 2003 Jul–Aug;23(4):951–963. PMID:12853670

17. Vaccaro JP, Brody JM. CT cystography in the evaluation of major bladder trauma. Radiographics. 2000 Sep–Oct;20(5):1373–1381. PMID: 10992026

18. Patel SJ, Reede DL, Katz DS, Subramaniam R, Amorosa JK. Imaging the pregnant patient for nonobstetric conditions: algorithms and radiation dose considerations. Radiographics. 2007 Nov–Dec;27(6):1705–1722. PMID: 18025513

19. Deurdulian C, Mittelstaedt CA, Chong WK, Fielding JR. US of acute scrotal trauma: Optimal technique, imaging findings, and management. Radiographics. 2007 Mar–Apr;27(2):357–369. PMID: 17374858

SECTION III Neuro

- Anatomy
- Technique
- CT Evaluation
- Head
- Neck
- Spine
- References

1. Anatomy

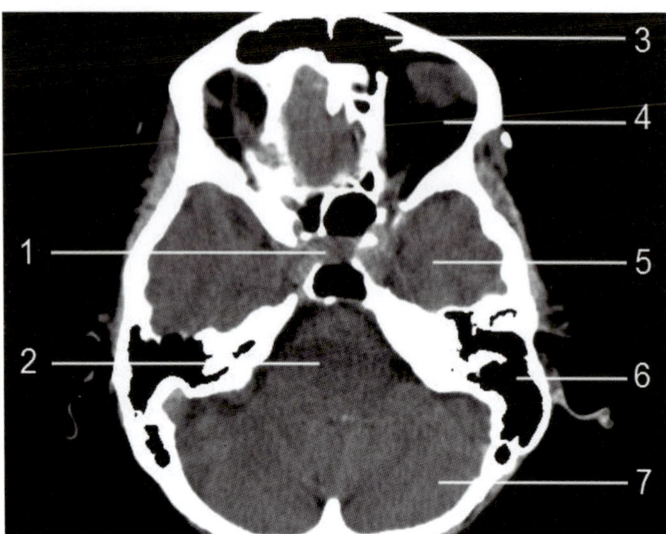

III-1

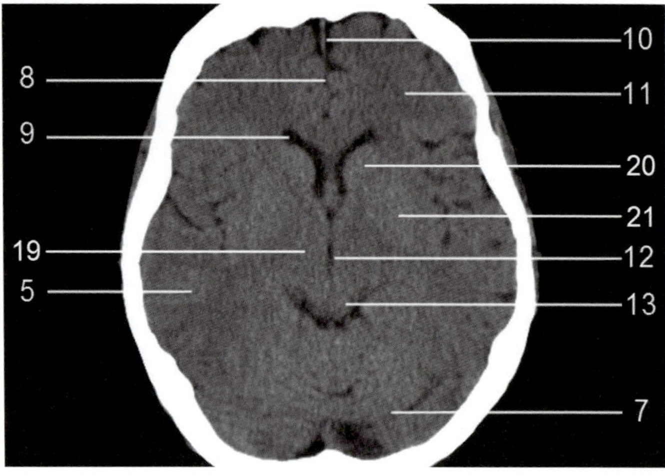

III-2

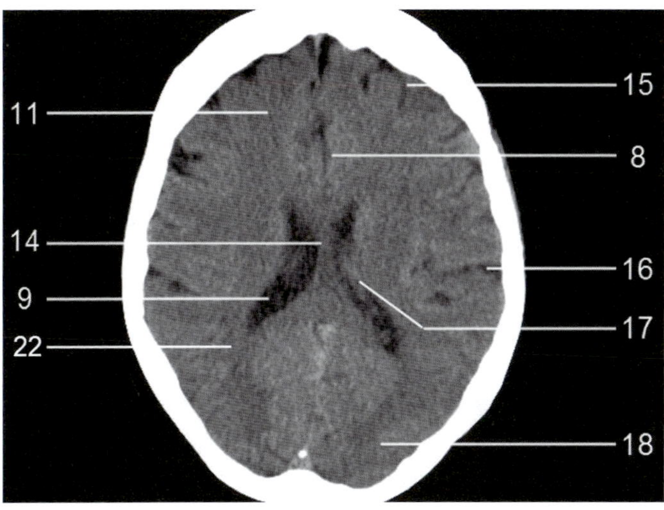

III-3

■ Table III-1. Anatomy of a Noncontrast Head CT   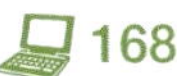 168

1. Chiasma	12. Third ventricle
2. Brainstem	13. Quadrigeminal plate
3. Frontal sinus	14. Septum pellucidum
4. Orbit	15. Sulci
5. Temporal lobe	16. Central sulcus
6. Mastoid air cells	17. Choroid plexus
7. Cerebellar hemisphere	18. Occipital lobe
8. Interhemispheric fissure	19. Thalamus
9. Lateral ventricle	20. Caudate nucleus
10. Falx cerebri	21. Basal ganglia
11. Frontal lobe	22. Parietal lobe

2. Technique

▊ TECHNIQUES   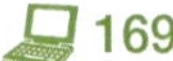 169

- Plain film radiography
- Ultrasonography
- Computed tomography (with or without contrast)
- MRI/MRA (with or without contrast)

Plain film radiography: Head – predominantly for fracture evaluation (eg, frontal and lateral skull views, mandibular "panorex" view); Neck – fracture, infection, airway compromise evaluation (AP, lateral views, odontoid view)

Ultrasonography: Evaluation of soft tissues and vasculature, especially in neck as well as head in neonates.

Computed tomography (CT): Evaluation for stroke, brain hemorrhage, intracranial pathology, facial bone and spine fractures.

Magnetic resonance imaging (MRI): Evaluation for stroke and head and neck vasculature (MRI/MRA), intracranial pathology (eg, infection and neoplasm), skull base pathology (which cannot be well evaluated by CT due to artifacts), and spine (soft tissues).

3. CT Evaluation

Table III-2. Evaluation of CT Without IV Contrast 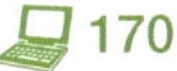 170

Structure	Finding (common etiology)
Brain parenchyma	• High attenuation (blood, calcification) • Low attenuation (cerebral edema, infarct) • CSF density (encephalomalacia)
Ventricles	• Midline position (normal) • Midline shift (mass effect) • Small (cerebral edema) • Large (cerebral atrophy, hydrocephalus)
Subarachnoid space	• Effaced or asymmetric (mass effect, filled with blood) • Filled with dense material (blood, pus)
Cortical sulci	• Effaced (mass effect, filled with hyper-/isodense fluid, eg, acute/remote blood)
Sinuses and mastoid air cells	• Opacified (mucus, pus, blood)
Skull	• Fracture
Scalp	• Air (laceration, infection)

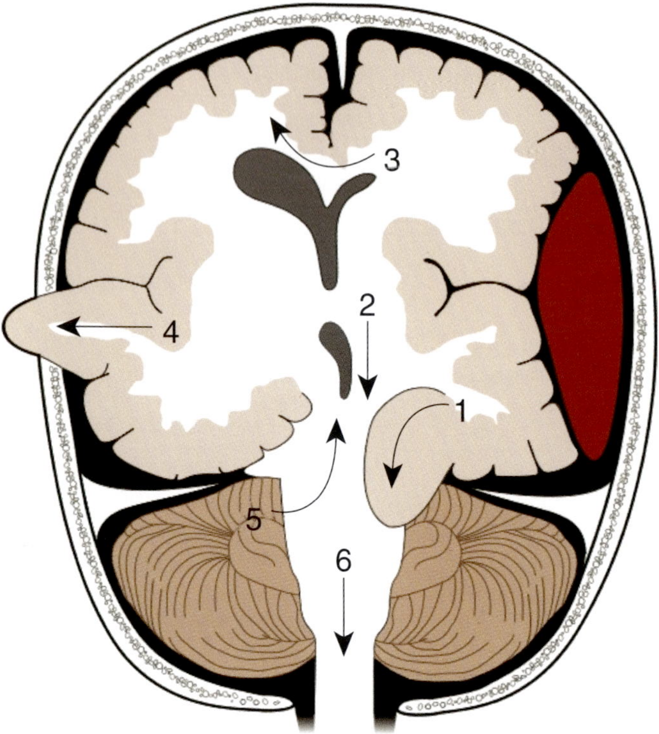

III-4

■ Table III-3. Types of Brain Herniation　　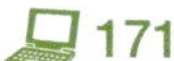171

Supratentorial herniation	Infratentorial herniation
1. Uncal	5. Upward (upward cerebellar or
2. Central (transtentorial)	upward transtentorial)
3. Cingulate (subfalcine)	6. Tonsillar (downward cerebellar)
4. Transcalvarial	

■ SOFT TISSUE AND BONE EVALUATION (NONCONTRAST CT)

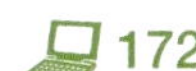 172

- Soft tissue swelling (scrutinize for skull fracture)
- Fracture (do not mistake sutures for fracture)
- If skull fracture check for pneumocephalus
- If temporal bone fracture check for inner ear integrity
- If facial bone fracture check for orbital, sinus, and anterior cerebral fossa involvement
- Lysis (bone metastasis, multiple myeloma)
- Sclerosis (chronic infection, slow growing tumor)

4. Head

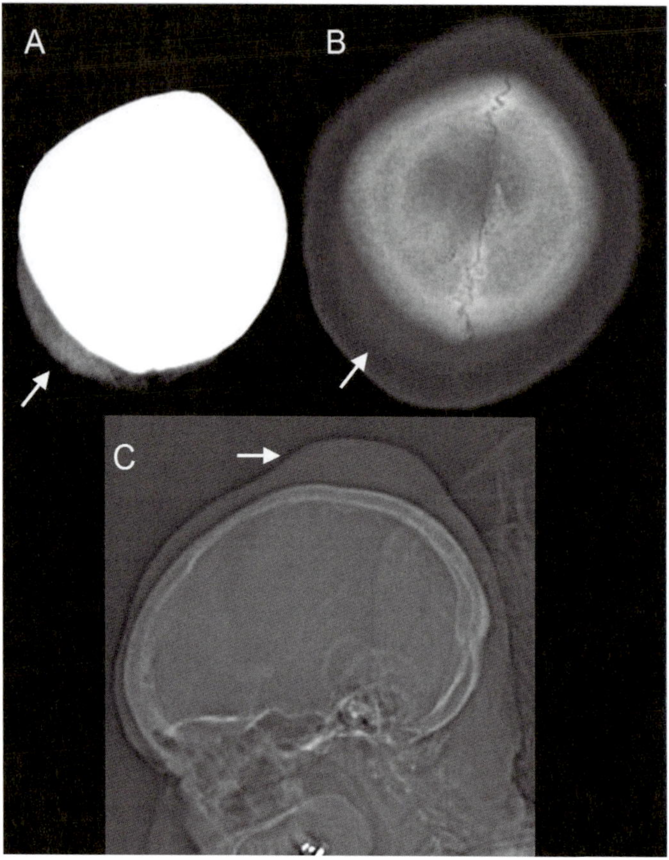

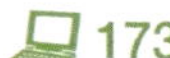

III-5

▪ SUBGALEAL HEMATOMA

Noncontrast CT of the head demonstrates a prominent subgaleal hematoma (arrows) over the vertex, measuring thickness of about 1 cm. No adjacent fracture is identified. A=brain window, B=bone window, and C=CT topogram.

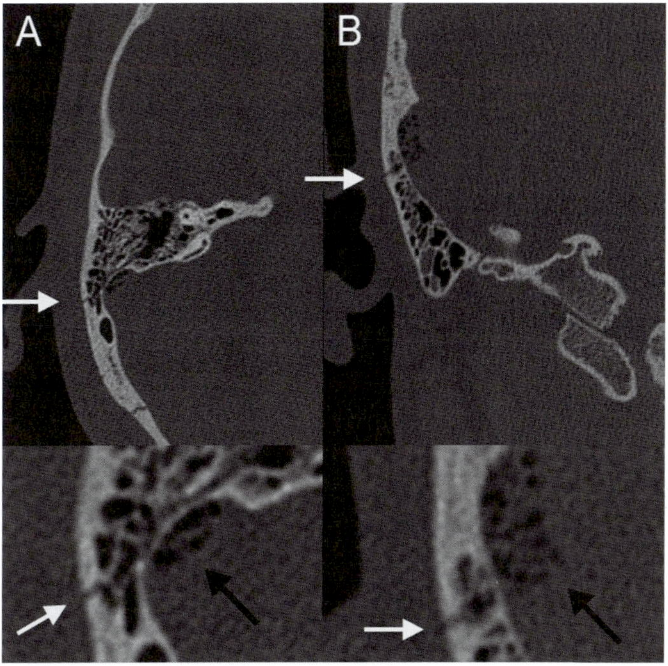

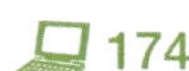

III-6

TEMPORAL BONE FRACTURE WITH PNEUMOCEPHALUS

174

Axial (A) and coronal reformatted (B) CT of the temporal bones demonstrate a nondisplaced fracture of the right temporal bone located posterior to the mastoid air cells (white arrows). This fracture line extends into mastoid air cells. Some mastoid air cells are fluid filled – likely from blood (best appreciated on panel B). About 1 cm focus of gas is present within the posterior cranial fossa adjacent to the right cerebellar hemisphere (black arrows).

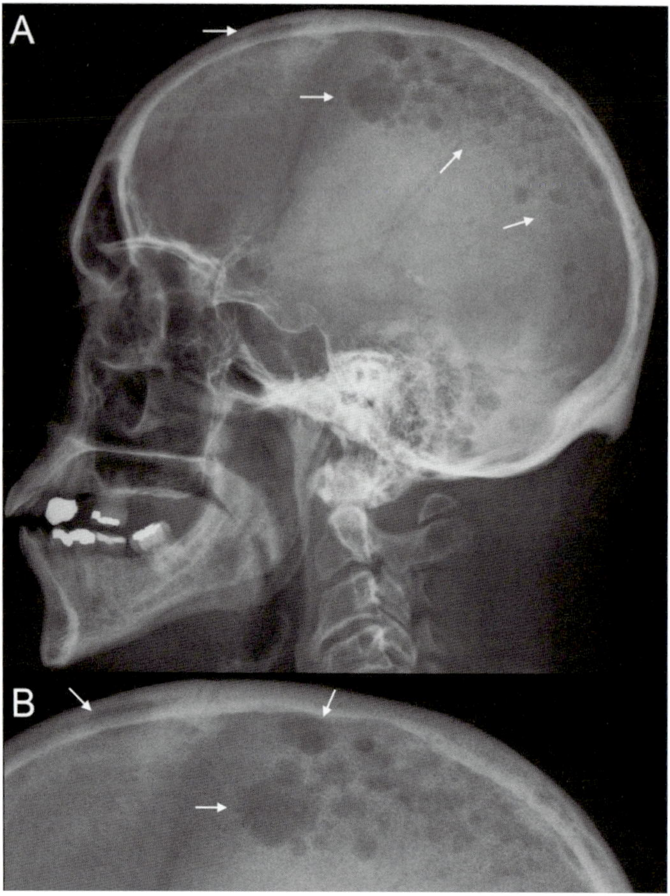

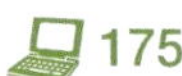

III-7

■ **MULTIPLE MYELOMA – RADIOGRAPH**   175

Lateral view of the skull demonstrates innumerable small "punched out" lytic lesions (arrows) consistent with myeloma. B=magnification.

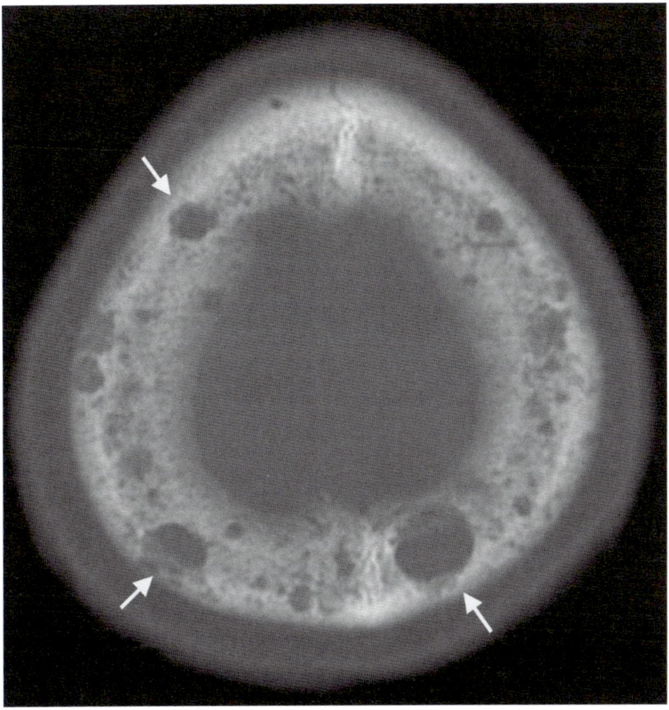

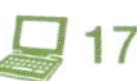

III-8

MULTIPLE MYELOMA – CT

176

Axial noncontrast CT of the head in bone window demonstrates innumerable well-defined, "punched out" lytic lesions within the skull (arrows) consistent with myeloma.

■ MIDFACE TRAUMA   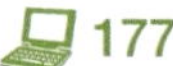 177

- CT is standard for evaluating midface trauma.
- Misinterpretation of facial suture lines can cause false positive diagnosis of facial fractures.
- Tripod fracture is the most common type of facial fracture (about 40% of midfacial fractures).
- Le Fort fractures make 10–20% of all facial fractures.

Le Fort facial fracture classification

Le Fort I fracture (horizontal)
- Only the lower maxilla
- Involves the inferior nasal aperture
- Guerin fracture or "floating palate"

Le Fort II fracture (pyramidal)
- The infraorbital rim

Le Fort III fracture (transverse)
- Complete detachment of the midface from the skull
- Involves the zygomatic arch
- Craniofacial dissociation

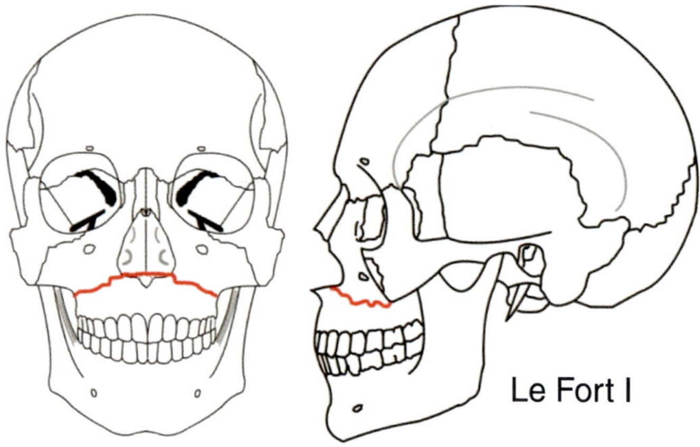

III-9

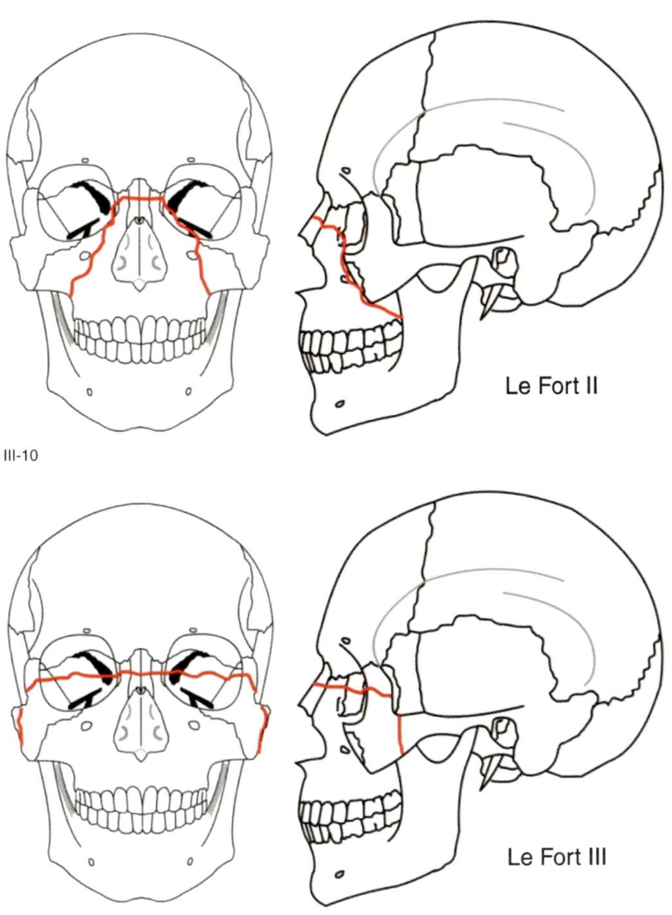

III-10

III-11

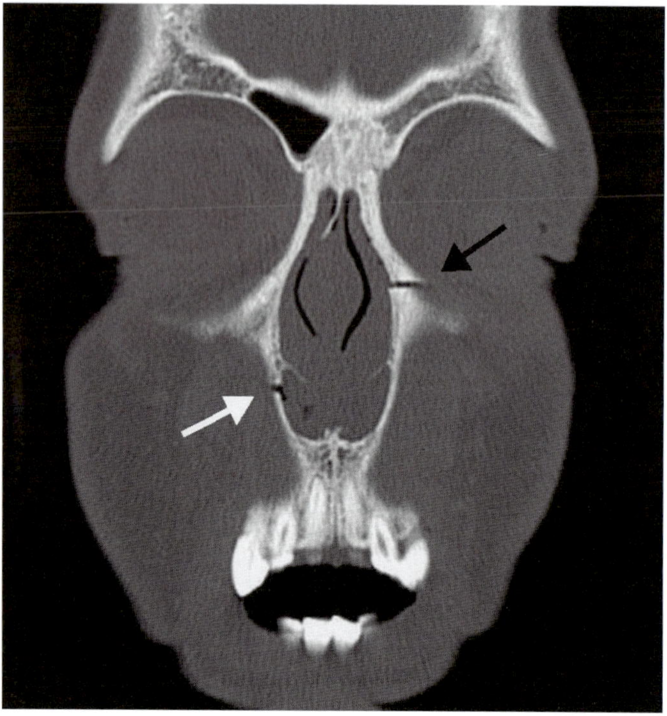

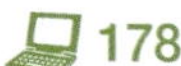

III-12

■ LE FORT I AND II FRACTURES   178

Coronal reformatted image from a facial CT in the bone window demonstrates bilateral horizontal facial fractures. On the right, the fracture plane is through the maxilla (white arrow), compatible with a Le Fort type I fracture. On the left, the plane traverses the medial orbital wall and orbital floor (black arrow), compatible with the Le Fort type II fracture.

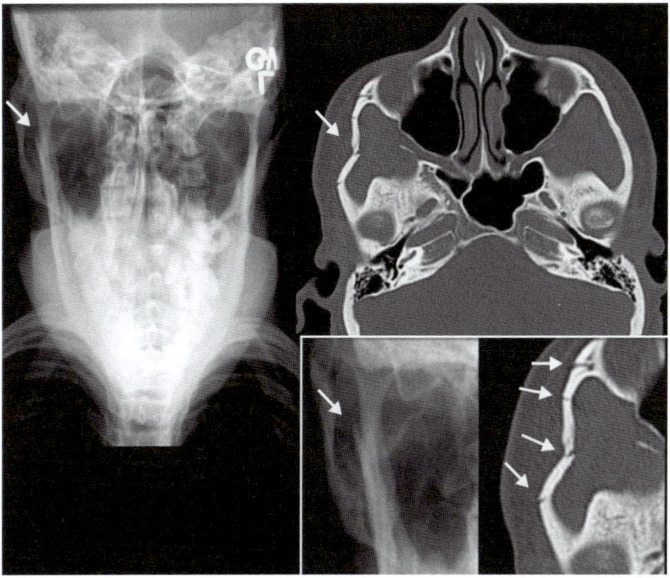

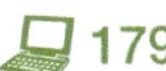

III-13

ZYGOMATIC ARCH FRACTURE   🖥 179

Frontal mandibular radiograph shows a depressed zygomatic arch fracture on the right (arrows). CT of the facial bones confirms a depressed fracture of the right zygomatic arch that has a concave contour (compared to the left arch which has a convex contour). Right lower corner = magnifications.

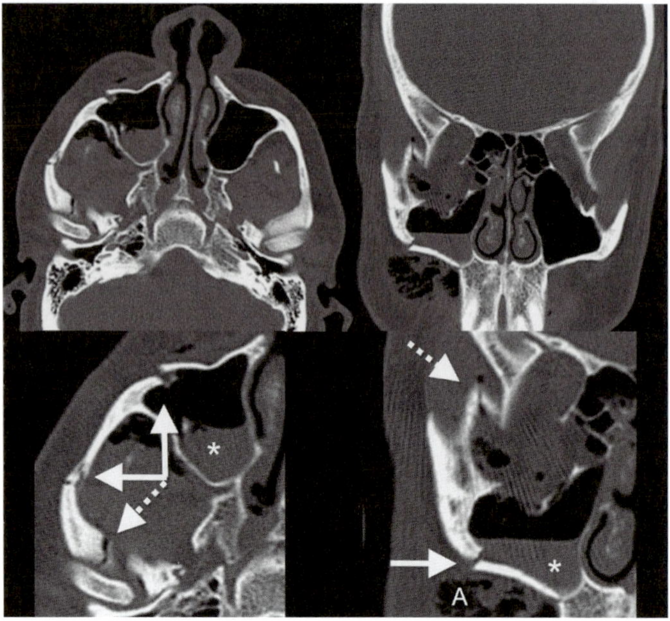

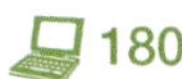

III-14

■ TRIPOD FRACTURE   □ 180

Axial (left) and coronal reformatted (right) CT of the orbits demonstrates a fracture of the zygomatic arch (arrows) with diastasis of the zygomaticofrontal suture (dotted arrows) as well as extensive subcutaneous emphysema (A). Air fluid level in the maxillary sinus represents hemorrhage (asterisk). The zygoma becomes a free-floating object because of separation of all three major attachments.

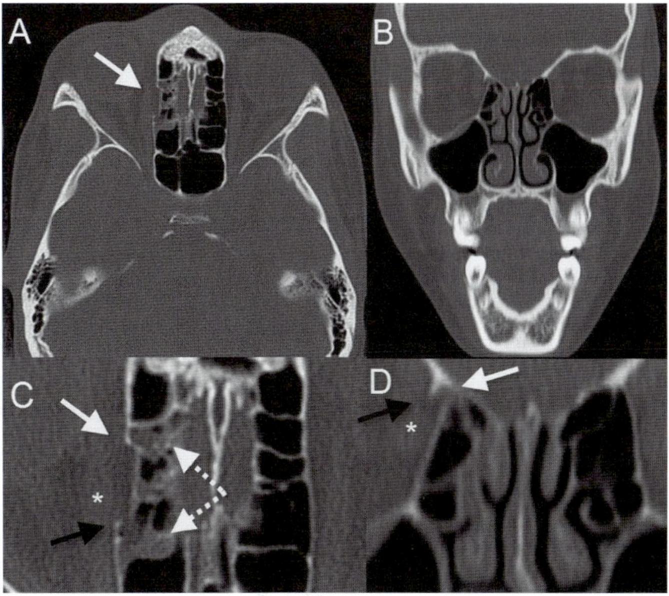

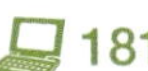

III-15

■ ORBITAL BLOW OUT FRACTURE – MEDIAL   181

Facial CT in bone window shows a mild comminuted fracture of the central aspect of the right medial orbital wall (white arrows), with displacement of a segment of the lamina papyracea medially about 2 mm into the underlying ethmoidal air cell. There is minimal herniation of orbital fat with the fracture fragment. The medial aspect of the medial rectus muscle (asterisk) appears to contact the fracture margin (black arrow), and to some degree entrapment cannot be excluded. There is fluid opacification of a few right ethmoid air cells (white dotted arrows).

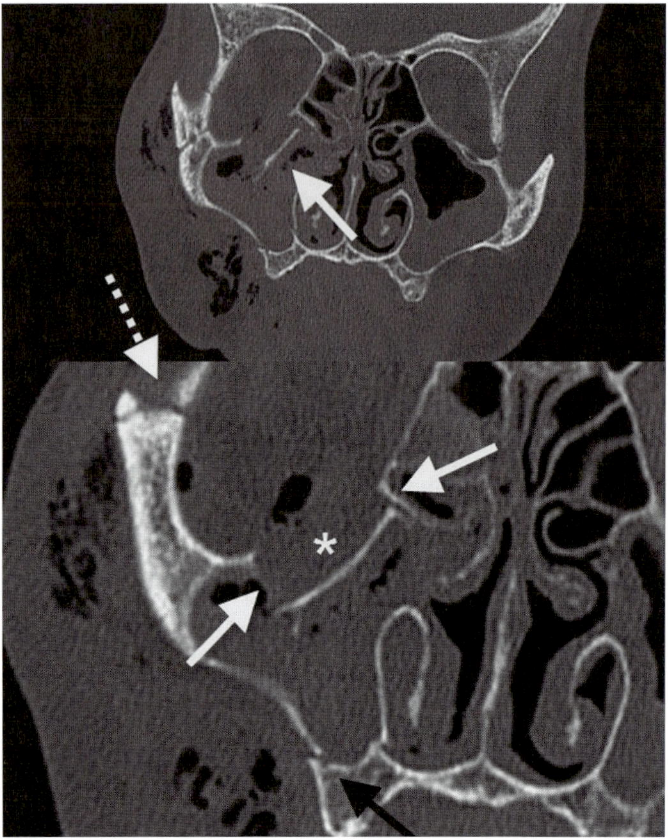

III-16

■ ORBITAL BLOW OUT FRACTURE – INFERIOR 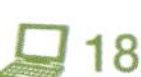 182

Coronal reformatted facial CT in bone window shows a blowout fracture of the inferior right orbital floor (white arrows), with a 1.7-cm fragment displaced inferiorly about 6 mm (white arrow upper image). A corresponding degree of orbital fat herniates inferiorly with the fragment (asterisk). There is marked soft tissue swelling and subcutaneous as well as orbital air. There is also minimally displaced fracture of the inferior maxilla just superior to the hard palate insertion (black arrow) as well as mild diastasis of the frontozygomatic synchondrosis (dotted white arrow). Upper and lower images are at slightly different levels.

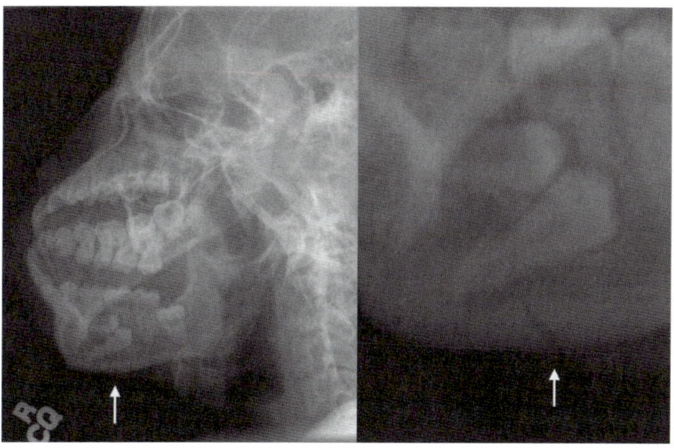

III-17

■ MANDIBULAR FRACTURE – RADIOGRAPH 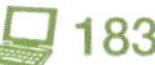 183

Lateral oblique mandibular radiograph (right=magnification) demonstrates a nondisplaced fracture through the right mandibular body.

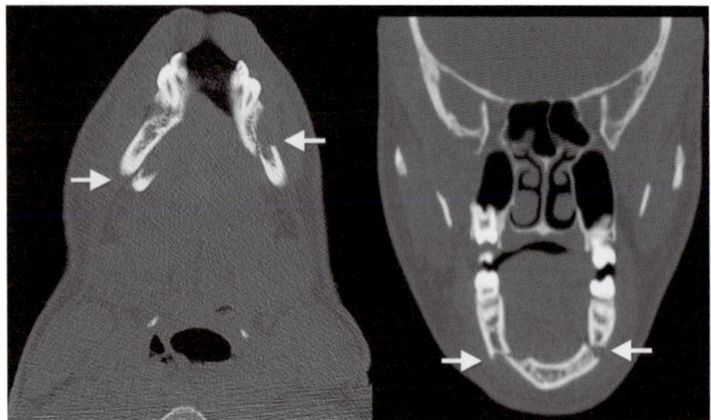

III-18

■ BILATERAL MANDIBULAR FRACTURE – CT  184

Facial CT in the bone window (axial left, coronal reformatted right) demonstrates a complete bilateral fracture of the mandibular body with separation of the anterior arch (arrows).

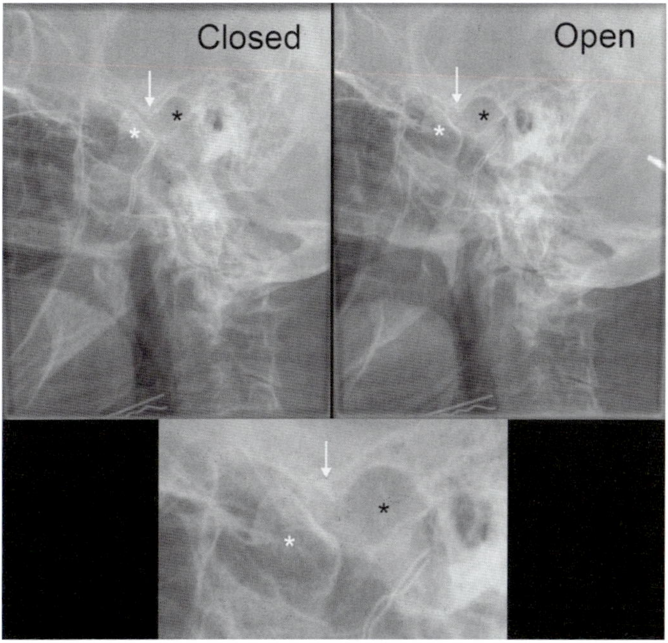

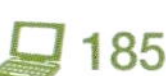

III-19

■ MANDIBULAR DISLOCATION   🖥 185

Mandibular views with mouth open (right) and attempt to close mouth (left) show that the right mandibular condyle (white asterisk) is displaced ante-riorly in respect to its mandibular fossa (black asterisk) in the temporal bone. The articular eminence (white arrow) prevents the relocation of the mandibular condyle into the mandibular fossa. It is Important to search for potential associated fractures (not in this case).

■ Table III-4. Different Types of Extraaxial Hemorrhage 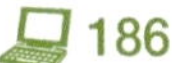 186

Type	Epidural	Subdural	Subarachnoid
Location	Between the skull and dura	Between the dura and arachnoid	Subarachnoid space
Involved vessel	Middle meningeal artery	Bridging veins	Ruptured aneurysm, AVM, brain contusion
Symptoms	Lucid interval followed by unconsciousness	Gradually increasing headache and confusion	Acute headache "worst headache of my life"
Appearance on CT	Biconvex	Crescent shaped	In sulci, fissures, ventricles, basal cisterns

■ BLOOD APPEARANCE ON CT 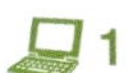 187

Blood changes its appearance over time. In the acute stage blood is bright (dense) and becomes less attenuating over time and becomes isodence to cerebrospinal fluid in the chronic stage (thus can be overlooked if small enough). If there is acute over chronic hemorrhage, a mixed pattern can be seen.

■ SKULL FRACTURE WITH EPIDURAL HEMATOMA – ACUTE  188

Axial noncontrast CT of the head demonstrates convex hyperdense fluid collections along both frontal lobes, compatible with acute epidural hematomas. Epidural hematomas are often associated with skull fractures – as in this case where we can see a temporal bone fracture (white arrow, right top image). Fracture line can also be seen on the CT topogram (lower image, arrows). The left hematoma is a coup hematoma and the right one a contracoup epidural hematoma.

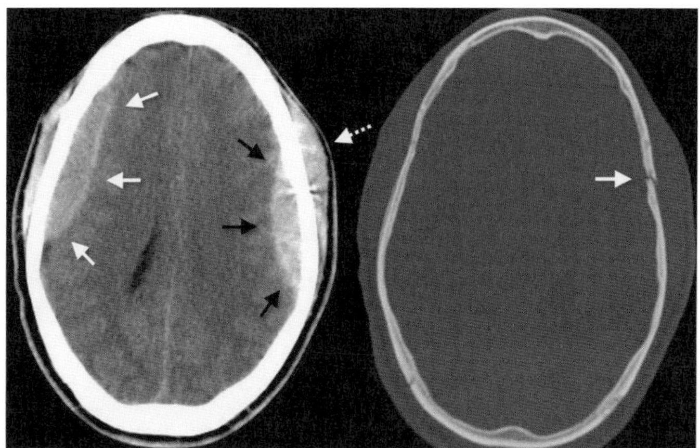

III-20

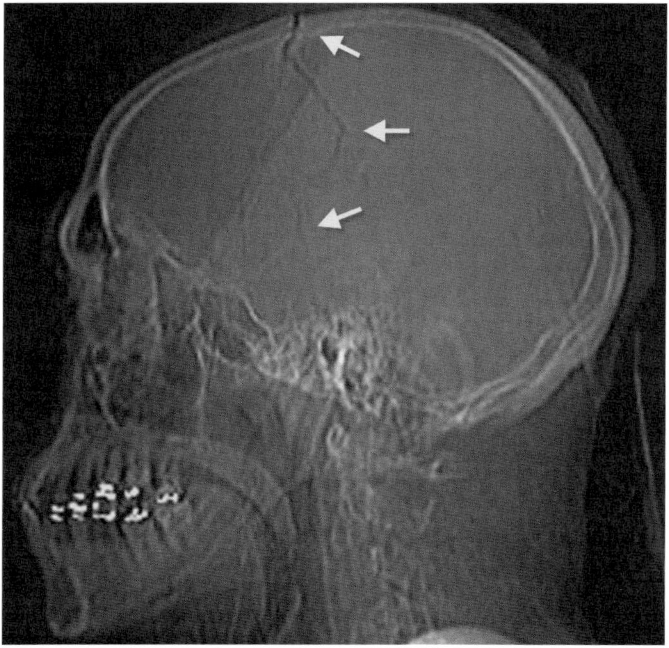

III-21

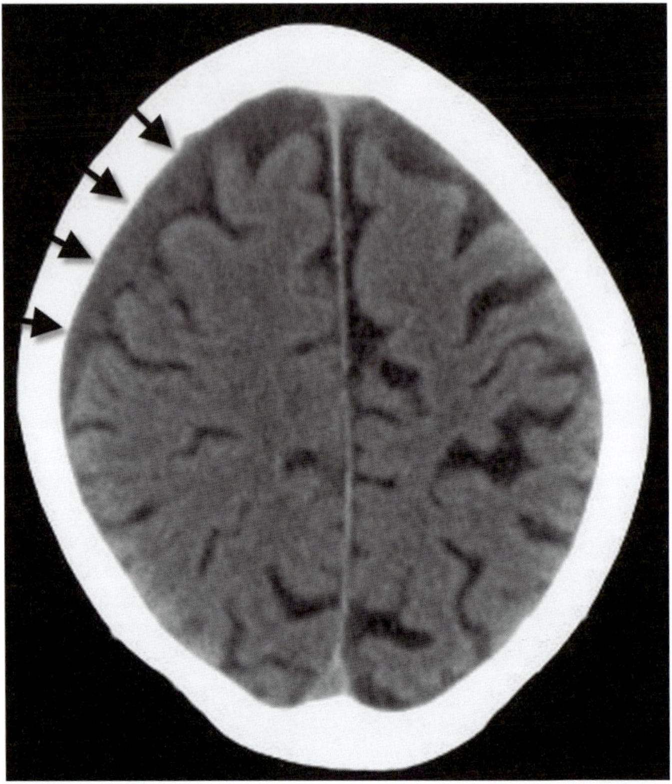

III-22

■ SUBDURAL HEMATOMA – CHRONIC   189

Axial noncontrats head CT shows a small mildly hyperdense extraaxial fluid collection over the right convexity, most prominent in the frontal region measuring 7 mm in the maximal diameter. There is minimal, if any underlying mass effect. The density is minimally more prominent than CSF, suggesting late subacute to early chronic subdural hematoma.

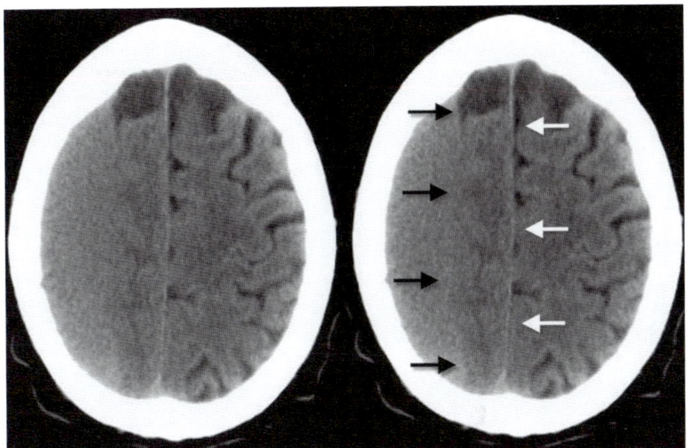

III-23

■ SUBDURAL HEMATOMA – SUBACUTE  190

Axial noncontrast head CT demonstrates a large crescentic extraaxial collection (black arrows), near isodense to gray matter, centered along the right cerebral convexity, with posterior extension to the right parietal are. The collection crosses the sutures indicative of a subdural nature. The density measures only 45 HU, suggestive of its subacute nature. It is homogeneous with no suspicion for active bleeding or recent clot. No midline shift is noted (white arrows).

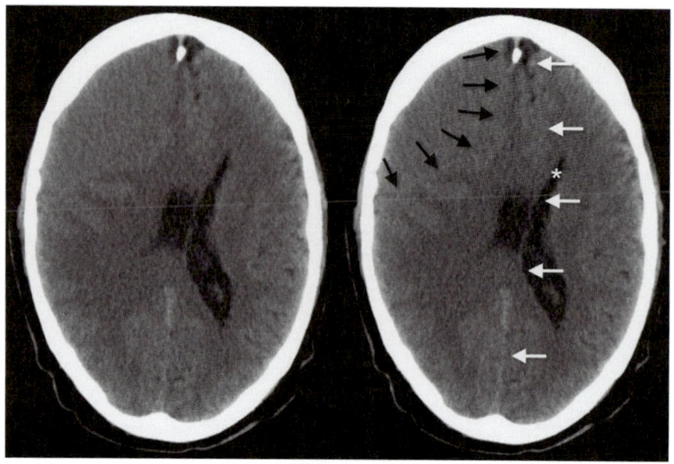

III-24

■ SUBDURAL HEMATOMA – SUBACUTE WITH MIDLINE SHIFT

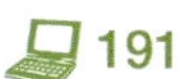 191

Axial noncontrast head CT of the same patient scanned a few centimeters more caudal demonstrates a large convex extraaxial collection extending from the previously seen crescentic collection, also near isodense to gray matter, centered along the right cerebral convexity, with posterior extension to the right parietal area. The collection crosses the sutures indicative of a subdural nature. The density measures only 45 HU, suggestive of its subacute nature. There is mass effect on the subjacent brain parenchyma (black arrows) which causes a midline shift (subfalcine herniation) of 1.3 cm (white arrows) that is most prominent at the right frontal horns. There is also compression of the anterior horn of the right as well as left ventricle (white asterisk).

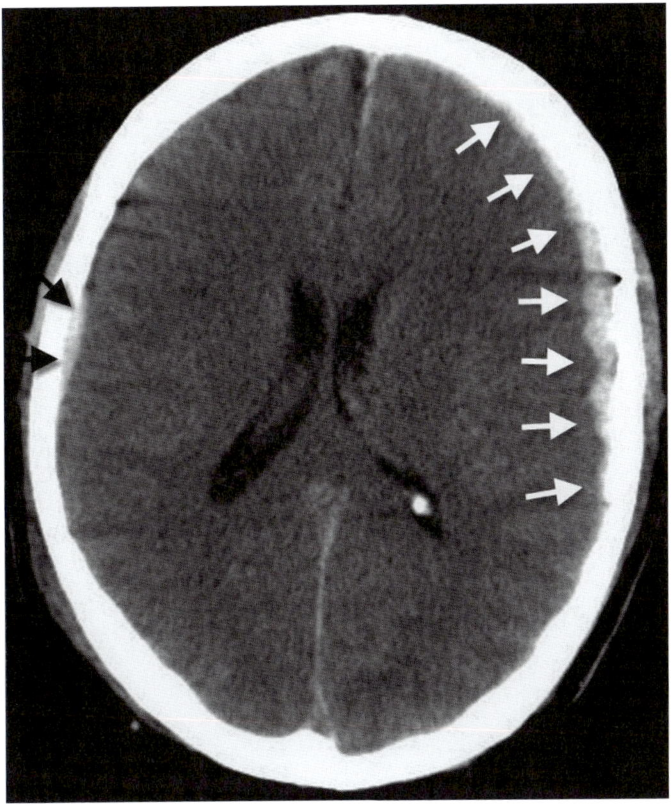

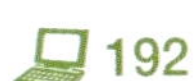

III-25

■ SUBDURAL HEMATOMA – ACUTE   🖥 192

There is a crescent-shaped hyperdense fluid collection overlying portions of the left frontal and parietal lobes (white arrows), compatible with an acute subdural hematoma. Subdural hematomas cross sutures – epidural hematomas do not. There is also present a small acute right posterior frontal/parietal subdural hematoma (black arrows).

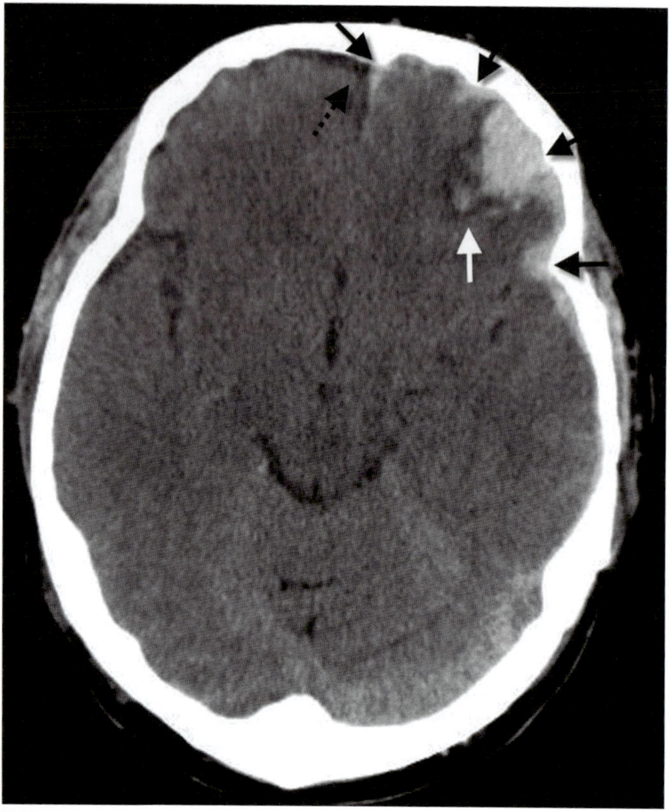

III-26

PARENCHYMAL HEMORRHAGE AND SUBDURAL HEMATOMA – ACUTE

193

This axial noncontrast head CT demonstrates an acute subdural hematoma overlying the left frontal lobe (black full arrows). The hematoma is subdural because it is contained by the falx cerebri and does not cross to the contralateral side (dotted black arrow). Also noticed is acute blood with associated edema in the left frontal brain parenchyma (white arrow).

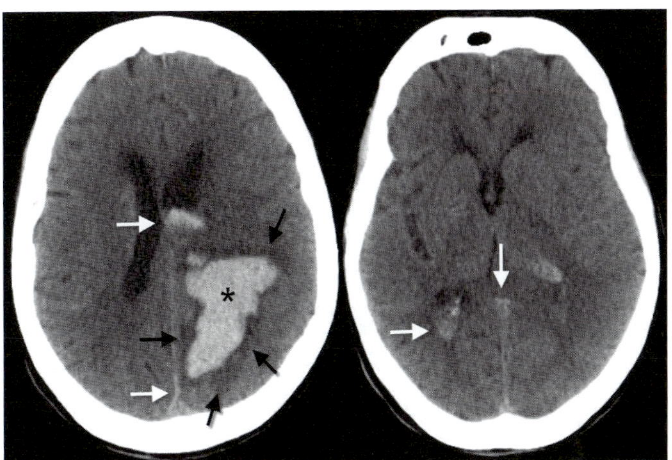

III-27

■ PARENCHYMAL HEMORRHAGE WITH INTRAVENTRICULAR EXTENSION

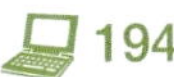 194

Noncontrast head CT shows an area of acute hemorrhage in the left occipital lobe (asterisk). There is mild edema (black arrows) with mild mass-effect surrounding the hemorrhage, without causing significant midline shift. Layering blood is also seen in the atrium of the left ventricle and posterior horn of the right ventricle, as well as blood in posterior falx and tentorium (white arrows). The ventricles are mildly dilated, which could suggest early trapping. Secondary intraventricular hemorrhage (IVH) may occur in one-third to one-half of the patients with spontaneous ICH as a result of arterial hypertension and/or small arteriolar degeneration. IVH is most often seen with thalamic, putaminal, or caudate nucleus hemorrhages, which can extend medially a short distance directly into the lateral or third ventricles.

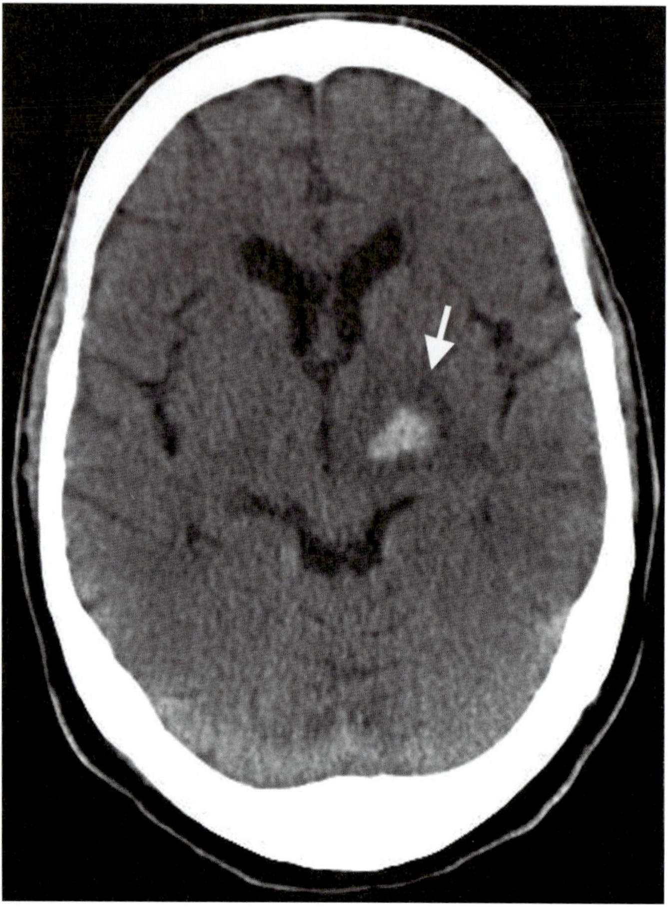

III-28

▨ THALAMIC HEMORRHAGE   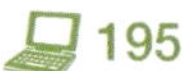 195

Noncontrast head CT demonstrates acute parenchymal hemorrhage centered at the left thalamus and posterior limb of the left internal capsule (arrow). This is a typical location for a hypertensive hemorrhage.

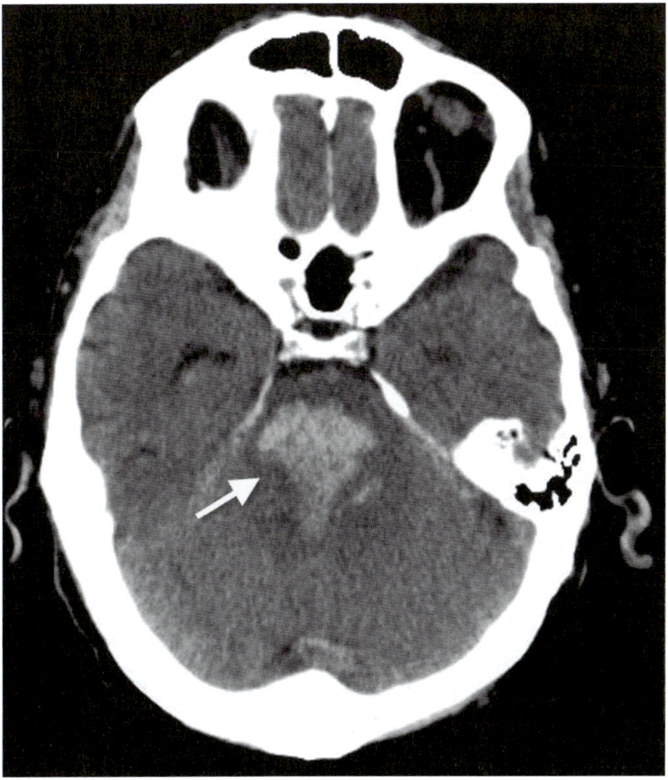

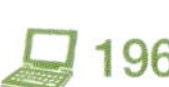

III-29

■ BRAINSTEM HEMORRHAGE   196

Noncontrast head CT shows an about 3 cm area of hyperattenuation in the brainstem (arrow) compatible with a focal hemorrhage which is centered within the pons. There is poor visualization of the fourth ventricle, which may be due to the presence of ventricular hemorrhage versus mass effect secondary to the focal hemorrhage.

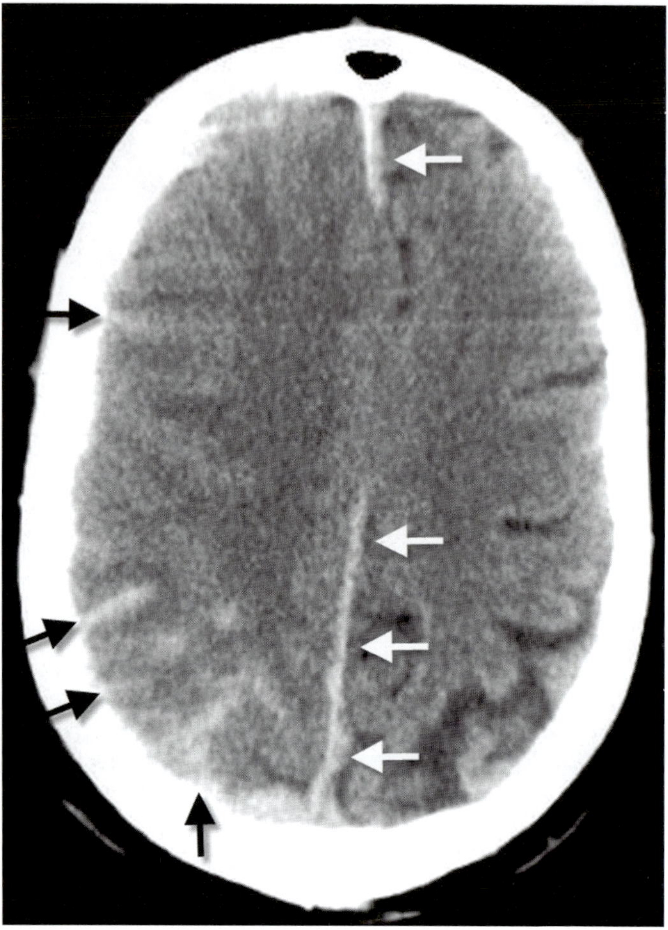

III-30

■ SUBARACHNOID HEMORRHAGE   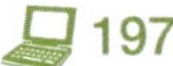 197

Axial noncontrast head CT demonstrates hyperdense material within sulci of the right frontal and parietal lobes (black arrows) as well as within the interhemispheric fissure (white arrows), compatible with an acute subarachnoid hemorrhage.

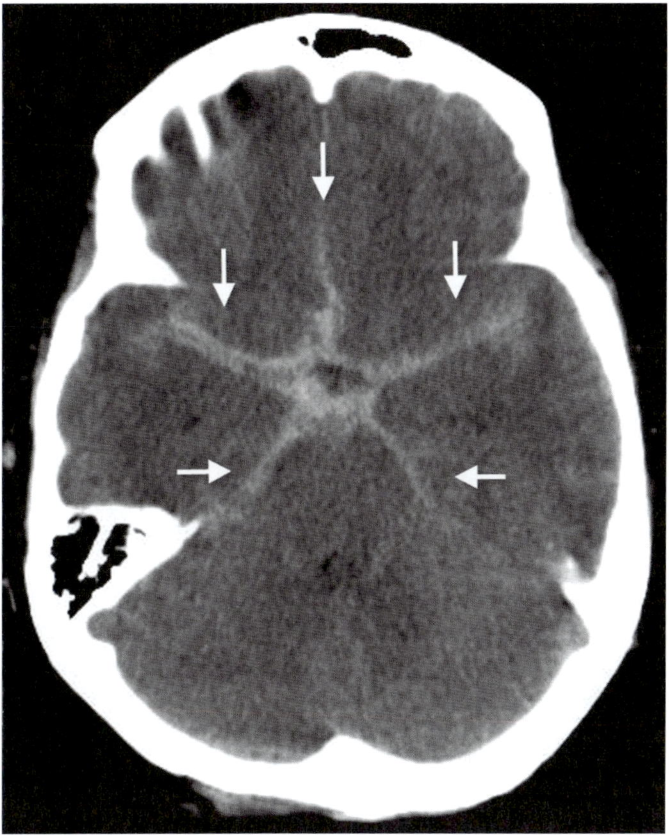

III-31

■ SUBARACHNOID HEMORRHAGE   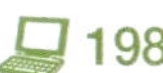 198

Axial noncontrast head CT demonstrates high attenuation material within the paramesencephalic cisterns, anterior and posterior interhemispheric fissure and also within the subarachnoid space of the mid and posterior cranial fossa bilaterally (arrows), consistent with subarachnoid hemorrhage.

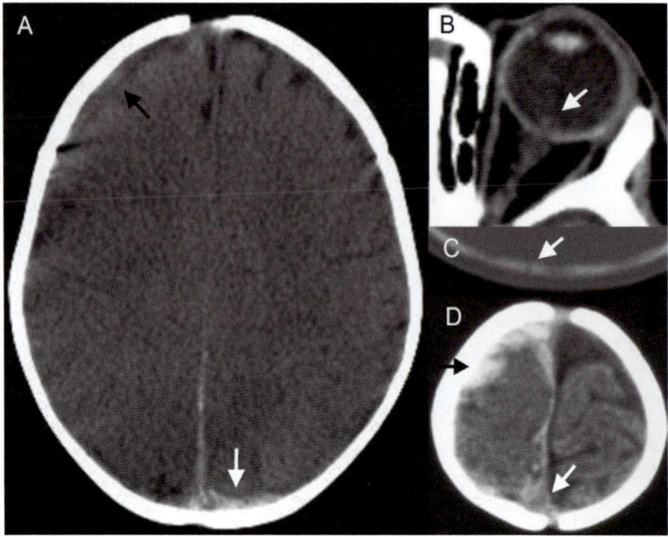

III-32

NONACCIDENTAL TRAUMA
(NAT, CHILD ABUSE) – HEAD INJURIES   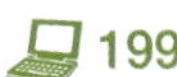 199

Axial noncontrast CT of the head in a young child demonstrates acute
blood in the interhemispheric fissure (A and D, white arrows) as well as
subdural and subarachnoid collections overlying the right frontal lobe
(A and C, black arrows). Furthermore, acute blood is seen in the posterior aspect of the left globe (B, arrow), consistent with acute retinal
hemorrhage. Bone window demonstrates also a nondisplaced linear skull
fracture in the occipital bone (C, arrow). Retinal hemorrhage and interhemispheric hemorrhage are most specific for child abuse. Other, less
specific abnormalities include subdural hematomas and edema in the
basal ganglia.

STROKE EVALUATION 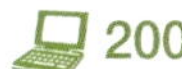 200

- Noncontrast head CT needs to be done first to exclude hemorrhage.
- Hyperacute stroke can appear normal.
- Early signs of stroke are ribbon sign (loss of gray – white matter differentiation).
- Later: effacement of sulci and hypoattenuation of brain parenchyma due to edema.
- Midline shift due to brain edema and subfalcine herniation.
- "Hyperdense MCA sign" can be seen on noncontrast CT if there is acute (dense) thrombus located in the MCA.
- Contrast enhanced CT shows hypoperfusion of affected area.
- CT or MR angiography shows the diminutive supplying vessel or cutoff (complete occlusion) of the vessel.
- Cerebral blood flow and time to peak (TTP) images can predict salvageable and at risk areas.
- MRI shows infarcted areas (restricted diffusion).
- MRI superior for evaluation of areas at skull base (brainstem, cerebellum).

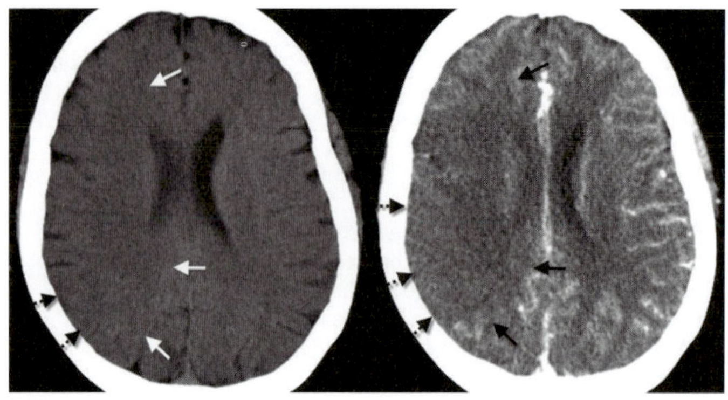

III-33

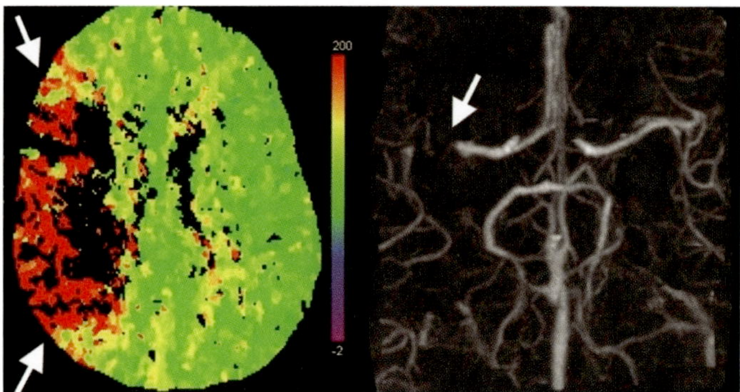

III-34

■ ACUTE RIGHT MCA INFARCT   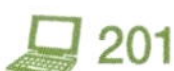 201

Noncontrast head CT (top left) shows in the right frontal lobe loss of corticomedullary (gray–white matter) differentiation, also known as the ribbon sign. There is also mild associated parenchymal swelling with effacement of the sulci and gyri (dotted black arrows). Contrast enhanced head CT (top right) demonstrates absent perfusion involving the right MCA territory. This appears to be larger than 1/3 of the MCA territory, which does not make it amendable anymore for lysis therapy. The time-to-peak (TTP) image (bottom left) demonstrates delayed perfusion to the right MCA territory. The maximum intensity projection (MIP) image shows an abrupt cutoff at the distal M1 segment of the right middle cerebral artery (MCA), consistent with occlusion.

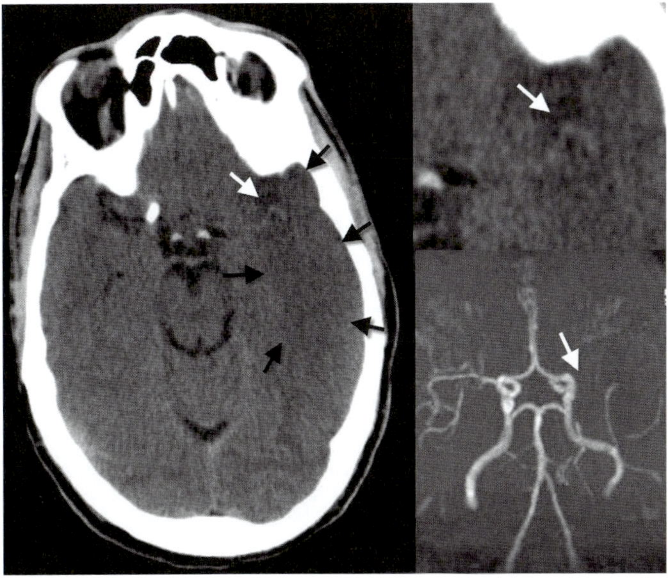

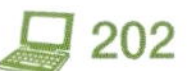

III-35

ACUTE LEFT MCA INFARCT – HYPERDENSE MCA SIGN

202

Noncontrast CT of the brain (left) demonstrates decreased attenuation with effacement of the cortical medullary junction along the left temporal lobe (black arrows), consistent with an acute infarct. The M2 and M3 segments of the left MCA are hyperdense, consistent with thrombus (white arrows, top right=magnification). Intracranial MRA demonstrates complete cutoff of the left M1 segment (bottom right).

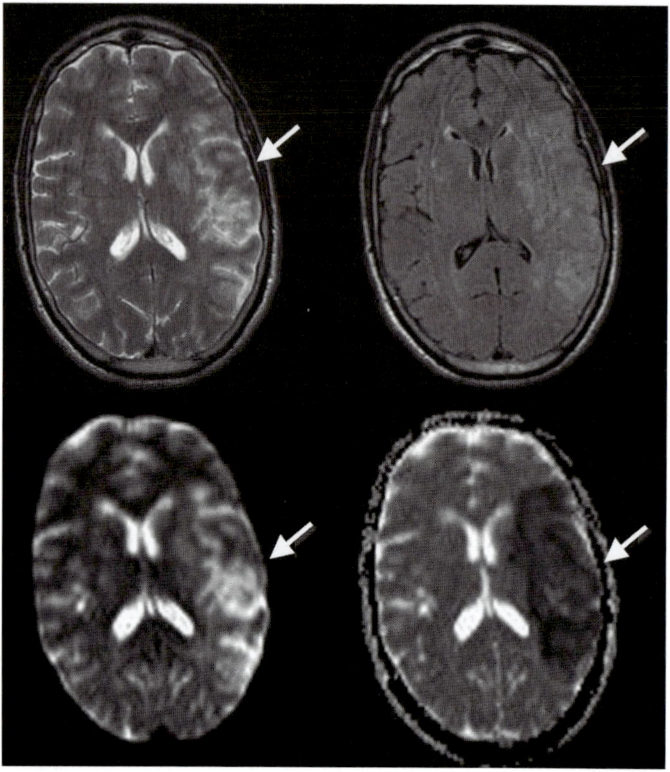

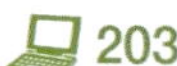

III-36

ACUTE LEFT MCA INFARCT – MRI   203

MRI of the brain demonstrates increased T2 (top left) and FLAIR (top right) signal in the left MCA territory. Diffusion weighted images (DWI, bottom left) and correlative ADC maps (bottom right) show restricted diffusion in that territory. Increased T2 signal on DWI could represent "T2 shine through" and has to be confirmed by ADC maps. Low signal on ADC map confirms restricted diffusion (compatible with infarct).

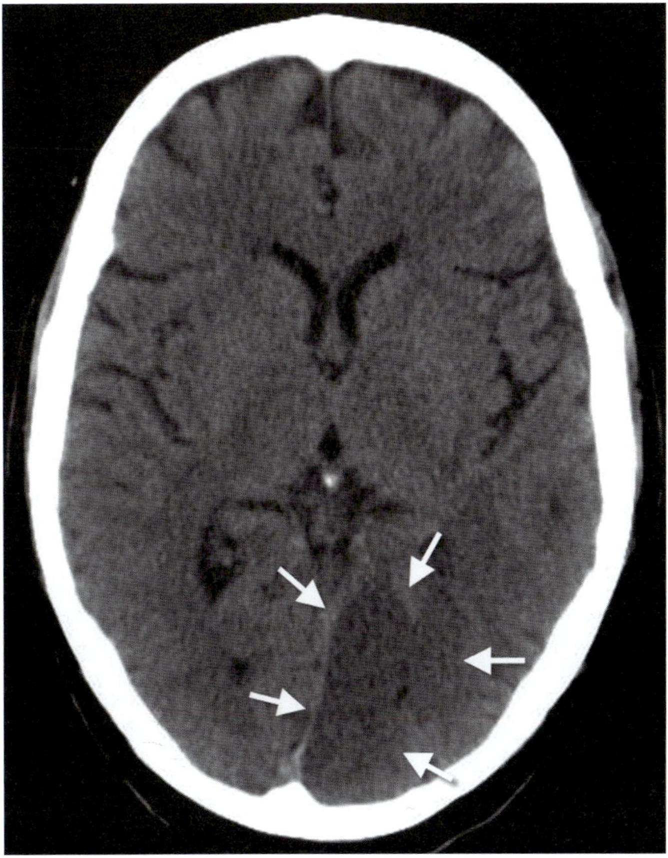

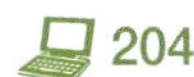

III-37

▪ ACUTE LEFT PCA INFARCT 💻 204

Noncontrast head CT demonstrates a well-defined wedge-shaped hypodensity (arrows) in the left occipital lobe medially extending to the occipital pole, representing acute ischemic infarct in left PCA territory, with involvement of the primary visual cortex.

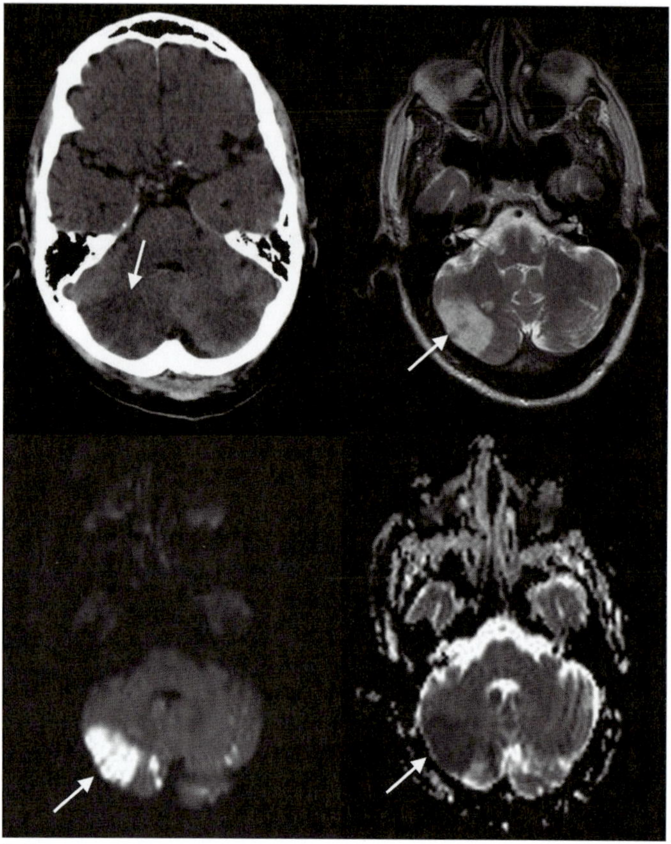

III-38

■ ACUTE RIGHT PCA INFARCT 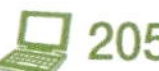 205

Noncontrast CT of the head (top left) shows an about 2 cm low attenuation area in the right cerebellar hemisphere. MRI of the brain demonstrates increased T2 signal (top right) and restricted diffusion (bottom row) corresponding to the abnormal hypodensity on CT scan.

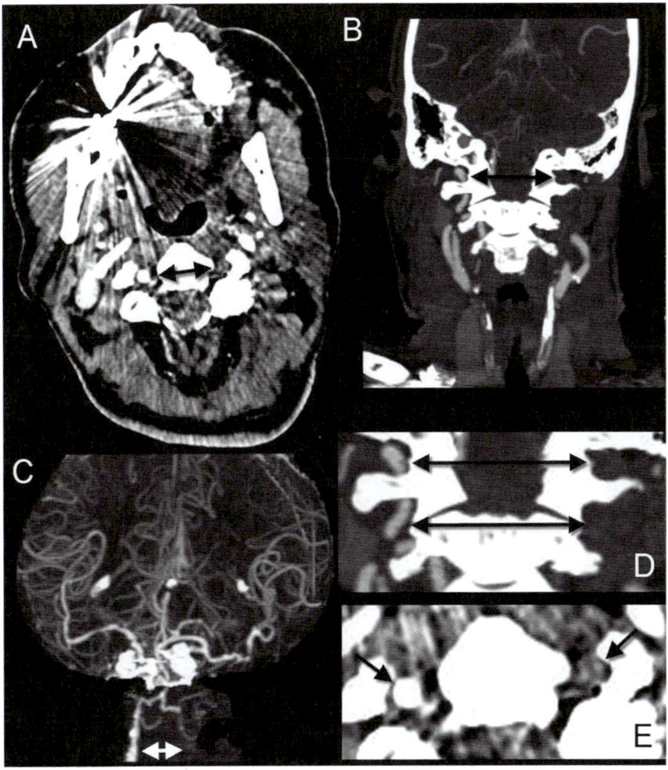

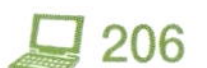

III-39

▪ LEFT VERTEBRAL ARTERY OCCLUSION   206

CT angiogram (CTA) of the head and neck: the left vertebral artery is not well seen proximal to the PICA origin when compared to the right vertebral artery (double arrows), compatible with occlusion. A=axial CTA (E=magnification), B=coronal reformatted CTA (D=magnification), and C=MIP of the CT angiogram.

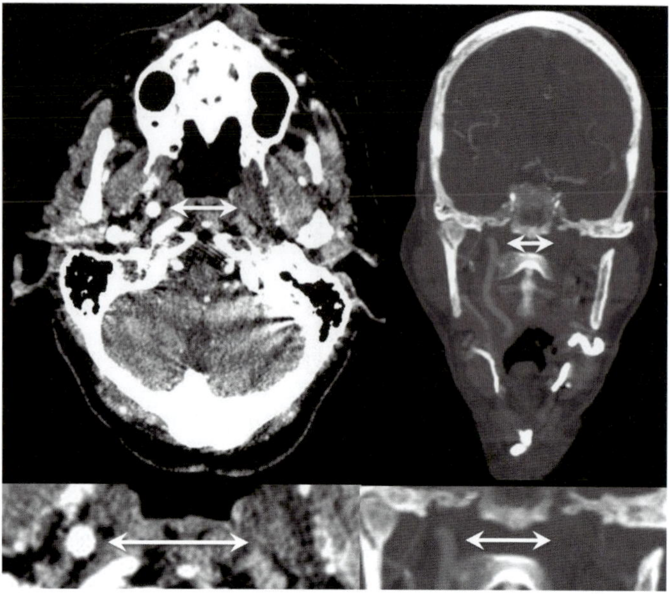

III-40

■ COMPLETE INTERNAL CAROTID ARTERY (ICA) OCCLUSION

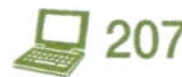 207

CTA of the head and neck (axial left; coronal reformatted right) show lack of contrast filling of the left internal carotid artery (ICA), compatible with complete occlusion. Compare normal appearance of the right ICA (double arrows, magnifications at bottom).

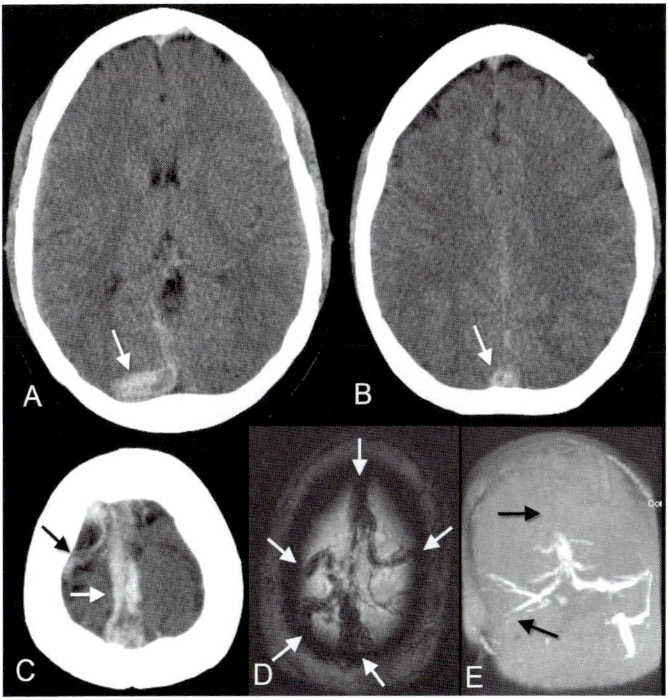

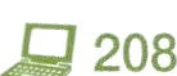

III-41

VENOUS SINUS THROMBOSIS – ON NON ENHANCED CT, MRI, AND MRV 📟 208

Noncontrast CT shows high density material throughout the superior sagittal sinus, right transverse sinus, and right sigmoid sinus (arrows in A–C), compatible with acute thrombus. MRI (gradient echo, D) demonstrates markedly abnormal signal within the cortical veins over frontal and parietal convexities bilaterally as well as within superior sagittal sinus, consistent with extensive thrombus. MR venogram (E) shows the total absence of signal within the superior sagittal sinus (total occlusion) and diminutive flow within the right transverse sinus (arrows in E).

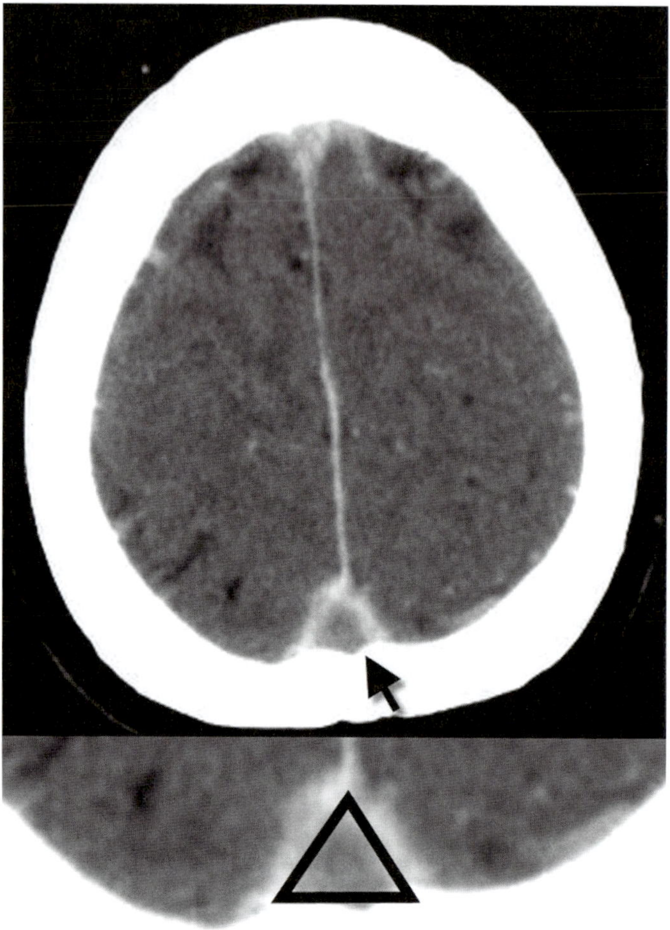

III-42

VENOUS SINUS THROMBOSIS – CONTRAST ENHANCED CT

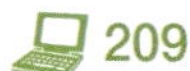 209

Contrast enhanced CT demonstrates the reverse delta sign (or empty triangle sign – lower image) which can be seen in the superior sagittal sinus from enhancement of the dural leaves surrounding the comparatively less dense thrombosed sinus.

■ NEOPLASM   ⬚ 210

- Usually focal low attenuation area
- Can contain areas of higher attenuation (hemorrhagic tumor)
- If multiple consider metastases
- Metastasis usually at corticomedullary (grey–white matter) junction
- Produce surrounding edema
- Contrast enhanced CT shows usually enhancement

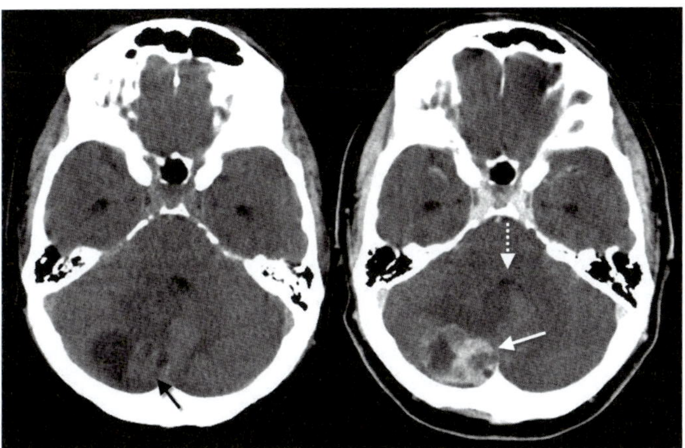

III-43

■ BRAIN METASTASIS TO CEREBELLUM   ⬚ 211

Noncontrast CT of the brain demonstrates a low attenuation area in the medial posterior aspect of the right cerebellar hemisphere. Also noted are higher attenuation foci within that area (black arrow), suggestive of acute blood and concerning for a hemorrhagic neoplasm. Contrast enhanced CT shows enhancement of that mass (white arrow). There is associated marked surrounding edema causing mass effect on the fourth ventricle (dotted white arrow).

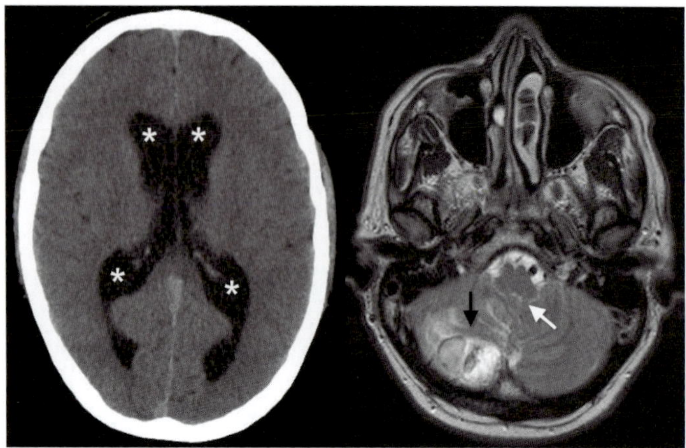

III-44

HYDROCEPHALUS – OBSTRUCTIVE 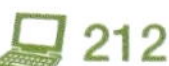 212

Noncontrast head CT (left) demonstrates mildly dilated lateral (asterisks) and third ventricles. T2 weighted MRI shows that reason for that is a right cerebellar mass (black arrow) causing mass effect on and obliteration of the fourth ventricle (white arrow).

INFECTION 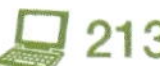 213

- Can often not be differentiated from neoplasm
- Usually focal low attenuation area
- Produce surrounding edema
- Contrast enhanced CT shows usually enhancement
- Abscess central area of fluid like attenuation
- Abscess produces ring enhancement on contrast CT
- If multiple consider septic emboli
- Meningitis: enhancement of the meninges (subarachnoid space)

In neck: evaluate for airway compromise!

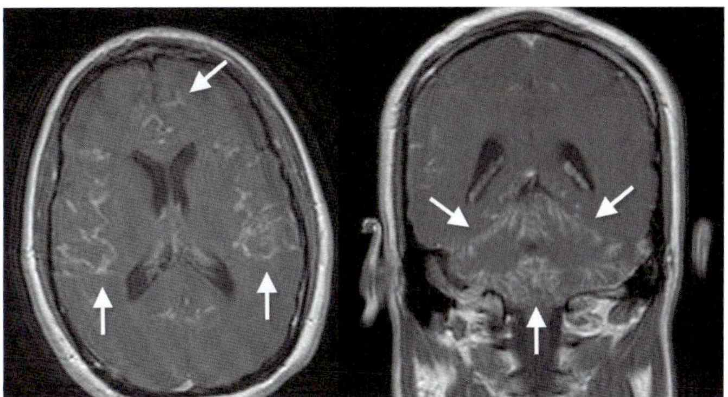

III-45

▪ MENINGITIS 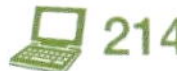 214

Postcontrast T1 weighted images (axial left, coronal right) demonstrate diffuse leptomeningeal enhancement which is most conspicuous in the posterior fossa, paramesencephalic and the basilar cisterns (right image), sylvian fissures, and interhemispheric fissure (left image), consistent with meningitis.

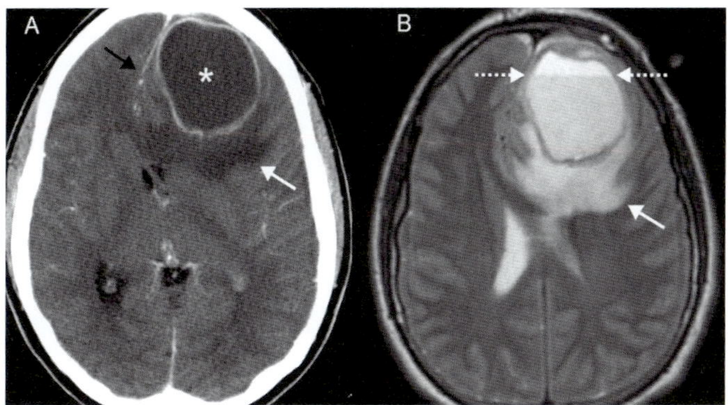

III-46

▪ BRAIN ABSCESS 215

Contrast enhanced CT (A) shows a ring-enhancing mass (asterisk) with a large amount of associated mass effect (black arrow) and surrounding edema (white arrows) in the left frontal lobe. T2 weighted axial MR image (B) demonstrates a fluid–fluid level (dotted white arrows) within this mass as well as extensive surrounding edema (white arrow).

5. Neck

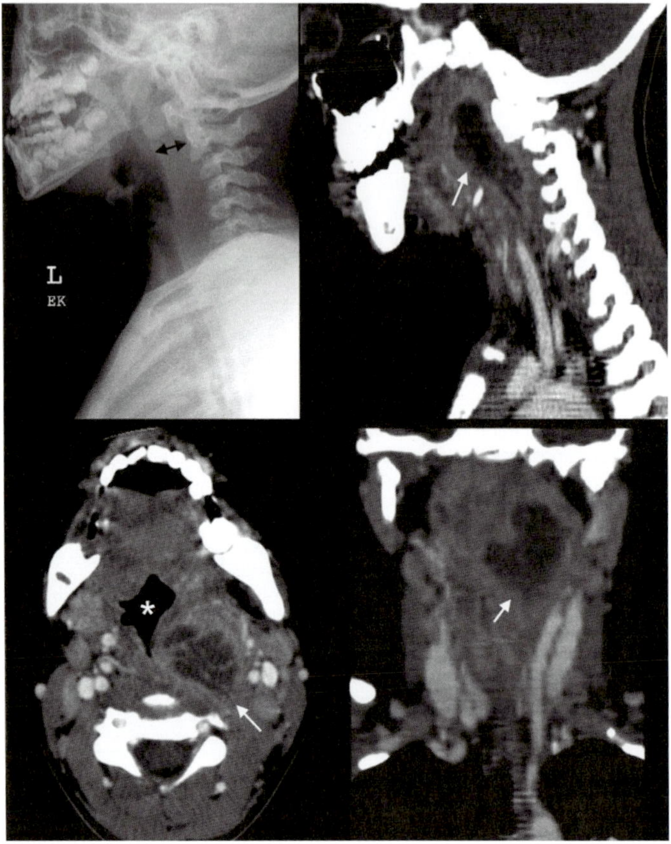

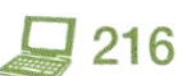

III-47

■ RETROPHARYNGEAL ABSCESS   216

Lateral airway film (top left) shows prominent upper cervical prevertebral soft tissue (double arrow). Contrast enhanced CT of the neck (top right and bottom row) demonstrates in the posterior oropharynx a large heterogeneous but predominantly low attenuation lesion with peripheral enhancement (arrows), compatible with a retropharyngeal abscess. Note also moderate narrowing of the airways (asterisk).

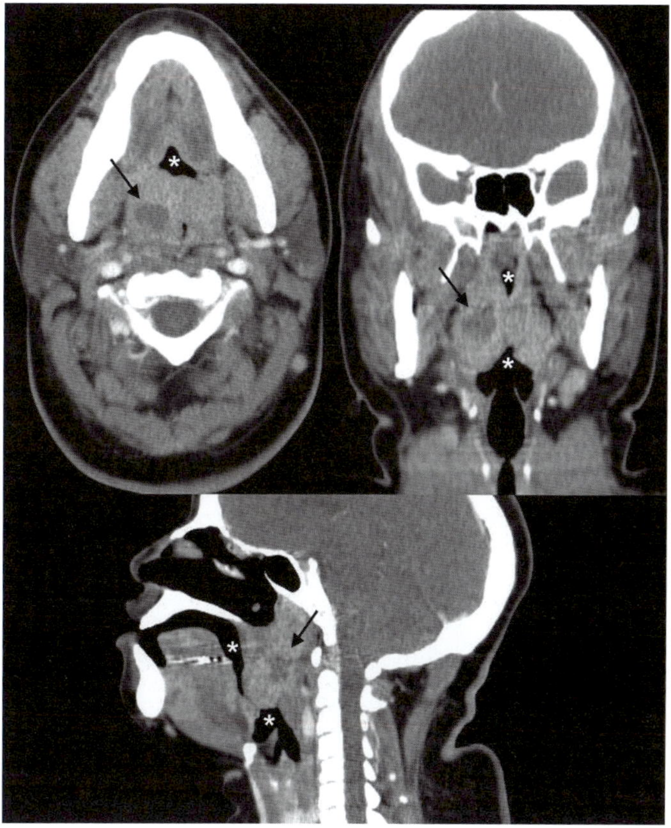

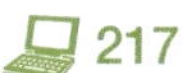

III-48

■ TONSILLAR ABSCESS   🖥 217

Contrast enhanced CT of the neck demonstrates an about 4 cm tonsillar soft tissue swelling, with an about 1.5 cm central area of low density on the right side (arrows), representing a tonsillar abscess. The soft tissue swelling causes luminal narrowing of the oro – and epipharynx (asterisks) bilaterally.

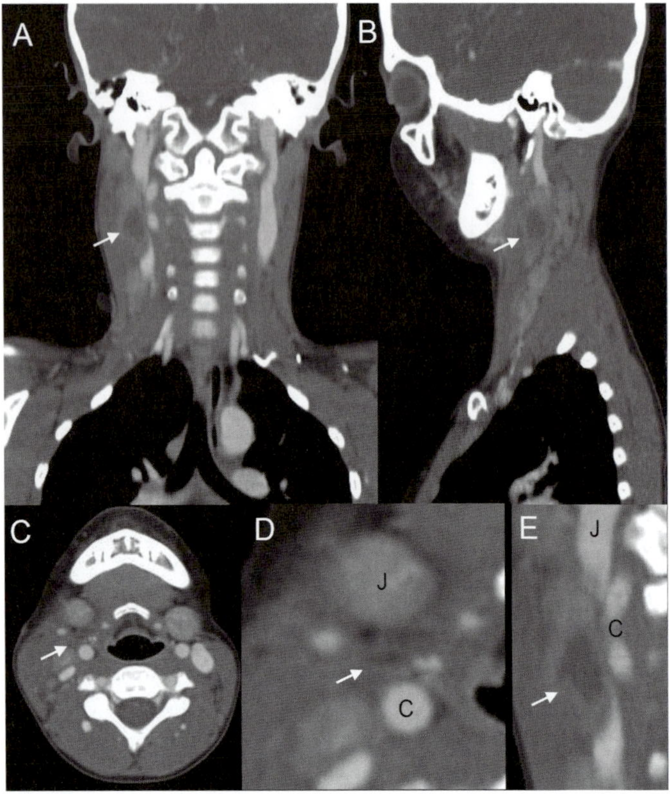

III-49

PRECAROTID ABSCESS   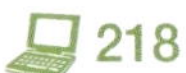 218

Contrast-enhanced CT of the neck demonstrates a 1.8×1.6×3.2 cm rim enhancing lesion with a low attenuation center in the right precarotid space (arrows), compatible with an abscess. Differential diagnosis would also include a necrotid lymph node. The abscess causes moderate mass effect on the right jugular vein (J) posteriorly. It is important to check if the carotid arteries (C) and jugular veins are patent and demonstrate normal contrast enhancement. (In this case they do.) D=magnification of the axial view (C) and E=magnification of the coronal view (A).

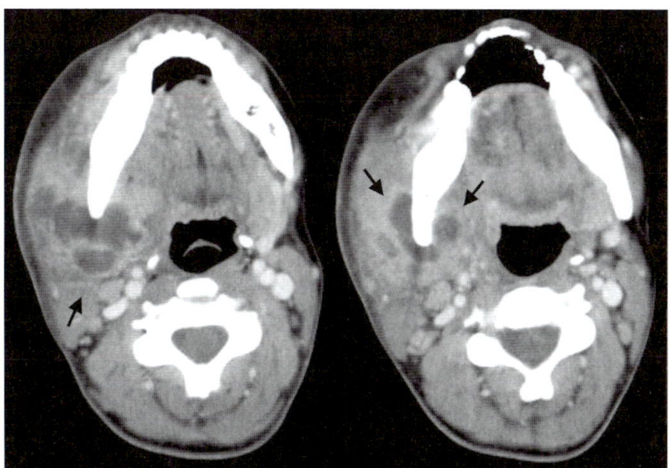

III-50

PERIODONTAL ABSCESS 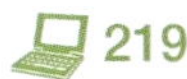 219

Contrast-enhanced axial CT of the neck shows inflammation of the right muscles of mastication and a fluid collection with septations and enhancing margins posterior to the right angle of the mandible (arrows), involving submandibular space.

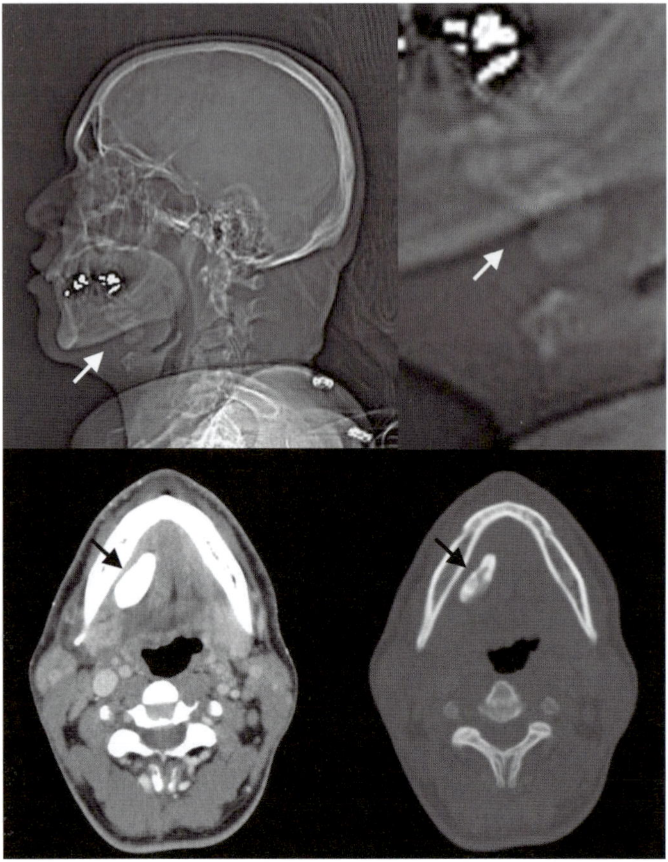

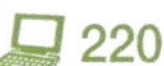

III-51

◼ SIALOLITHIASIS   📖 220

CT topogram (upper row, with magnification to the right) and contrast enhanced CT of the neck demonstrate a large ovoid shaped calcification in the right sublingual space, representing a sialolith within Wharton's duct. About 80–95% of sialoliths occur within the submandibular gland or duct.

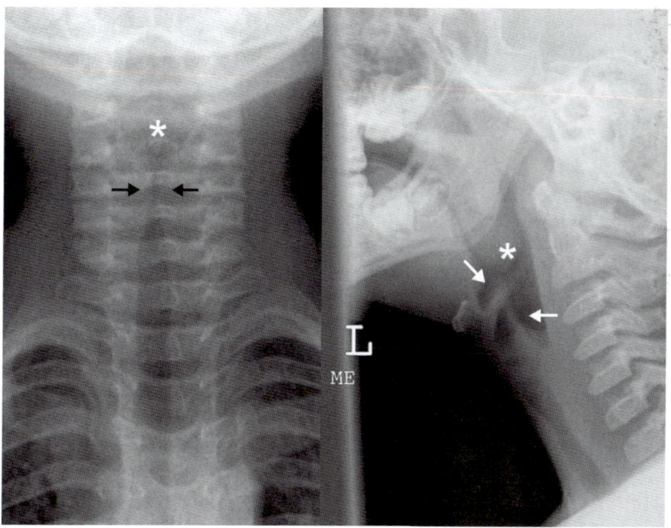
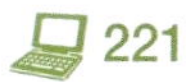

III-52

■ CROUP (LARYNGOTRACHEOBRONCHITIS) 💻 221

Frontal radiograph (left) of the upper airways demonstrates symmetric subglottic narrowing (black arrows) with loss of normal shouldering giving it a "steeple sign." There is also mild associated ballooning of the hypopharynx (asterisk). Note the normal epiglottis and aryepiglottic folds (white arrows) on the lateral view. Croup is the most common cause of upper airway obstruction in children with peak age between 6 months and 3 years). Croup is viral in etiology (usually caused by parainfluenza or RSV).

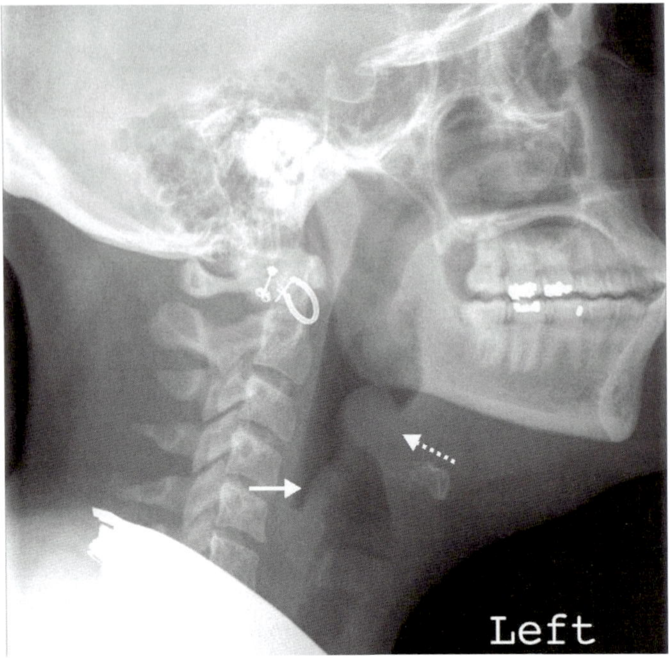

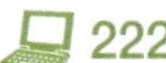

III-53

◼ EPIGLOTITIS   💻 222

Lateral view of the upper airways demonstrates marked thickening of the epiglottis (dotted arrow) and aryepiglottic folds (full arrow).

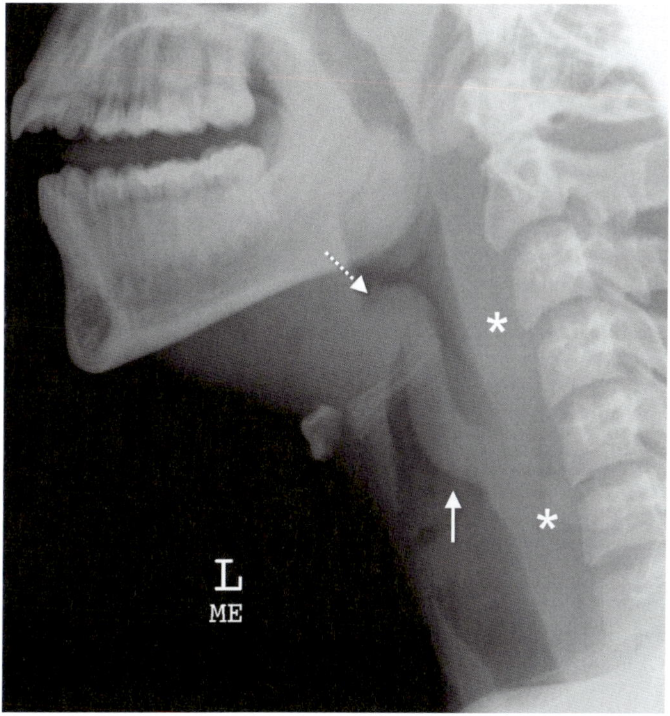

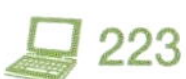

III-54

EPIGLOTITIS   223

Lateral view of the upper airways demonstrates thickening of the epiglottis (dotted arrow) and marked thickening of the aryepiglottic folds (full arrow). Also noticed is mild prominence of the prevertebral soft tissues (asterisks).

6. Spine

■ EVALUATION OF THE SPINE
ON RADIOGRAPH

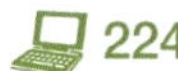 224

General
- Cervical lordosis
- Thoracic kyphosis
- Lumbar lordosis
- Vertebral alignment
- Vertebral height
- Intervertebral disc height
- Spinous process
- Fractures
- Lucencies (neoplasm, infection)
- Paravertebral soft tissue shadows (infection, neoplasm)

Cervical spine
- Evaluate spinal (anterior, posterior, spinolaminar) lines
- Make sure that cervical radiograph includes C7–T1 junction
- Predental space (adults <=3 mm, children <=5 mm)
- Retropharyngeal space (anterior to C3 vertebral body <=7 mm in adults and children)
- Retropharyngeal space (anterior to C6 vertebral body <=22 mm in adults, <=14 mm in children)

CT is the superior modality for bone evaluation.

MRI is the superior modality for soft tissue and spinal canal evaluation (eg, cord compression).

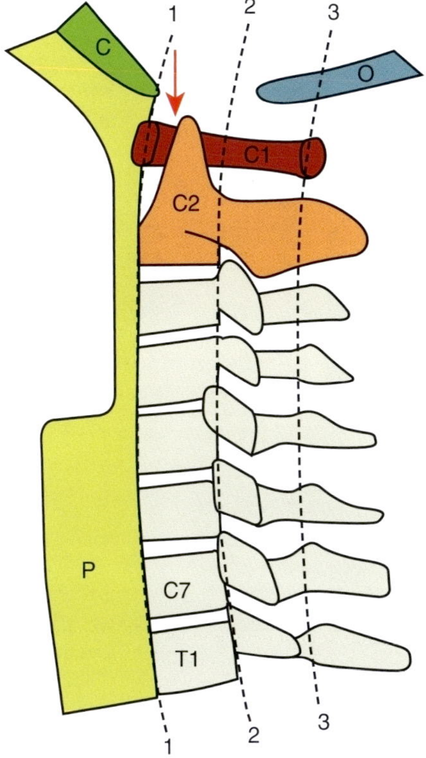

CERVICAL SPINE ON LATERAL VIEW

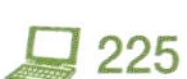 225

- C = Clivus
- O = Occiput
- C1 = Atlas (C1 vertebral body)
- C2 = Axis (C2 vertebral body)
- Red arrow = Atlanto-axial articulation/predental space
- C7 = C7 vertebral body (last cervical vertebra)
- T1 = T1 vertebral body (first thoracic vertebra)
- P = Prevertebral space
- 1 = Anterior spinal line
- 2 = Posterior spinal line
- 3 = Spinolaminar line

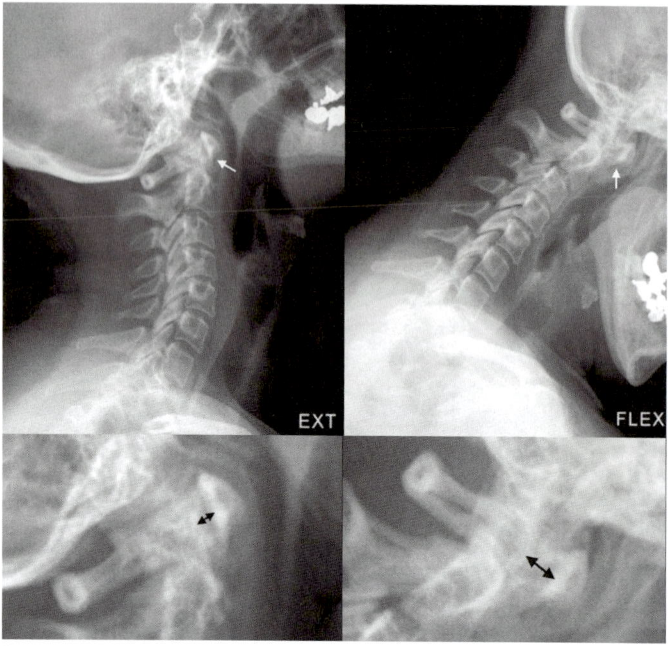

III-56

ATLANTO-AXIAL SUBLUXATION   226

The lateral view of the cervical spine obtained in flexion (right) demon-strates a 9 mm gap at the atlanto-axial articulation (arrows, right), which is reduced in extension (arrows, left). Atlanto-axial subluxation is called if the distance between the dens and the anterior arch of C1 exceeds 2.5 mm in adults or 4.5 mm in children.

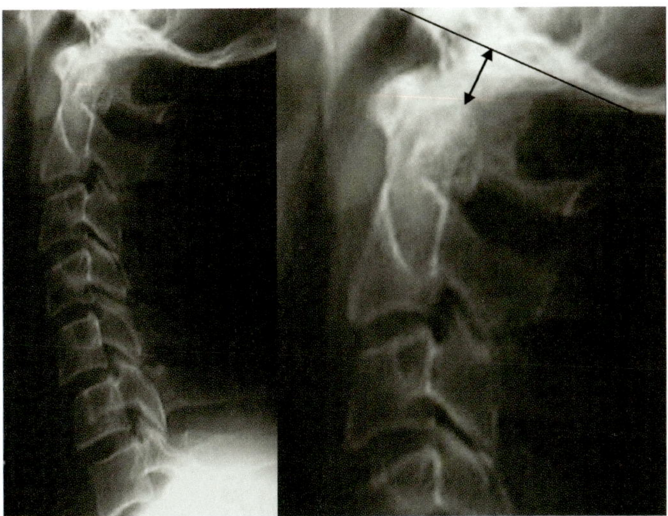

III-57

■ ALANTO-OCCIPITAL DISSOCIATION 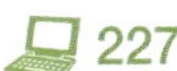 227

Lateral radiograph of the cervical spine shows distraction of the atlanto-occipital junction (double arrow) with superior displacement of the calvarium. The black line demonstrates the inferior margin of the occiput. Atlanto-occipital dissociation can be missed up to 50% of initial radiographs.

■ TYPES OF DENS FRACTURE 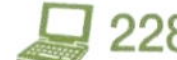

- Type I = avusion fracture of the tip of the dens
- Type II = fracture through the base of the dens at the junction with the C2 body (most common)
- Type III = fracture extending through the upper body of C2

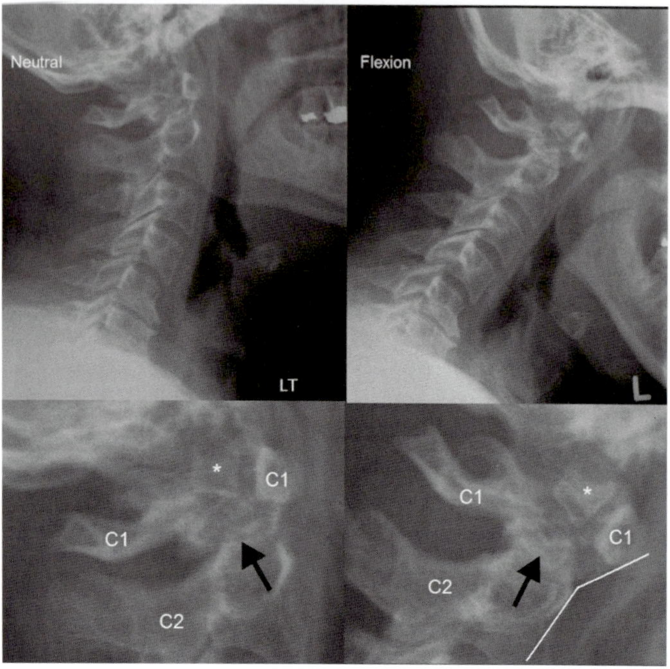

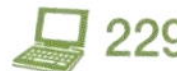

III-58

■ DENS FRACTURE – TYPE II RADIOGRAPH

Lateral radiograph of the cervical spine shows a horizontal lucency extending through the base of the dens with sclerotic margins (black arrows), indicating a chronic dens fracture. There is mild retrolisthesis of the dens fragment (asterisk) in neutral position. In flexion, there is anterolisthesis and anterior angulation of the dens fragment (indicated by the white angle lines).

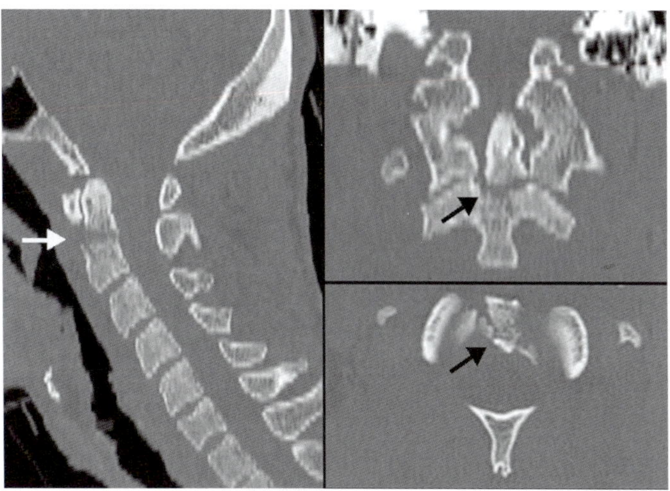

III-59

DENS FRACTURE – TYPE II CT 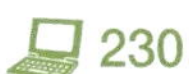 230

Cervical spine CT in sagittal (left), coronal (top right) and axial (bottom right) planes demonstrate a slightly oblique, nondisplaced fracture through the base of the dens. There is mild fragmentation of the fracture (best seen on the axial view).

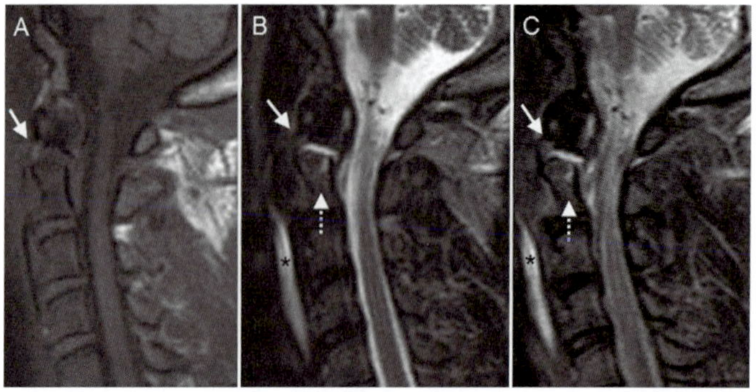

III-60

■ DENS FRACTURE – TYPE II MRI 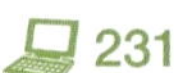 231

Cervical MRI (A = T1, B = T2, C = STIR) in the sagittal plane demonstrates a slightly oblique, mildly posteriorly displaced and angulated fracture through the base of the dens (full arrow). There is associated adjacent bone marrow edema (dotted arrow) confirming the acute state of injury. Prevertebral fluid collection extending from the level of the dens to C4 (asterisk) is secondary to ligamentous injury.

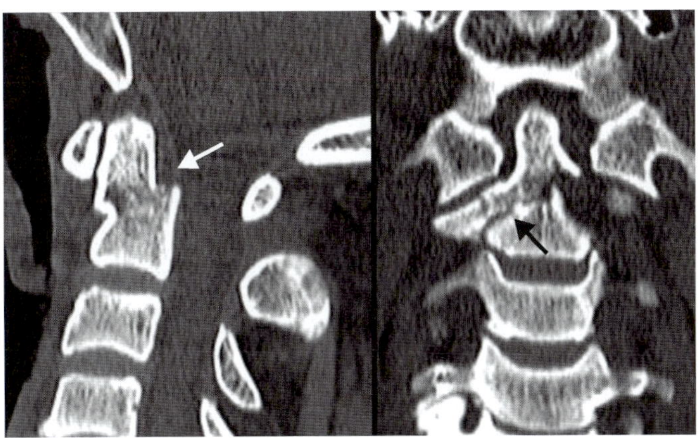

III-61

DENS FRACTURE – TYPE III 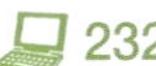 232

CT of the cervical spine in bone window shows an odontoid fracture that extends into the C2 body (seen on the coronal view to the right, black arrow). The dens is displaced anteriorly (seen on sagittal view to the left.)

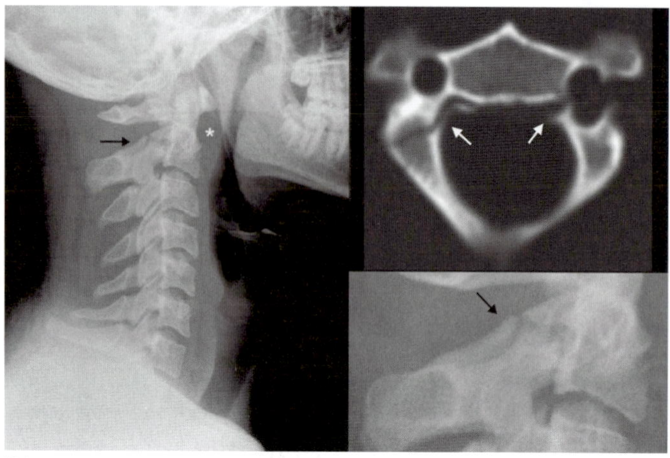

III-62

■ HANGMAN'S FRACTURE   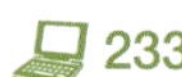 233

Lateral cervical radiograph of the cervical spine (left and bottom right = magnification) shows an irregular, linear lucency through the posterior elements of C2. There seems to be mild angulation at C2/C3 and the spinolaminal line is slightly offset at C2. Furthermore, there is thickening of the upper prevertebral soft tissues (asterisk), measuring about 10 mm at the level of the base of the dens. Axial CT image (top right) through the level of C2 shows a fracture through the bilateral pedicles, with the left pedicle fracture extending through the left foramen transversarium.

Hangman's fracture is an unstable bilateral pedicle fracture of C2, typically with traumatic spondylolisthesis of C2–3. Common mechanism is hyperextension.

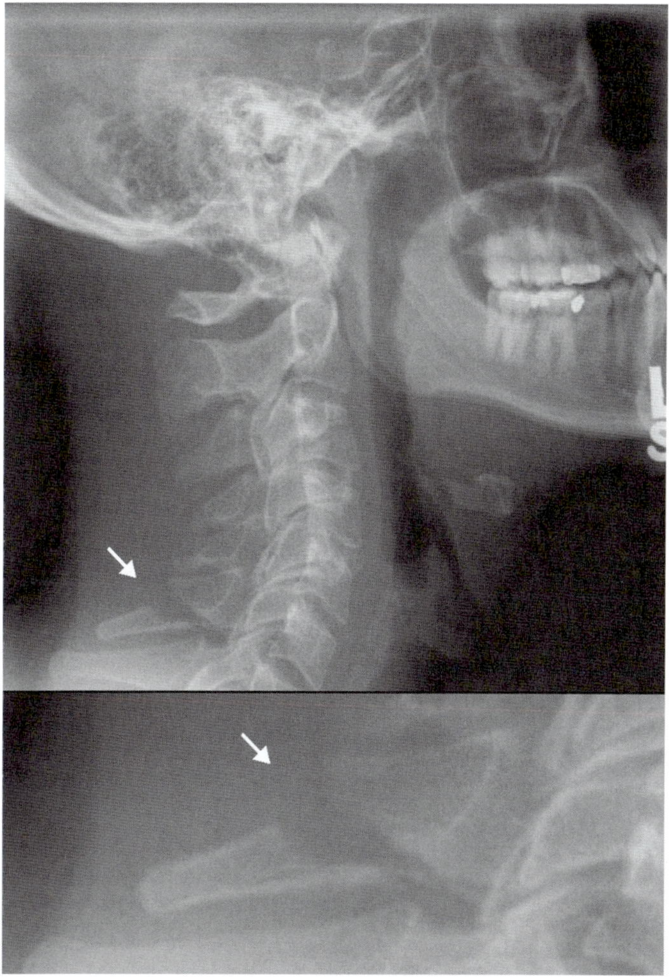

III-63

CLAY SHOVELER'S FRACTURE 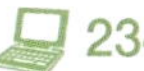 234

Lateral radiograph of the cervical spine demonstrates a distracted oblique fracture of the C6 spinous process (arrow).

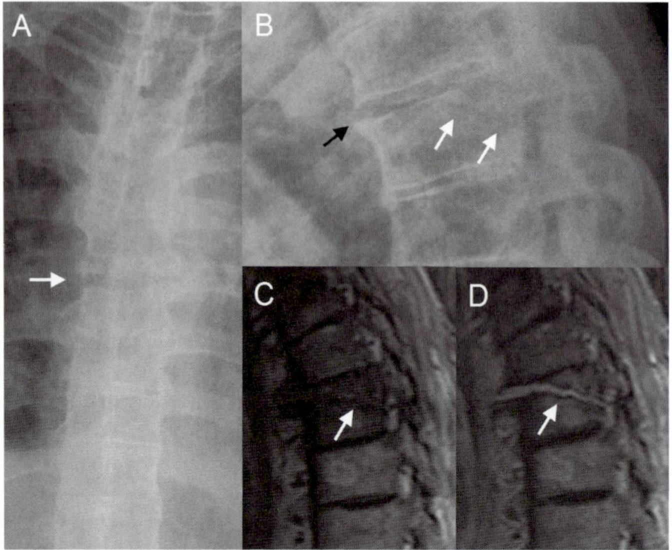

III-64

CHANCE FRACTURE (SEATBELT FRACTURE) – RADIOGRAPHY AND MRI

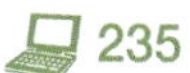 235

Frontal (A) and lateral (B) radiographs of the thoracic spine demonstrate ankylosis at all levels due to calcified syndesmophytes with an abnormal horizontal hyperlucent line just below the superior endplate of T7 vertebral body (anterior view) and an oblique lucent line through the posterior T7 vertebral body (lateral view, white arrows). In addition, a fracture of the anterior syndesmophyte between T6 and T7 is also identified on the lateral view (black arrow). T1 (C) and T2 (D) weighted sagittal MR images confirm the fracture of T7 vertebral body extending through to the posterior elements. This type of injury (hyperflexion, eg, due to seatbelt compression while decelerating) is frequently associated with injuries to internal organs (eg, pancreas, duodenum).

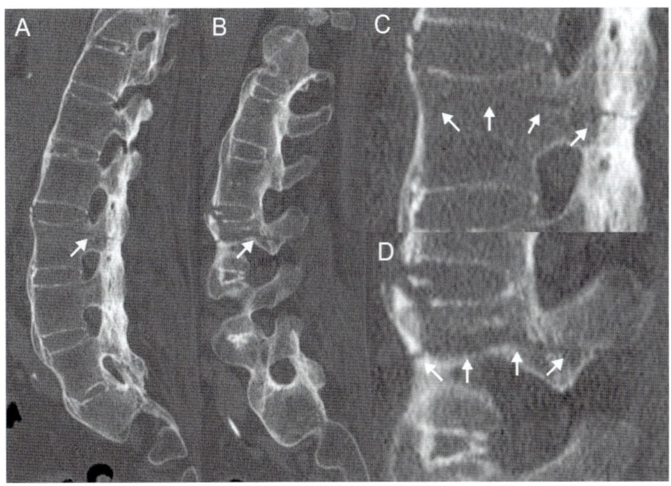

III-65

CHANCE FRACTURE (SEATBELT FRACTURE) – CT

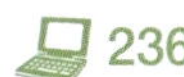 236

Sagittal CT of the lumbar spine in bone window demonstrates ankylosis of the vertebral bodies at all visualized levels due to calcified syndesmophytes, with squaring of the vertebral bodies, which is a typical feature of ankylosing spondylitis. A horizontal fracture line is seen extending through the upper L3 vertebral body, the left L3 pedicle, and superior right L3 facet. The ankylosed spine in ankylosing spondylitis is prone to fracture even in minor traumas. (C and D = magnified views of A and B)

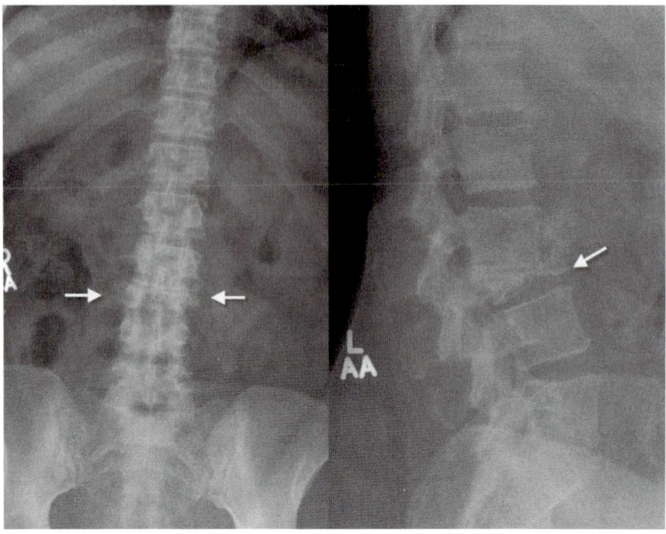

III-66

COMPRESSION FRACTURE (BURST FRACTURE)

 237

AP and lateral views of the lumbar spine demonstrate a burst fracture of L3 with resulting gibbus deformity of the lumbar spine. There appears to be retropulsion of bony fragments into the spinal canal.

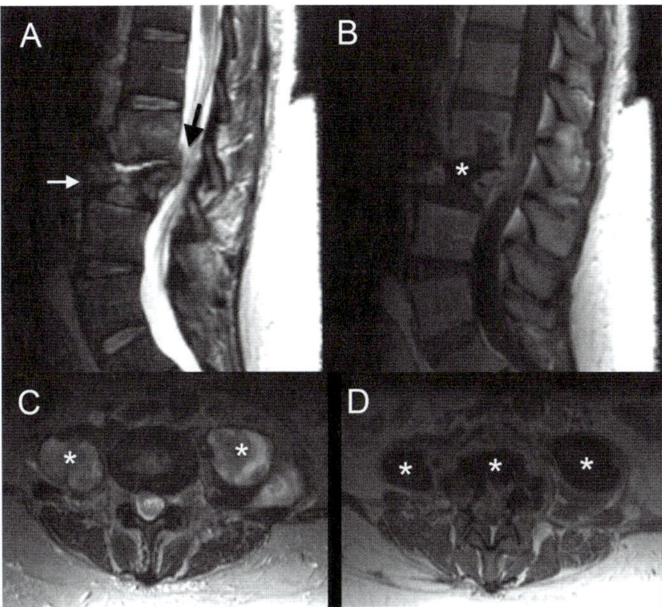

III-67

▣ BURST FRACTURE FROM SPINAL TUBERCULOSIS   🖥 238

Sagittal (A, B) and axial (C, D) T2 (A, C) and post contrast T1 (B, D) weighted images of the lumbar spine demonstrate destruction of the L3 vertebral body (A, white arrow) with gibbus formation and retropulsion of bony fragments with compromise of the central canal at that level (A, black arrow). There is fluid signal within the disc space that communicates with bilateral psoas abscesses (B, C, D, white asterisks), and pathologic enhancement is noted following contrast administration (B, D). These are typical features of spinal tuberculosis (Pott's disease).

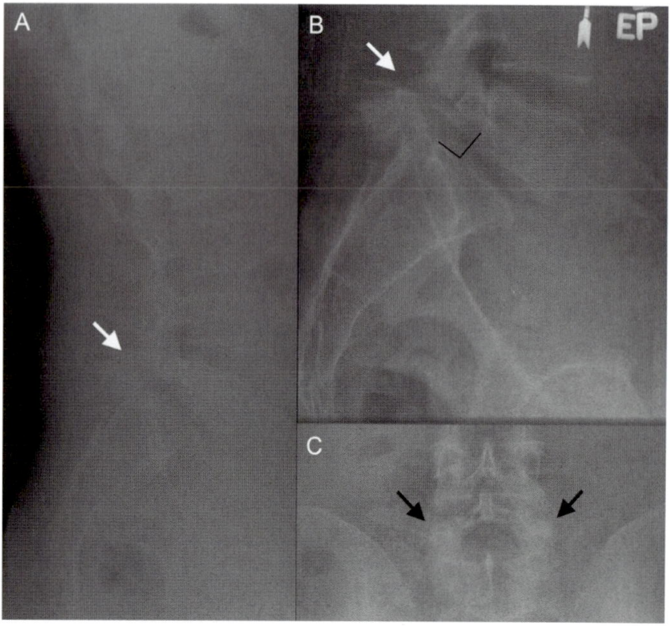

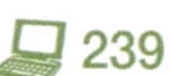

III-68

■ SPONDYLOLYSIS WITH SPONDYLOLYSTHESIS

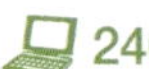 239

Lateral (A), coned down (B), and frontal (C) radiographs of the lumbar spine show bilateral pars defects (white and black arrows) with anterior displacement of the L5 vertebral body in relation to S1 vertebral body of less than 25% of the total superior vertebral body length (=grade I spondylolysthesis).

■ SPONDYLOLISTHESIS (MEYERDING) GRADING SYSTEM

240

- Grade 1 is 0–25%
- Grade 2 is 25–50%
- Grade 3 is 50–75%
- Grade 4 is 75–100%
- Over 100% (Spondyloptosis)

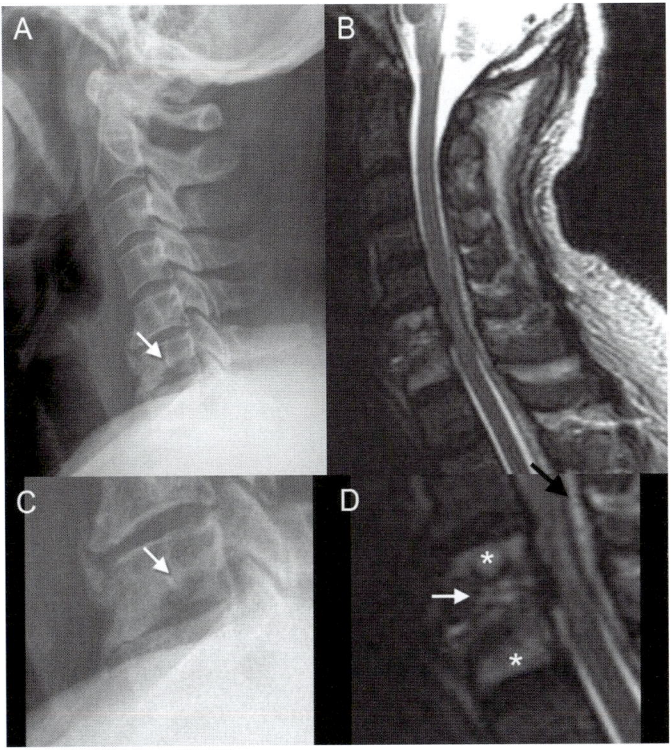

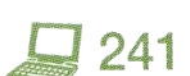

III-69

VERTEBRAL DISCITIS/OSTEOMYELITIS WITH EPIDURAL ABSCESS

241

Lateral radiograph of the cervical spine (A, C=magnification) demonstrates a scalloped area of erosive changes at the inferior endplate of C6 with loss of disc space height at C6–C7. Sagittal T2 weighted MRI of the cervical spine (B, D=magnification) shows marked bone marrow edema signal change within the C6 and C7 vertebral bodies (asterisks) along with increased fluid signal in the disc space (D, white arrow). This is compatible with discitis/osteomyelitis. An abnormal dorsal epidural fluid collection (D, black arrow) extends from C5 through T4 (here only visualized till T2 level) with narrowing of the central canal and compatible with an epidural abscess. There is associated increased T2 signal in the cord (myelomalacia) at C6–C7 as sign of significant cord compression.

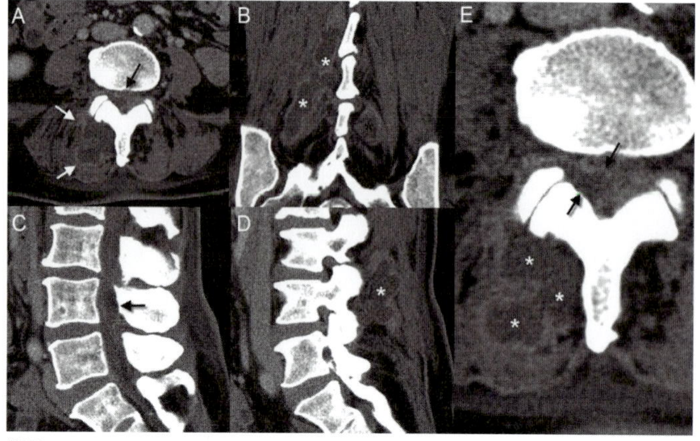

III-70

EPIDURAL AND PARAVERTEBRAL ABSCESS WITH SEPTIC FACET JOINT

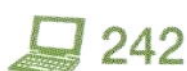 242

Contrast enhanced CT of the lumbar spine shows multiple connected enhancing lobulated fluid collections within the right paravertebral musculature at the level of L3–L4 disc base which extends inferiorly to the level of mid aspect S2 vertebral body (white arrows and asterisks). This is consistent with a paravertebral abscess. Fluid collection abuts the facet joint on the right at level of L4–L5 (panel A and magnification panel E). At the level of L4 vertebral body, there is a 2 cm enhancing epidural fluid collection representing an epidural abscess (black arrows, panel C, and magnification panel E). This epidural abscess results in moderate to severe mass effect on the thecal sac. Smaller collection is present in the left paravertebral soft tissues at the level of L5–S1 (black asterisk, panel B).

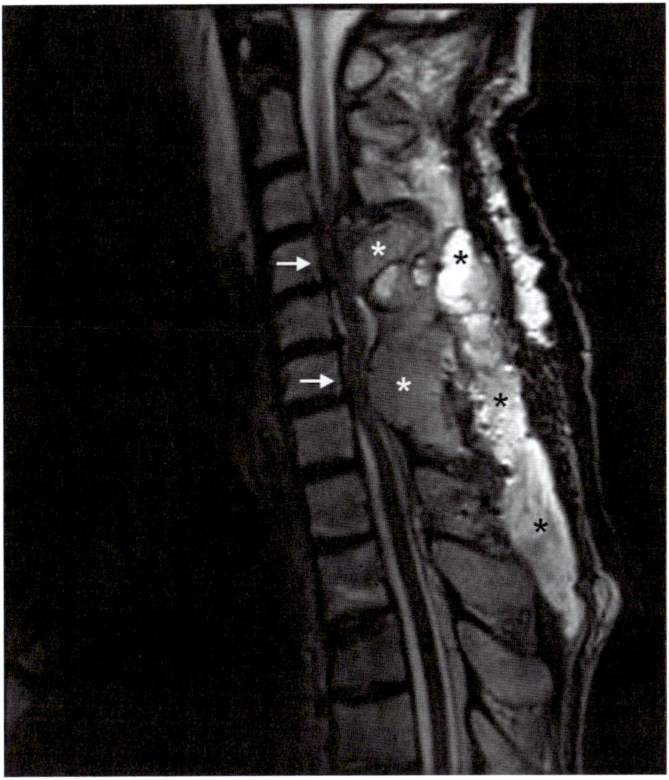

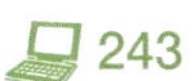

III-71

■ CORD COMPRESSION – DUE TO POSTOPERATIVE HEMATOMA

243

This patient is status post posterior fusion of C3 to T2 and experienced weakness after the spine surgery. Sagittal T2 weighted image of the cervical spine demonstrates substantial dorsal fluid in the paraspinal soft tissues (asterisks). These collections are most prominent at C4–C5 and C6–C7 where they cause severe compression on the spinal cord (arrows). The overall appearance of this heterogeneous fluid collection (white and black asterisks) suggests a mixture of seroma and loculated hematomas, which are responsible for the dorsally applied mass effect.

References

There are many freely available high quality review articles available about specific topics discussed in this book. These selections of references are only references to high quality journal articles that are freely and directly available.

How to get access to these articles?

Each reference has a so-called PMID at the end. Please use that number and go on the following hyperlink by exchanging "PMID" with that respective number. *http://www.ncbi.nlm.nih.gov/pubmed/PMID*

That hyperlink provides the abstract and further links to direct access to these full text articles.

1. de Lucas EM, Sánchez E, Gutiérrez A, Mandly AG, Ruiz E, Flórez AF, Izquierdo J, Arnáiz J, Piedra T, Valle N, Bañales I, Quintana F. CT protocol for acute stroke: tips and tricks for general radiologists. Radiographics. 2008 Oct;28(6):1673–1687. PMID: 18936029

2. Clinch CR. Evaluation of acute headaches in adults. Am Fam Physician. 2001 Feb 15;63(4):685–692. PMID: 11237083

3. Wintermark M, Sincic R, Sridhar D, Chien JD. Cerebral perfusion CT: technique and clinical applications. J Neuroradiol. 2008 Dec;35(5):253–260. PMID: 18466974

4. Rhea JT, Novelline RA. How to simplify the CT diagnosis of Le Fort fractures. AJR Am J Roentgenol. 2005 May;184(5):1700–1705. PMID: 15855142

5. Walid MS, Zaytseva NV. Upper cervical spine injuries in elderly patients. Aust Fam Physician. 2009 Jan–Feb;38(1–2):43–45. PMID: 19283235

6. Chang W, Alexander MT, Mirvis SE. Diagnostic determinants of craniocervical distraction injury in adults. AJR Am J Roentgenol. 2009 Jan;192(1):52–58. PMID: 19098179

7. Kubal WS. Imaging of orbital trauma. Radiographics. 2008 Oct;28(6):1729–1739. PMID: 18936032

8. Alcalá-Galiano A, Arribas-García IJ, Martín-Pérez MA, Romance A, Montalvo-Moreno JJ, Juncos JM. Pediatric facial fractures: children are not just small adults. Radiographics. 2008 Mar–Apr;28(2):441–461. PMID: 18349450

9. Valencia MP, Castillo M. Congenital and acquired lesions of the nasal septum: a practical guide for differential diagnosis. Radiographics. 2008 Jan–Feb;28(1):205–224. PMID: 18203939

10. Donovan WH. Donald Munro Lecture. Spinal cord injury—past, present, and future. J Spinal Cord Med. 2007;30(2):85–100. PMID: 17591221

11. Girard N, Confort-Gouny S, Schneider J, Chapon F, Viola A, Pineau S, Combaz X, Cozzone P. Neuroimaging of neonatal encephalopathies. J Neuroradiol. 2007 Jul;34(3):167–182. PMID: 17590440

12. Adams SM, Knowles PD. Evaluation of a first seizure. Am Fam Physician. 2007 May 1;75(9):1342–1347. PMID: 17508528

13. Nguyen ET, Silva CI, Seely JM, Chong S, Lee KS, Mueller NL. Pulmonary artery aneurysms and pseudoaneurysms in adults: findings at CT and radiography. AJR Am J Roentgenol. 2007 Feb;188(2):W126–W134. PMID: 17242217

14. Wolffsohn JS, Peterson RC. Anterior ophthalmic imaging. Clin Exp Optom. 2006 Jul;89(4):205–214. PMID: 16776728

15. Rao SK, Wasyliw C, Nunez DB Jr. Spectrum of imaging findings in hyperextension injuries of the neck. Radiographics. 2005 Sep–Oct;25(5):1239–1254. PMID: 16160109

16. Sliker CW, Mirvis SE, Shanmuganathan K. Assessing cervical spine stability in obtunded blunt trauma patients: review of medical literature. Radiology. 2005 Mar;234(3):733–739. PMID: 15734929

17. Núñez DB Jr, Torres-León M, Múnera F. Vascular injuries of the neck and thoracic inlet: helical CT-angiographic correlation. Radiographics. 2004 Jul–Aug;24(4):1087–1098. PMID: 15256630

18. Slack SE, Clancy MJ. Clearing the cervical spine of paediatric trauma patients. Emerg Med J. 2004 Mar;21(2):189–193. PMID: 14988345

19. Lustrin ES, Karakas SP, Ortiz AO, Cinnamon J, Castillo M, Vaheesan K, Brown JH, Diamond AS, Black K, Singh S. Pediatric cervical spine: normal anatomy, variants, and trauma. Radiographics. 2003 May–Jun;23(3): 539–560. PMID: 12740460

20. el-Khoury GY, Whitten CG. Trauma to the upper thoracic spine: anatomy, biomechanics, and unique imaging features. AJR Am J Roentgenol. 1993 Jan;160(1):95–102. PMID: 8416656

1. Technique

TECHNIQUES 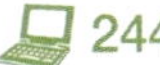 244

- **Plain film radiography** (first line modality, "bread and butter," for fractures, dislocation, soft tissue swelling/air, foreign bodies)

- **Computed tomography** (ideal for further evaluation of bony structures, eg, fracture, masses containing bone, or chondroid matrix)

- **Ultrasonography** (for superficial soft tissue lesions, evaluation of joint effusion)

- **Magnetic resonance imaging** (ideal for evaluation of soft tissues and bone marrow involvement, usually second line modality)

2. Radiograph Evaluation

▪ EVALUATE FOR   💻 245

- Fracture
- Soft tissue swelling
- Periosteal reaction
- Effusion
- Joint congruence

■ FRACTURE DESCRIPTION 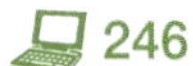 246

- Complete versus incomplete
- Fracture plane (transverse, oblique, spiral, avulsion)
- Displacement of distal fragment
- Angulation (direction of fracture angle apex)
- Comminution
- Overriding fragments, limb shortening
- Articular relation (intra-articular)
- In pediatric population: involvement of physis
- Associated subluxation/dislocation

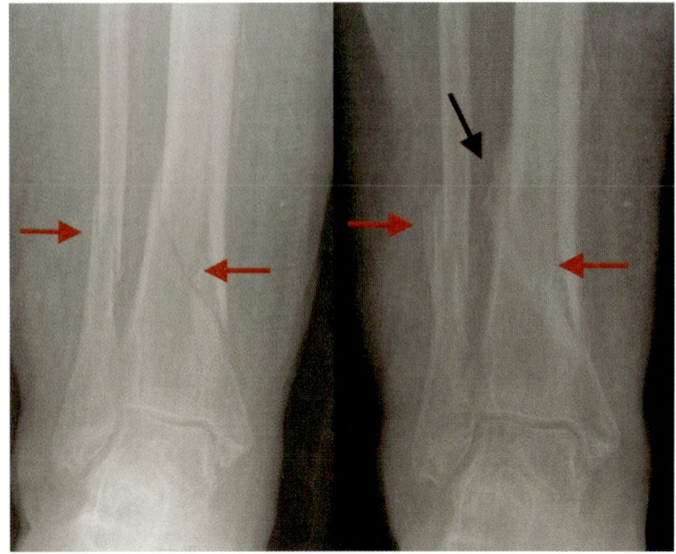

IV-1

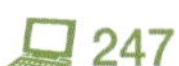 FRACTURE – ACUTE VERSUS REMOTE   247

AP radiographs of the right tibia and fibula demonstrate to the left acute oblique and complete fractures of the distal tibia and fibula (red arrows). The fibular fracture is mildly displaced laterally. Both acute fractures show clean cut lucent fracture lines through both bones, while the right radiograph has been obtained 4 months later, showing callus formation (black arrow) around the fractures and bony sclerosis adjacent to fracture lines. The fracture lines are also not that "clean" lucent anymore as those in the acute stage.

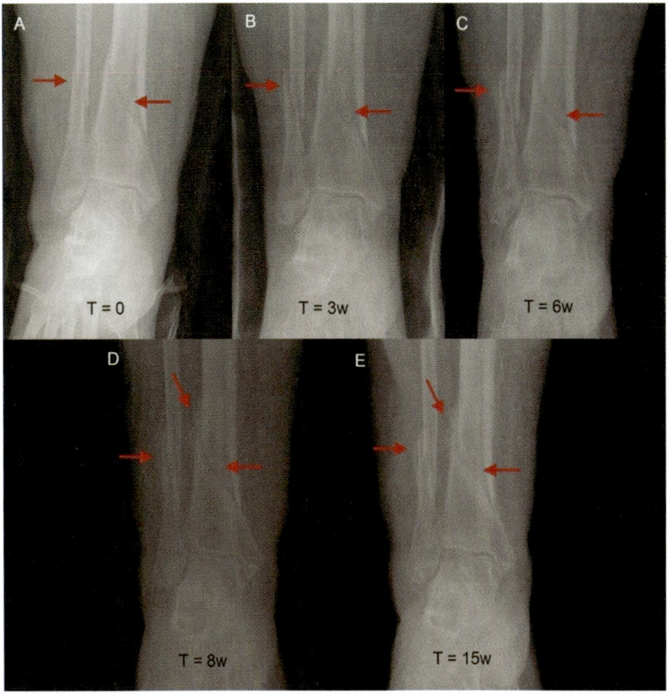

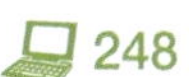

IV-2

■ FRACTURE – HEALING PROCESS   248

Chronologic healing progress of a distal tibial and fibular fracture on AP radiographs is seen. (A) is at the time of fracture. Radiograph (B) has been taken 3 weeks later, (C) 6 weeks later, (D) 8 weeks later, and (E) 15 weeks after the fracture occurred. Note the progression of callus formation. Healing process is however dependent on many variables (eg, underlying metabolic conditions, physical activity, age etc).

■ **Table IV-1.** Associated Injuries with Common Fractures 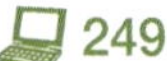 249

Fracture	Associated trauma
Clavicle	Lungs and neurovascular (pneumothorax, hematothorax), scapula
Upper ribs	Aorta, great vessels
Lower ribs	Spleen, liver, kidneys
Pelvis	Genitourinary tract, neurovascular
Femur	Hip
Calcaneus	Spine (vertical deceleration trauma), contralateral foot and ankle

■ **Table IV-2.** Easily Missed Traumata 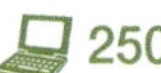 250

Region	Best diagnostic view/modality
Shoulder	Scapular (Y) view for dislocation. Type of dislocation determined by AP relation of humeral head to glenoid
Clavicle	Apical lordotic view
Sternoclavicular joint	CT with coronal reconstructions
Elbow	Lateral view shows displaced fat pad suggestive of effusion. In adults look for the radial head fracture, in children look for the supracondylar fracture
Scaphoid	Scaphoid views (MRI or repeat radiograph in 1 week)
Carpal bones	Lateral wrist radiograph
Osteochhondral defect	CT or MRI
Sacral joints	Sacroiliac views, CT, Scintigraphy

NONACCIDENTAL TRAUMA (NAT/CHILD ABUSE) – INTRODUCTION   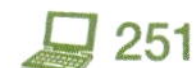 251

- If nonaccidental trauma (NAT) is suspected, then skeletal survey is indicated (babygram is not adequate).

Injuries virtually pathognomonic of NAT
- Metaphyseal corner fracture
- Multiple fractures of various age
- Interhemisperic subdural hematoma

Fractures suggestive of NAT
- Ribs (especially first rib and posterior rib ractures)
- Skull (especially multiple, cross sutures, bilateral fractures)
- Scapula, sternum, spinous process fractures
- Spiral fractures around long bones (before toddler age)
- Subdural hematoma

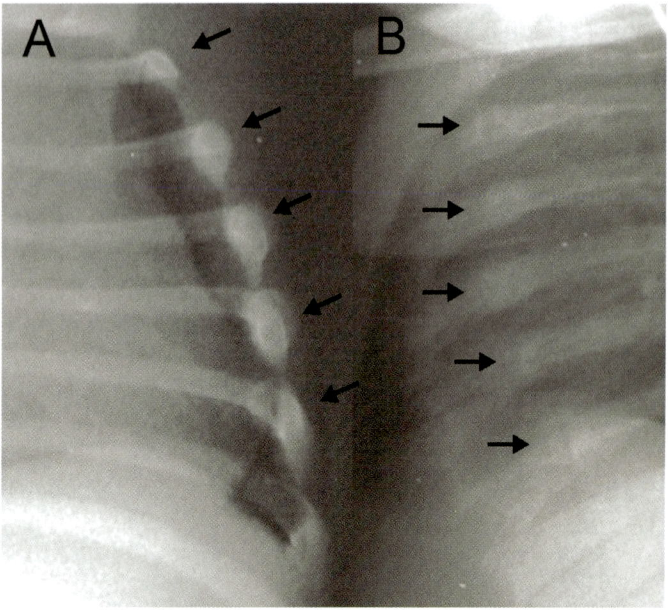

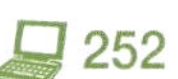

IV-3

NAT (CHILD ABUSE) – RIB FRACTURES   252

AP (A) and lateral (B) radiographs of this 2-month-old girl show multiple healing left-sided rib fractures with callus formation (arrows).

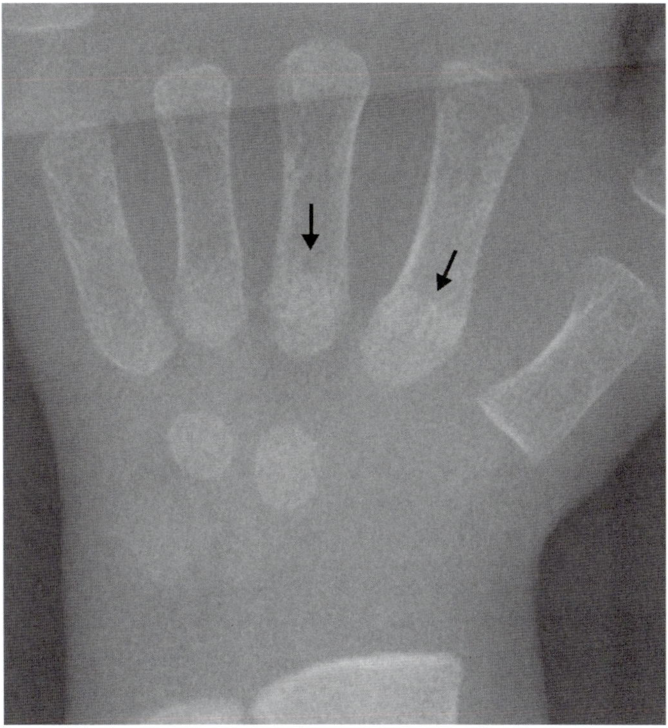

IV-4

■ NAT (CHILD ABUSE) – METACARPAL FRACTURES   253

AP radiograph of the hand of this 7-month-old boy demonstrates healing fractures at the bases of the second and third left metacarpal bones (arrows).

3. Shoulder Girdle

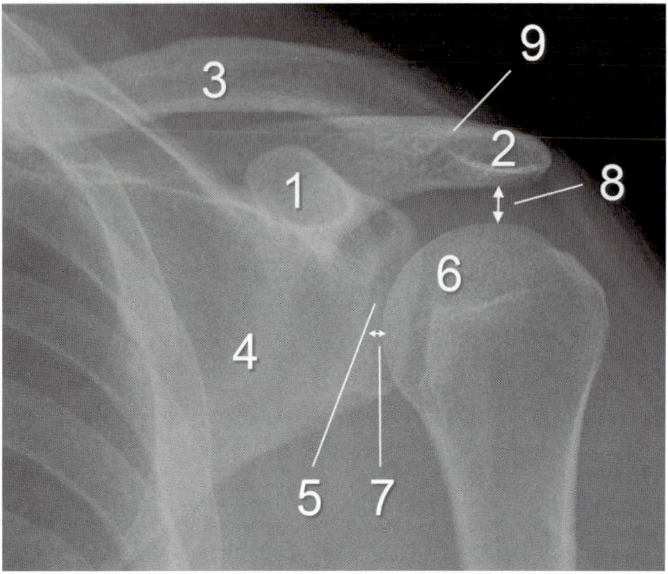

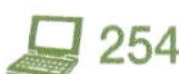

IV-5

■ NORMAL AP SHOULDER RADIOGRAPH   💻 254

1. Coracoid process
2. Acromion
3. Clavicle
4. Scapula
5. Glenoid
6. Humeral head
7. Glenohumeral joint
8. Acromiohumeral interval (normal 1 to 1.5 cm)
9. Acromioclavicular (AC) joint

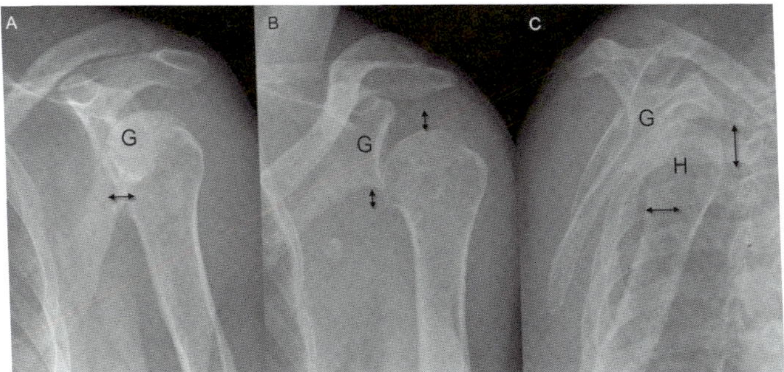

IV-6

■ ANTERIOR SHOULDER DISLOCATION 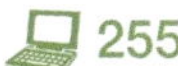 255

AP (A), true AP (B), and Y (C) views of the left shoulder demonstrate that the humeral head (H) is anteriorly and inferiorly displaced (arrows) in relation to the glenoid (G), compatible with an anterior shoulder dislocation. Normally, on the Y view (C) the humeral head should project nearly over the glenoid (H over G).

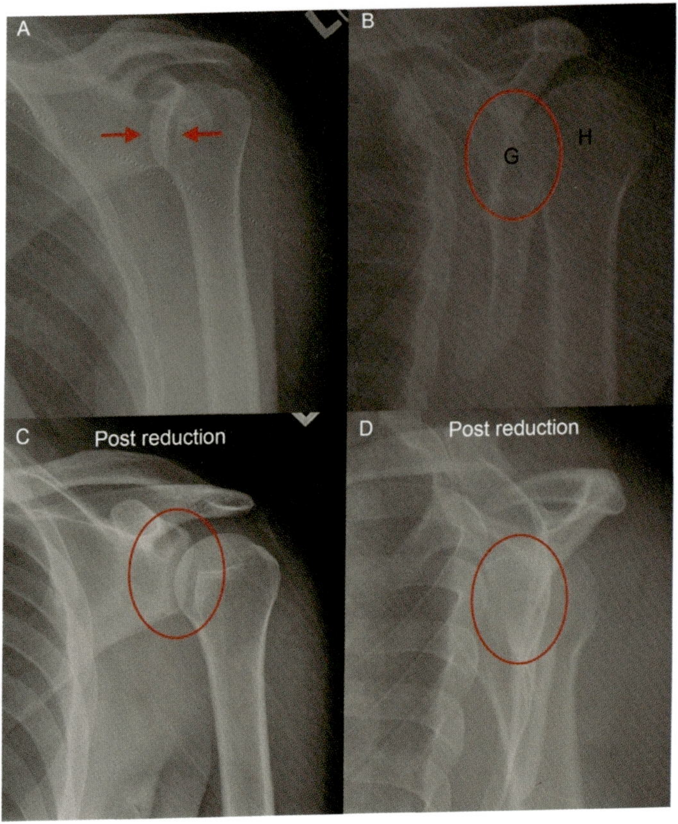

IV-7

POSTERIOR SHOULDER DISLOCATION 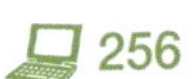 256

True AP and Y views of the left shoulder demonstrate an empty glenoid sign (G and circle in B) with the humeral head (H in B) in malposition in relation to the glenoid (arrows, A). Repeat radiographs (C, D) are post reduction, demonstrating the humeral head in anatomic position with the glenoid, (circles), forming a so-called crescent sign (C, circle).

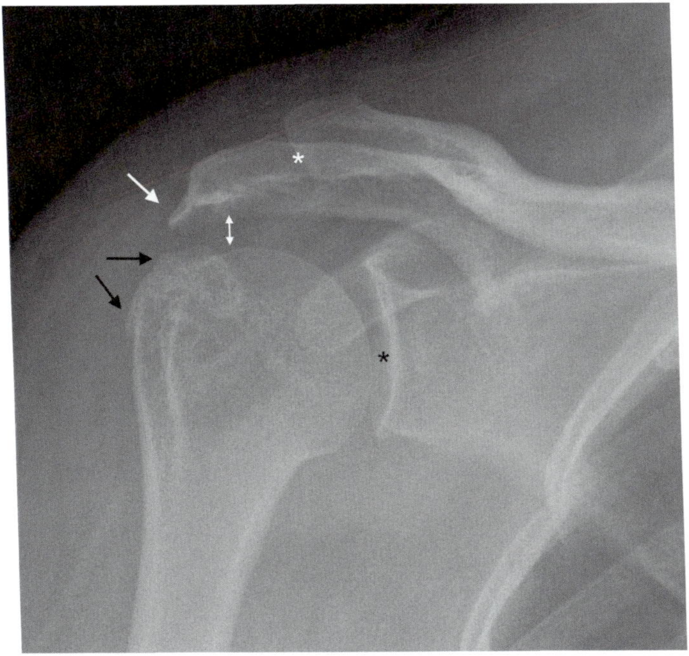

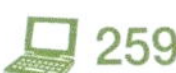

IV-8

IMPINGEMENT SYNDROME   259

True AP radiographs of the right shoulder demonstrate an acromial enthesophyte (white arrow) with hypertrophic changes involving the greater tuberosity of humerus (black arrows). These findings are suggestive of impingement syndrome in this patient with shoulder pain. The acromioclavicular (white asterisk) and glenohumeral (black asterisk) joints are intact and the acromiohumeral interval (white double arrow) is also normal.

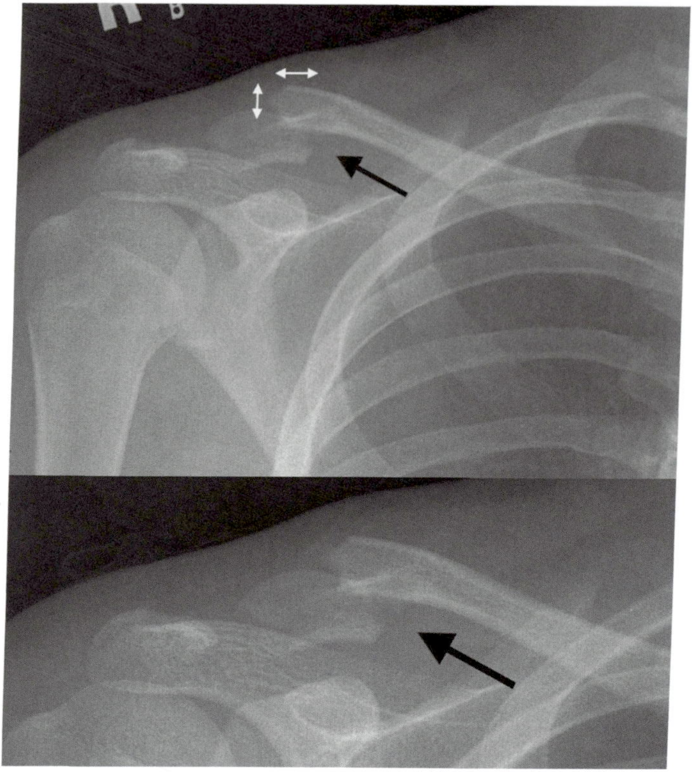

IV-9

CLAVICULAR FRACTURE (BAYONET FRACTURE)

 257

AP radiograph of the right shoulder demonstrates a complete transverse fracture approximately 3 cm medial to the distal end of the clavicle (black arrow). The distal fracture end is inferiorly and medially displaced (white arrows) in bayonet apposition.

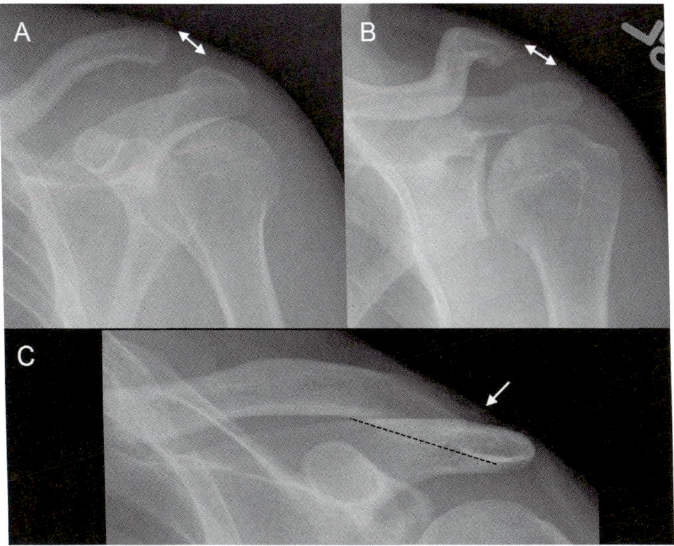

IV-10

■ ACROMIOCLAVICULAR LIGAMENT TEAR   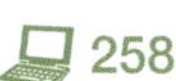 258

AP (A) and true AP (B) radiographs of the left shoulder show widening of
the acromioclavicular (AC) interval (double arrows), compatible with AC
ligament tear. (C) is an AP shoulder radiograph demonstrating a normal
AC interval (arrow). Normally the inferior margin of the clavicle and acromion should be both aligned (dotted line).

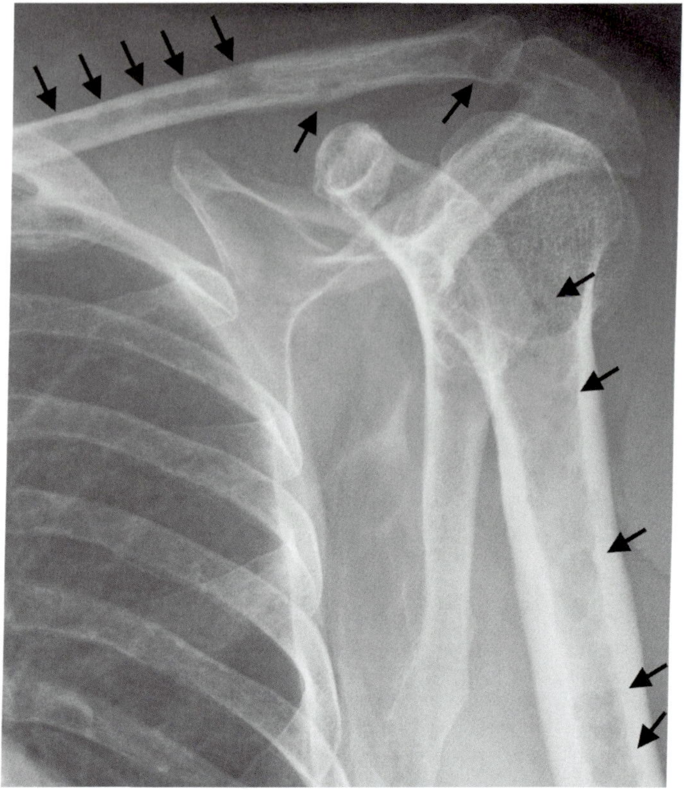

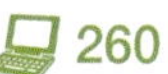

IV-11

■ MULTIPLE MYELOMA   260

Frontal radiograph of the left shoulder demonstrates innumerable focal lucent lesions involving the shoulder girdle and proximal humerus, and visualized ribs. These lesions have a "punched out" appearance that favors multiple myeloma rather than metastatic disease.

4. Upper Extremities

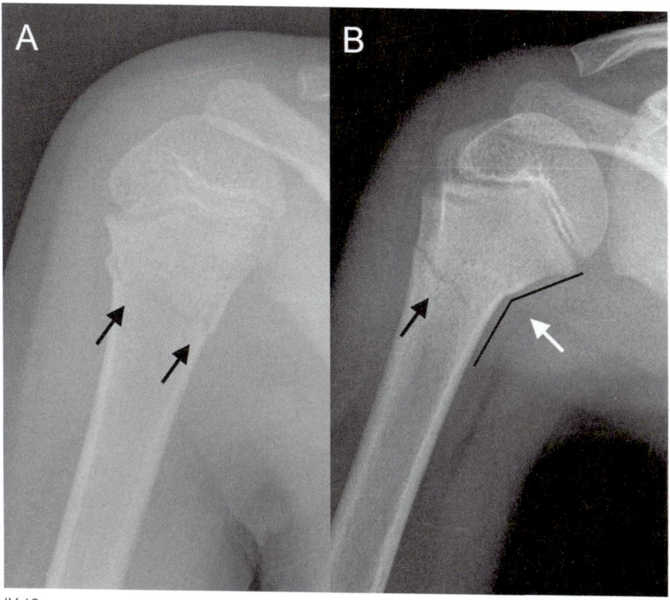

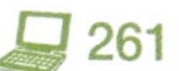

IV-12

PROXIMAL HUMERUS FRACTURE   261

AP (A) and lateral (B) radiographs of the right humerus demonstrate a horizontal lucent line in the proximal humeral metadiaphysis (black arrows). The line traverses throughout the entire diameter of the shaft, consistent with a complete fracture. The fracture is nondisplaced; however, there is mild posterior angulation noticed on the lateral view (white arrow and black angle lines).

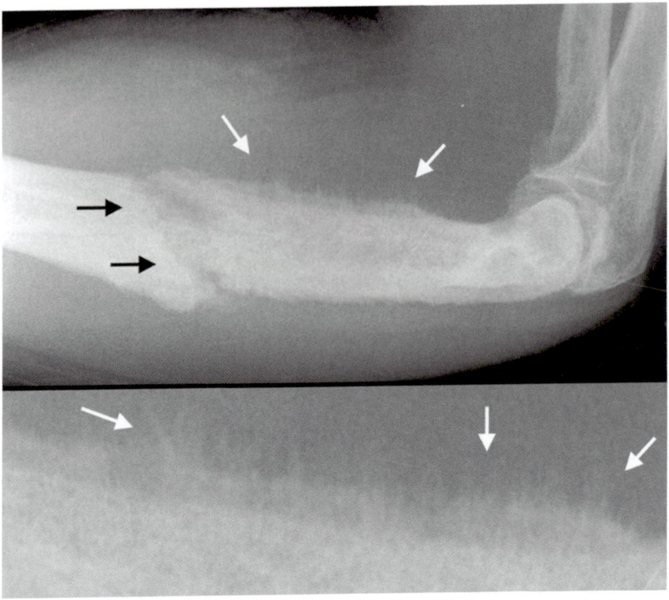

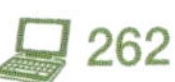

IV-13

PATHOLOGIC HUMERUS FRACTURE FROM METASTASIS

262

Lateral radiograph of the left upper arm demonstrates an oblique nondisplaced fracture (black arrows) of the distal humerus with surrounding hair-on-end pattern periosteal reaction (white arrows). This type of periostal reaction suggests a very aggressive process – as in this case due to a prostate metastasis.

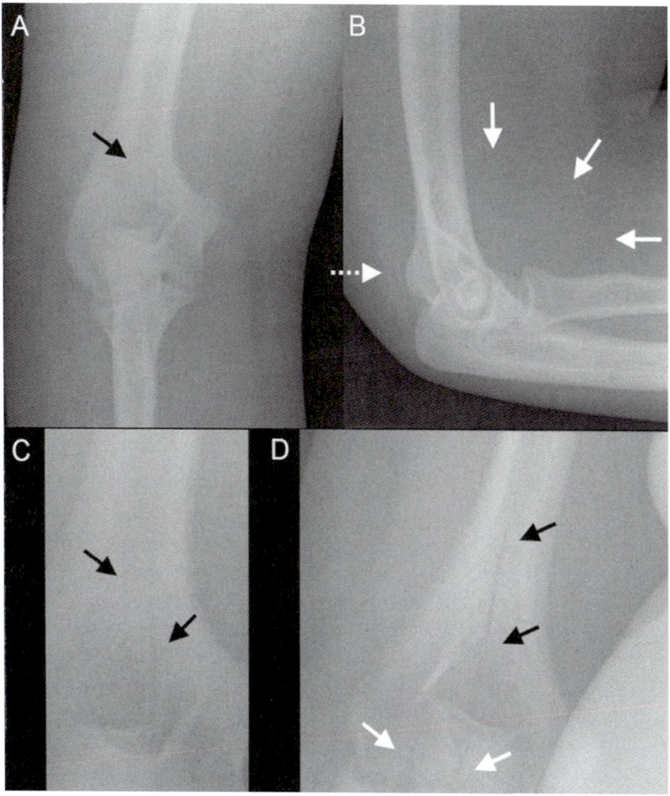

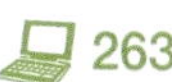

IV-14

■ DISTAL HUMERUS FRACTURE   💻 263

AP (A) and lateral (B) views of the elbow demonstrate a anterior (B, white arrows) and posterior (B, dotted arrow) fat pad, consistent with a joint effusion. The frontal images (A, C = magnification) demonstrate a vertical lucent line within the distal humeral metaphysis, which likely extends to the articular surface, even though definite intra-articular extension is not confirmed. This is consistent with a nondisplaced sagittal fracture. Lateral radiograph (B) does not identify any fracture line. A follow up radiograph obtained 9 days later (D) shows the fracture line better and also confirms the extension to the articular surface at two locations (D, white arrows).

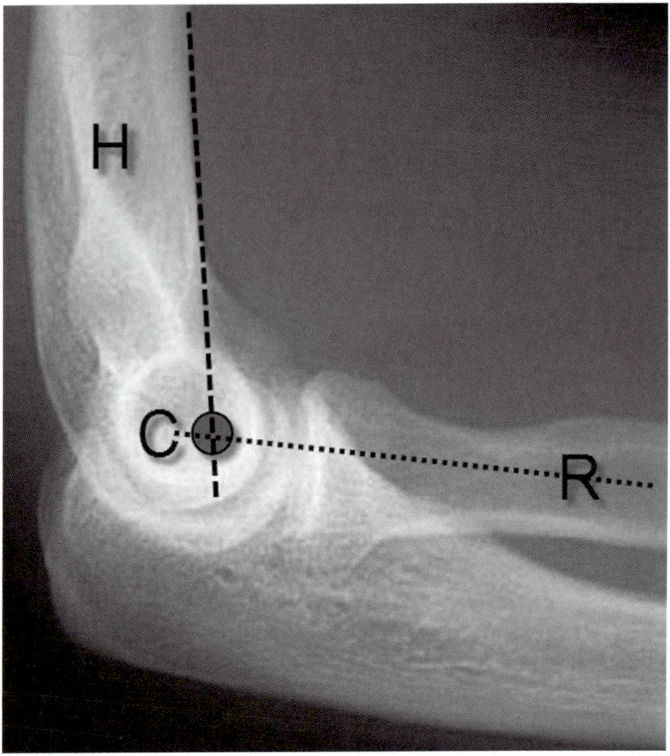

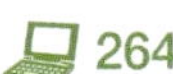

IV-15

■ NORMAL ANTERIOR HUMERAL AND RADIOCAPITELLAR LINES

The anterior humeral line (dashed line) is drawn along the anterior cortex of the humeral shaft (H) and extends to the capitellum (C). This line should pass through the middle third of the capitellum (circle).

The radiocapitellar line is drawn through the midradial shaft (R) and passes through the capitellum on any radiographic view.

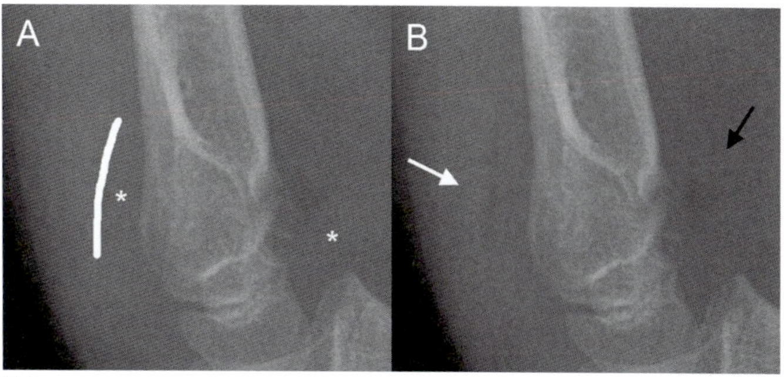

IV-16

ELBOW JOINT EFFUSION – POSTERIOR FAT PAD SIGN

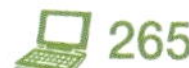 265

The fat pad sign or sail sign is seen on a lateral elbow radiograph if a joint effusion is present and where the more lucent fat pad is displaced by the more dense fluid (asterisks) either anteriorly (anterior fat pad/sail sign, black arrow) or posteriorly (posterior fat pad/sail sign, white arrow) providing the impression of a blown sail (A, white line).

If an elbow joint effusion is present, especially the supracondylar area in children and the radial head in adults should be scrutinized because adults fracture most commonly the radial head while children present with a supracondylar fracture.

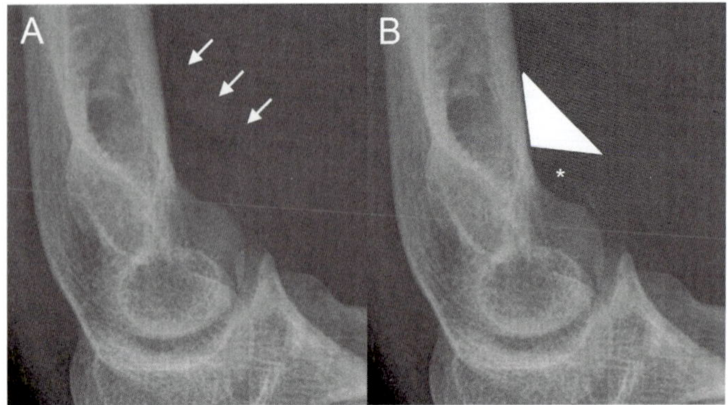

IV-17

■ ELBOW JOINT EFFUSION – ANTERIOR FAT PAD SIGN

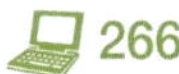 266

Lateral radiograph of the elbow demonstrates an anterior fat pad sign where the anterior fat pad (triangle) has been displaced anteriorly and superiorly (arrows) by the joint effusion (asterisk).

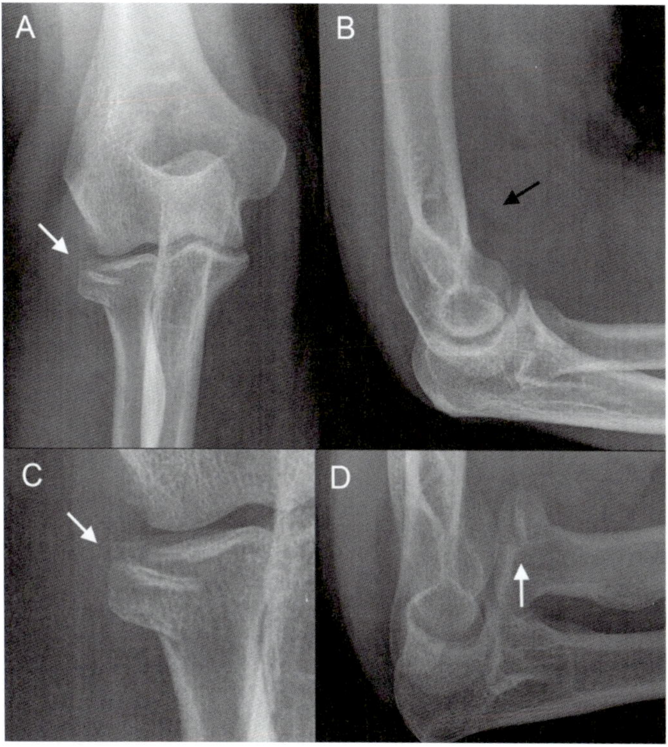

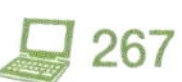

IV-18

■ RADIAL HEAD FRACTURE   267

AP (A) and lateral (B) and lateral pronation (D) radiographs of the right elbow demonstrate an elbow joint effusion with an anterior sail sign (B, black arrow) and a fracture of the radial aspect of the radial head depressed up to 3 mm which extends to the radiocapitellar articular surface (A, C, D, white arrows). Again if an elbow joint effusion is present, especially the supracondylar area in children and the radial head in adults should be scrutinized because adults fracture most commonly the radial head (as in this case) while children present with a supracondylar fracture.

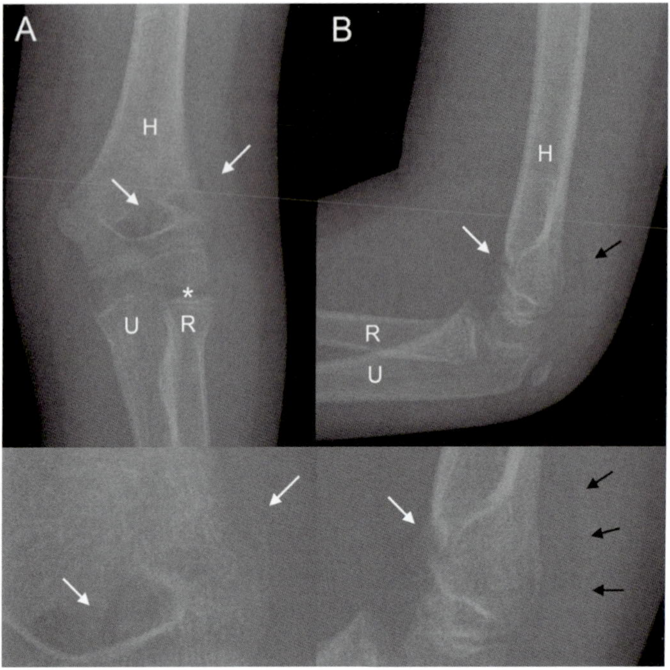

IV-19

■ SUPRACONDYLAR FRACTURE WITH ELBOW EFFUSION

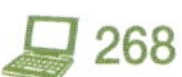 268

AP (A) and lateral radiographs of the left elbow (lower row respective magnifications) in a child (growth plates are not closed yet) demonstrate a distal humeral supracondylar fracture through the lateral aspect with minimal dorsal displacement of the distal fracture fragment (white arrows). Radiocapitellar alignment (asterisk) is preserved on all images. There is a marked joint effusion (see posterior and upward displacement of the posterior fat pad – black arrows). Soft tissue swelling is also seen at the elbow joint and along the medial aspect of the distal upper arm. H=humerus, R=radius, U=ulna.

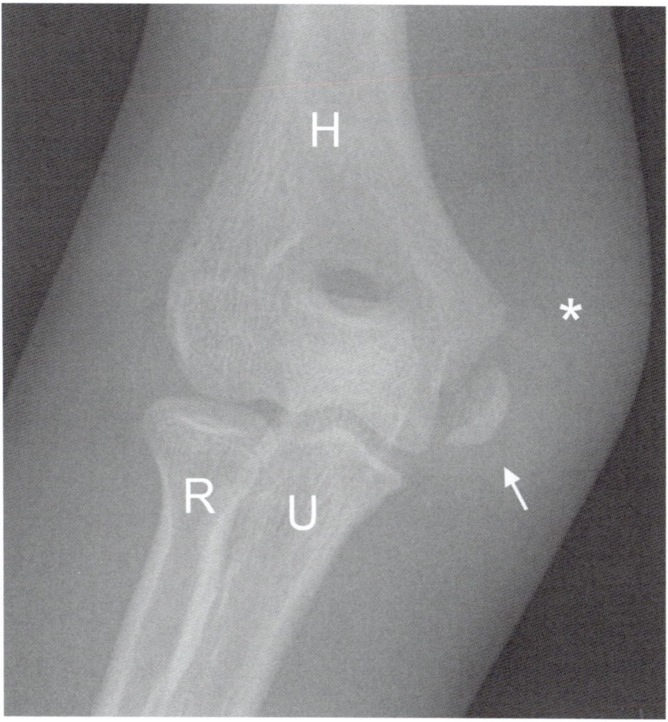

IV-20

MEDIAL EPICONDYLE AVULSION – ADULT   269

AP radiograph of the right elbow in an adult shows a fractured and avulsed medial humeral epicondyle (arrow). There is also marked associated soft tissue swelling (asterisk). H=humerus, U=ulna, R=radius.

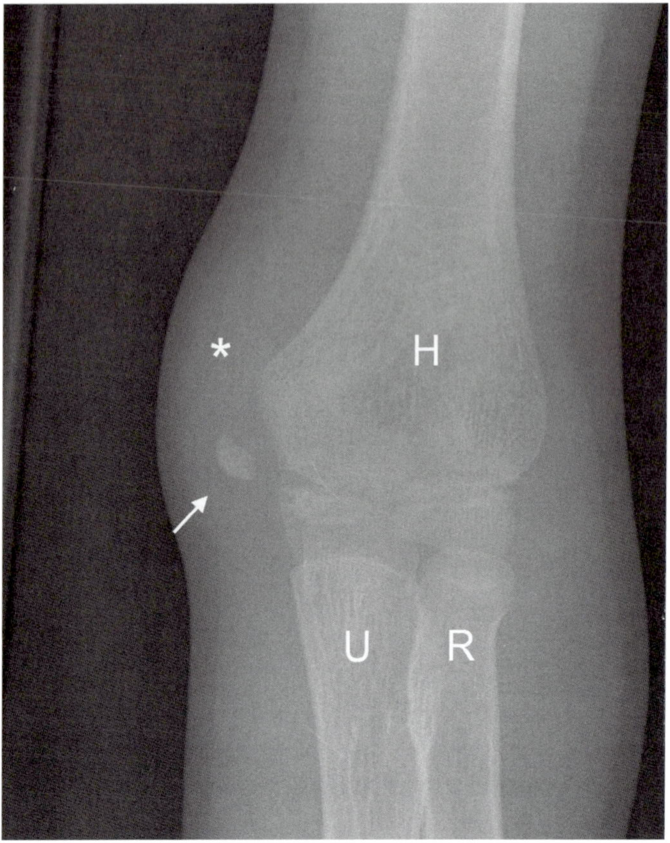

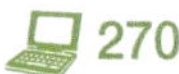

IV-21

■ MEDIAL EPICONDYLE AVULSION - CHILD   270

AP radiograph of the left elbow in a child (growth plates not closed yet) shows a medial humeral epicondyle dissociated from its normal location (arrow), consistent with an avulsion. This is an example of a Salter–Harris I fracture. Associated soft tissue swelling is also marked (asterisk). H = humerus, U = ulna, R = radius.

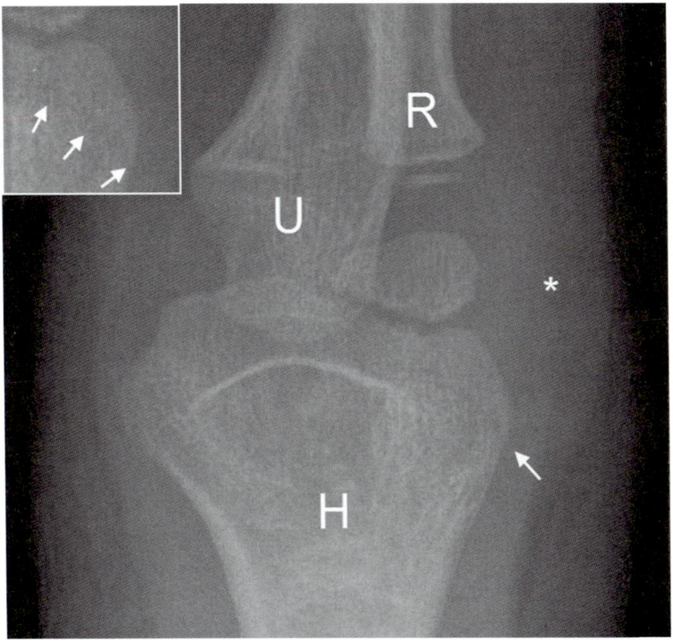

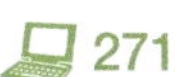

IV-22

LATERAL EPICONDYLE FRACTURE 271

Anterior radiograph of the right elbow in a child demonstrates a linear lucency along the lateral epicondyle (arrows, top left=magnification), consistent with a nondisplaced lateral epicondylar fracture. There is associated soft tissue swelling adjacent to the lateral epicondyle (asterisk). H=humerus, U=ulna, R=radius.

■ SPECIAL FRACTURES IN CHILDHOOD 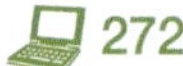 272

- Growth plate fractures
- Avulsion injuries
- Greenstick
- Buckle/torus fractures

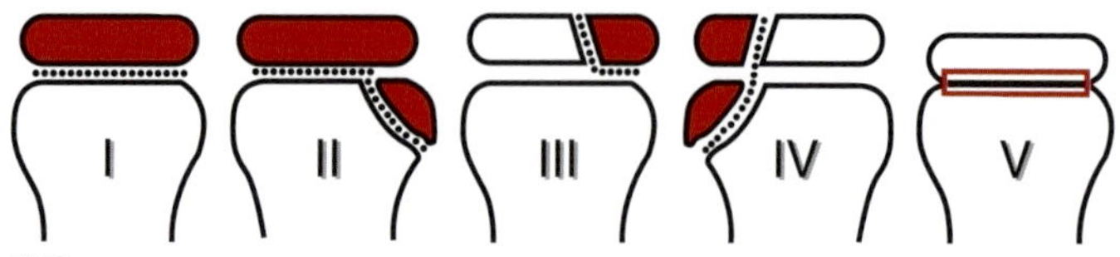

IV-23

■ GROWTH PLATE FRACTURES – SALTER–HARRIS CLASSIFICATION 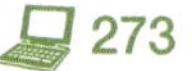 273

Type I – A transverse fracture through the growth plate: 6% incidence.

Type II – A fracture through the growth plate and the metaphysis, sparing the epiphysis: 75% incidence.

Type III – A fracture through growth plate and epiphysis, sparing the metaphysis: 8% incidence.

Type IV – A fracture through all three elements of the bone, the growth plate, metaphysis, and epiphysis: 10% incidence.

Type V – A compression fracture of the growth plate (resulting in a decrease in the perceived space between the epiphysis and diaphysis on X-ray): 1% incidence.

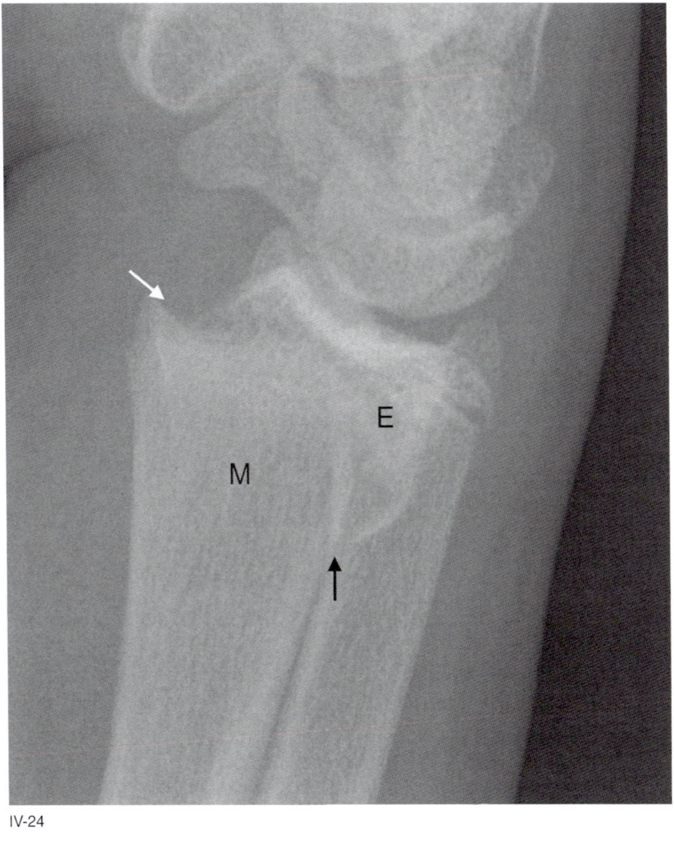

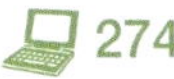

IV-24

DISTAL RADIAL HEAD FRACTURE – SALTER–HARRIS II FRACTURE

274

Radiograph of the right forearm show a fracture (black arrow) that involves the growth plate (white arrow) of the distal radius that goes through the growth plate and the metaphysis (M) while sparing the epiphysis (E), consistent with a Salter–Harris II fracture.

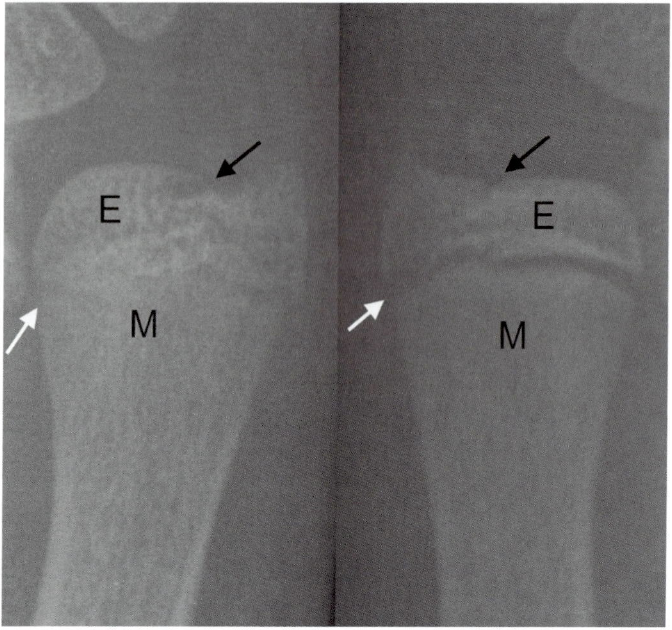

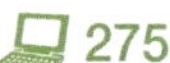

IV-25

DISTAL ULNAR HEAD FRACTURE – SALTER–HARRIS III FRACTURE   275

Two radiographs of the right forearm in different projections demonstrate a fracture (black arrows) that goes through the distal ulnar growth plate (white arrows) and the epiphysis (E) while sparing the metaphysis (M), consistent with a Salter–Harris III fracture.

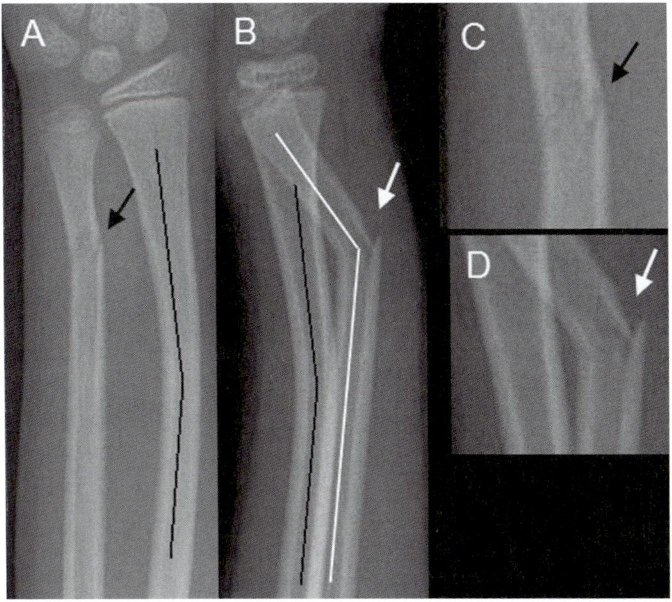

IV-26

GREENSTICK FRACTURE   276

AP (A, C) and lateral (B, D) radiographs of the left forearm demonstrate an incomplete fracture involving the distal ulnar diaphysis (arrows) with ventral angulation (white angle lines). The distal radius is abnormally bowed with a ventral and mild ulnar convexity (black angle lines). Greenstick fractures occur when the fracture line does not propagate through the bone with plastic deformation occurring on the compression side.

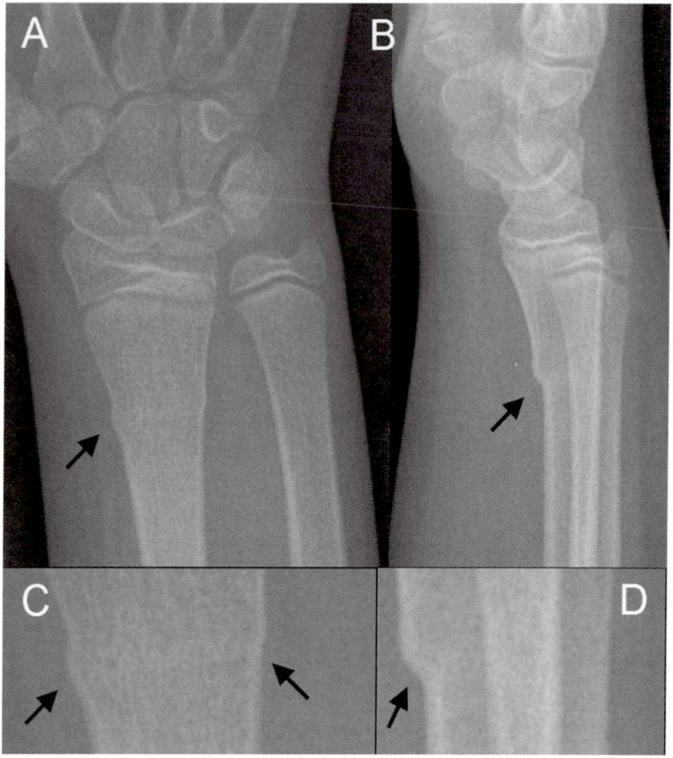

IV-27

TORUS FRACTURE (BUCKLE FRACTURE) 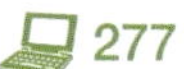 277

AP (A, C) and lateral (B, D) radiographs of the right forearm demonstrate a buckle fracture (arrows) of the distal radial metaphysis without significant angulation. Buckle fractures (or torus fractures) are an impaction type of fracture identified by a focal widening (or outward buckling) of the cortex.

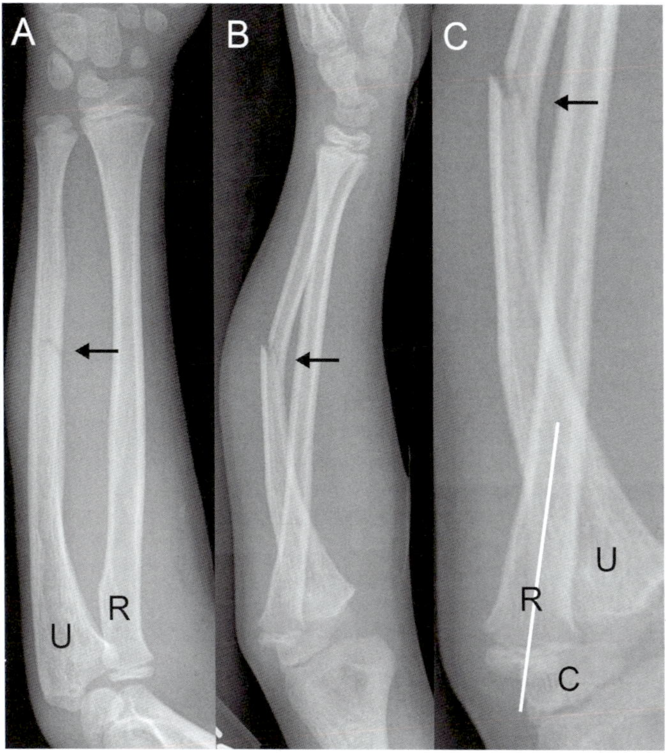

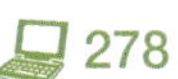

IV-28

■ MONTEGGIA FRACTURE   💻 278

AP (A) and lateral (B, C) views of the forearm demonstrate a greenstick single-cortex fracture of the ulna (arrows) with lateral dislocation of the radial head and loss of normal radiocapitellar alignment. The radiocapitellar alignment is a virtual line that goes through the axis of the radius (white line, C) and should pass through the center of the capitellum (C). The Monteggia fracture is a fracture of the proximal third of the ulna with dislocation of the head of the radius. U = ulna, R = radius.

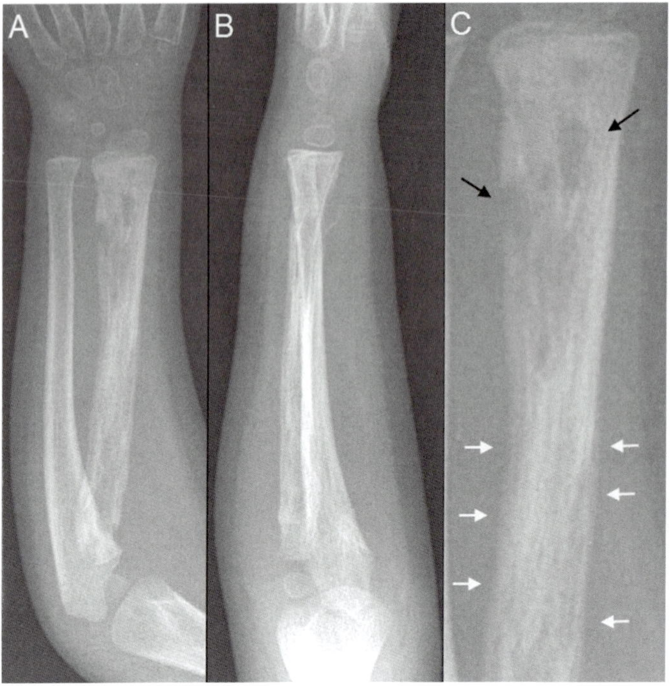

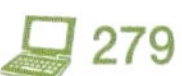

IV-29

OSTEOMYELITIS – RADIUS   279

AP (A, C) and lateral (B) radiographs of the right forearm of a 2-year-old girl demonstrate a diffuse, permeative mixed lytic, and sclerotic process (black arrows) involving the entire radius. Also noticed is marked laminated periosteal thickening along the radius (white arrows). *S. aureus* accounts for 85% of organisms in osteomyelitis in the first 2 years of life.

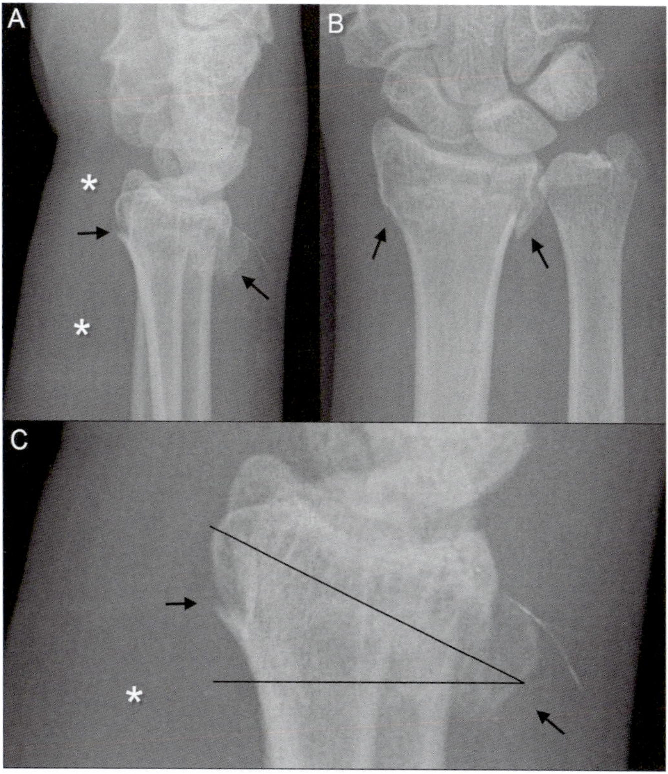

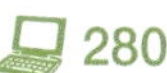

IV-30

■ COLLES' FRACTURE   280

Lateral (A, C) and AP (B) radiographs of the right forearm show a complete fracture of the distal radius (arrows) with dorsal angulation of the fracture fragment (angle lines). There is marked surrounding soft tissue swelling (asterisk). Colles' fracture is a distal fracture of the radius with dorsal (posterior) displacement of the wrist. This fracture is sometimes referred to as a "dinner (or silver) fork deformity" due to the shape of the resultant forearm.

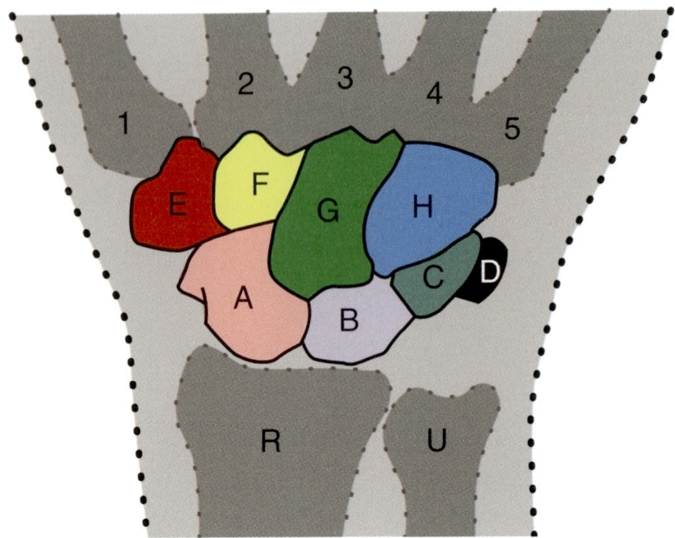

IV-31

■ CARPAL BONE ANATOMY (ADAPTED FROM WIKIPEDIA)

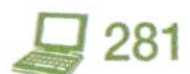 281

Carpal bones highlighted, as seen on the right hand of an AP view. (R = radius, U = ulna, 1–5 = metacarpals 1–5.)

Proximal arch
- A – Scaphoid
- B – Lunate
- C – Triquetrum (Triangular)
- D – Pisiform

Distal arch
- E – Trapezium
- F – Trapezoid
- G – Capitate
- H – Hamate

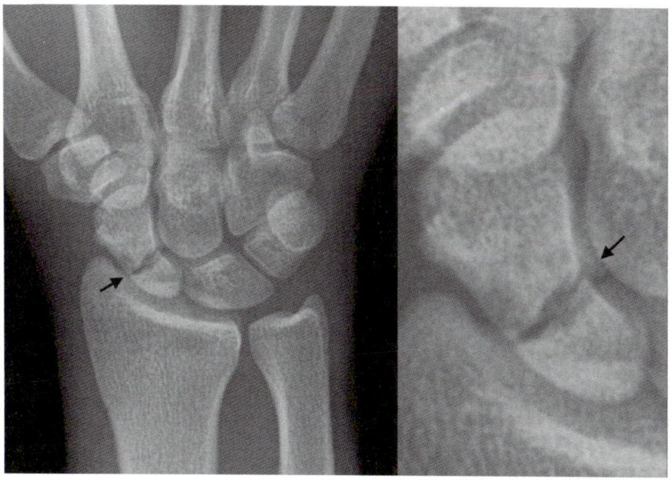

IV-32

SCAPHOID FRACTURE 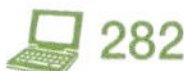 282

AP radiograph of the right wrist demonstrates a linear lucency (arrows) crossing the waist of the scaphoid consistent with an acute scaphoid fracture. The scaphoid is the most frequently fractured carpal bone. The proximal pole of the scaphoid is at high risk of AVN in fractures of the mid- and proximal pole.

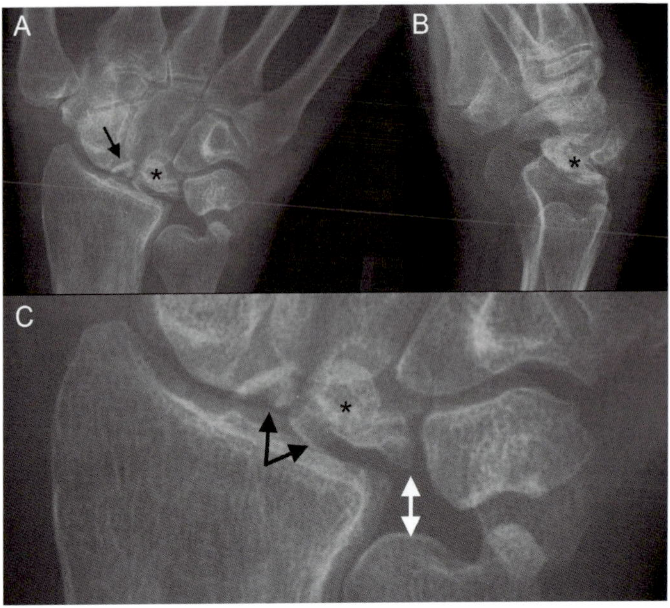

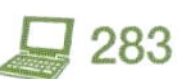

IV-33

■ LUNATE AVASCULAR NECROSIS (KIENBOECK'S DISEASE)

283

AP (A, C) and lateral radiographs of the left wrist show collapse of the left lunate (asterisk) with fragmentation (black arrows), from remote avascular necrosis. Also noticed is foreshortening of the ulna (white arrow). A shorter ulna, or negative ulnar variance, may lead to increased load across the radiolunate articulation with an increased risk of lunate avascular necrosis.

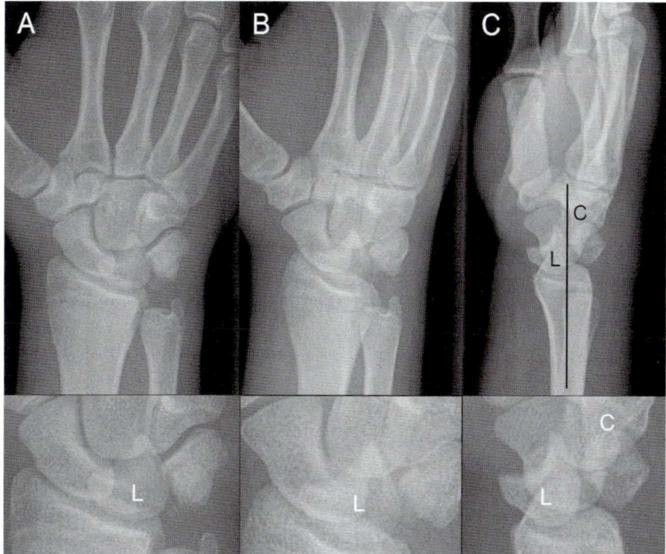

IV-34

■ PERILUNATE DISLOCATION 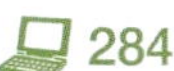 284

AP (A), oblique (B), and lateral (C) radiographs of the right wrist show volar angulation of the lunate bone (L). The lunate maintains its relation with the distal radius (intersects with black line) while the capitate (C) has dislocated posteriorly relative to the lunate, consistent with a perilunate dislocation. With a perilunate dislocation, the capitate is dislocated and lie, along with the metacarpals, dorsal to the line drawn through the radius and the lunate.

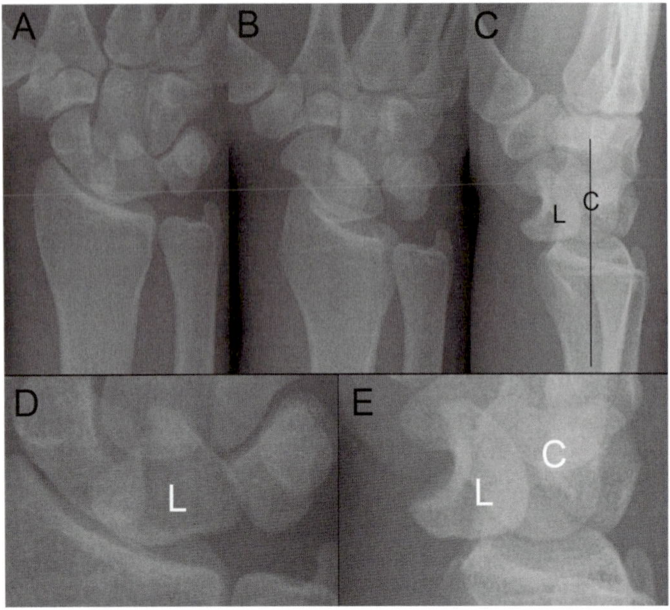

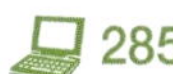

IV-35

LUNATE DISLOCATION   285

AP (A, D), oblique (B), and lateral (C, E) radiographs of the left wrist show a pie-shaped lunate (L) on the AP view. On the lateral view, the lunate is located volar to the radius, but the capitate appears normally aligned with the radius (C, vertical line). These findings are consistent with a lunate dislocation. In lunate dislocation the lunate is volarly displaced and a line through the axis of the radius goes through the capitate.

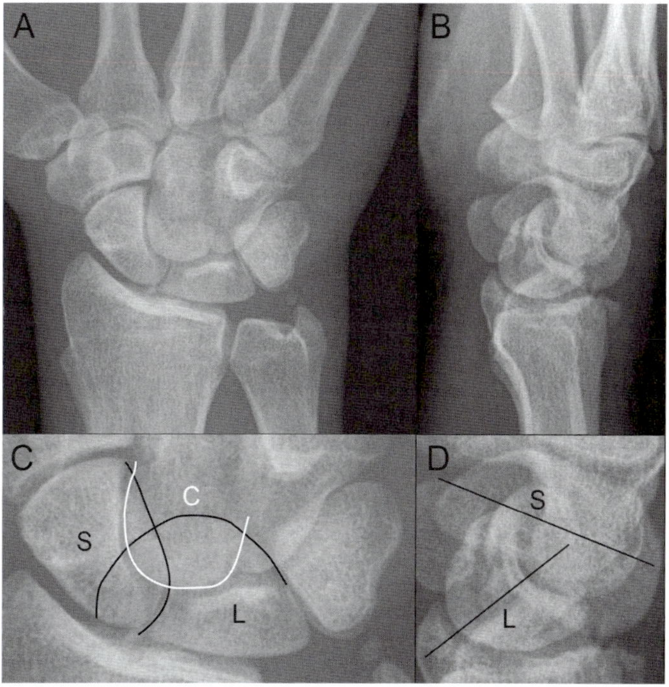

IV-36

DORSAL INTERCALATED SEGMENTAL INSTABILITY (DISI)

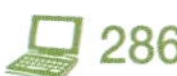 286

AP (A, C) radiographs of the right wrist demonstrate disruption of the carpal arcs and abnormal contour of the lunate (L). The lateral (B, D) radiograph shows carpal instability with dorsal tilt of the lunate (L) and volar flexion of the scaphoid (S), consistent with DISI. DISI = scapholunate angle greater than 60° and lunate is tilted dorsally with capitatolunate angle greater than 10° to 20°.

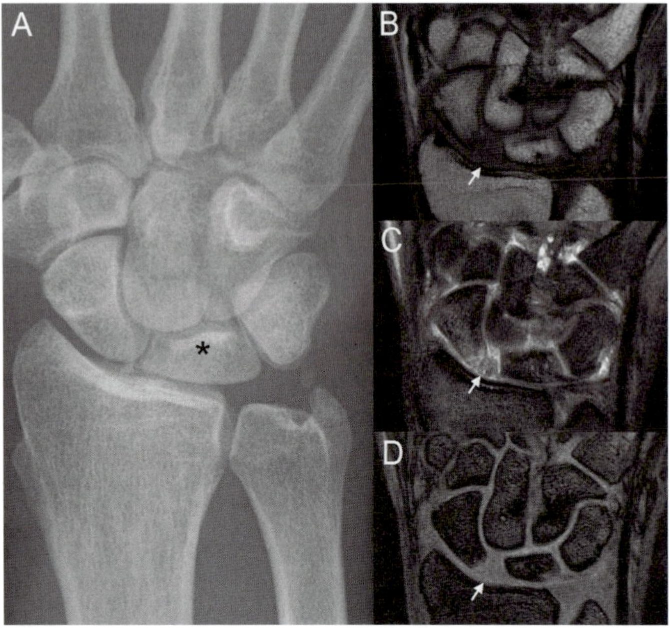

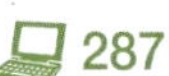

IV-37

■ SCAPHOLUNATE LIGAMENT TEAR   287

AP (A) radiographs of the right wrist demonstrate disruption of the carpal arcs and abnormal contour of the lunate (L). T1 (A), fat saturated T2 (C) and gradient echo (D) MR images of the same wrist show widening of the scapholunate interval and abnormal signal within the scapholunate ligament (best seen on the T2 sequence), consistent with complete scapholunate ligament tear.

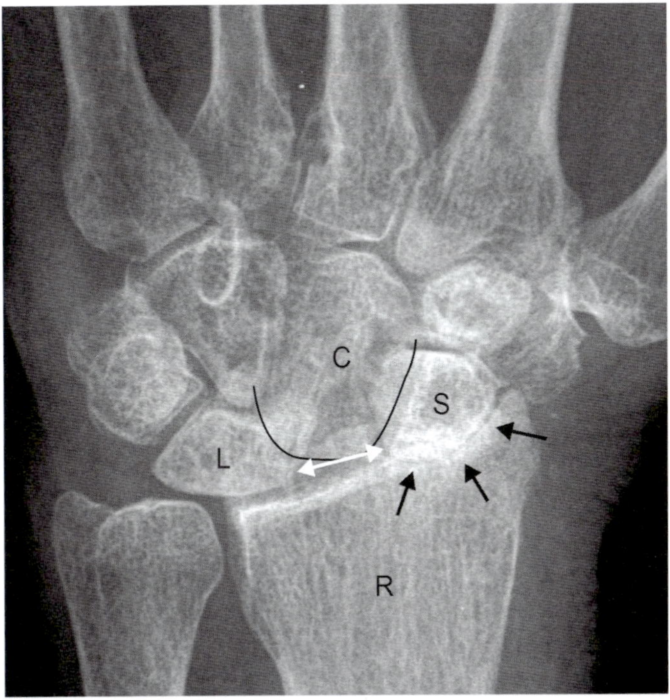

IV-38

SCAPHOLUNATE ADVANCED COLLAPSE (SLAC WRIST)

 288

AP radiograph of the wrist shows a widened scapholunate interval (white double arrow) with proximal migration of the capitate (C) into the resulting space. Carpal osteoarthritis is identified as narrowing of the radioscaphoid joint space (black arrows) with associated subchondral sclerosis and cyst formation. L=lunate, S=scaphoid, and R=radius.

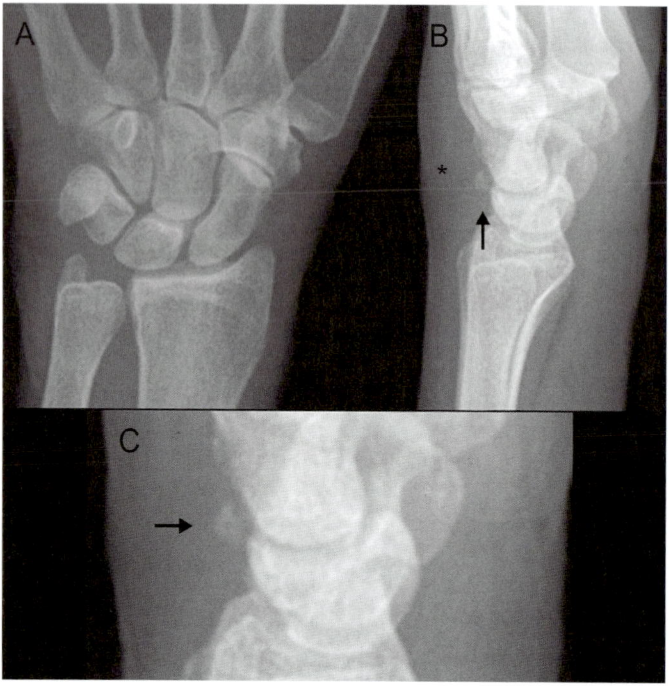

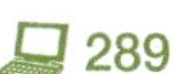

IV-39

▪ TRIQUETRAL FRACTURE   🖥 289

AP (A) and lateral (B, C) views of the left wrist demonstrate a small bony fragment dorsal to the proximal carpal row (arrows). There is a moderate amount of associated soft tissue swelling in adjacent tissues (asterisk). The triquetral fracture is best seen on lateral films because it is usually a small avulsion fracture of the attachments of the perilunate ligaments.

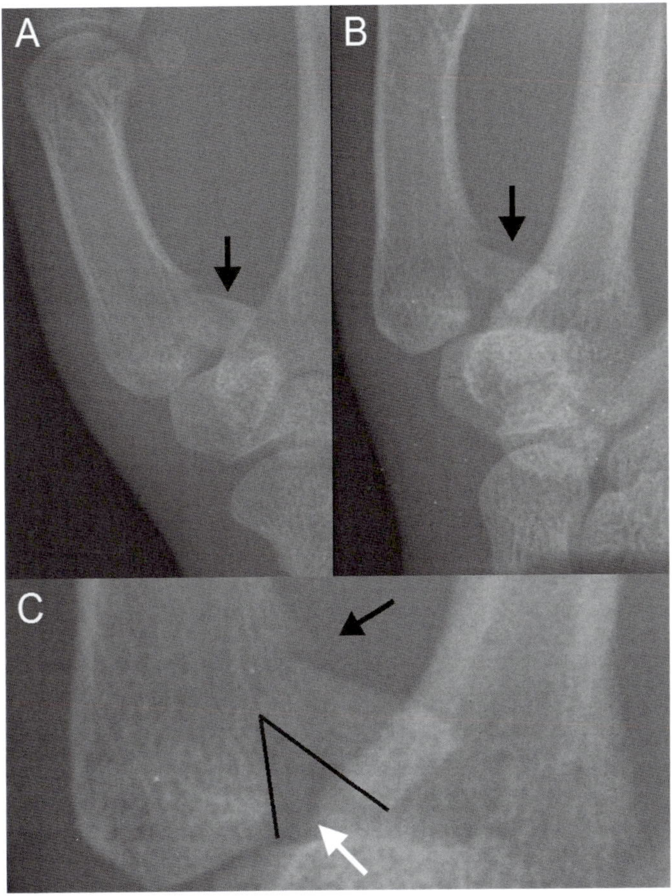

IV-40

BENNETT'S FRACTURE 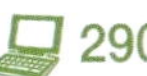 290

AP thumb view (A, C) and AP view of the left wrist (B) demonstrate a fracture of the base of the first metacarpal (arrows). The fracture extends into the intra-articular surface of the first carpometacarpal joint (white arrow). There is medial distraction of the proximal portion of the bony fragment (C, indicated by arrow and angle lines). Bennett's fracture is characterized by an intra-articular fracture/dislocation of the base of the first metacarpal at the ulnar aspect.

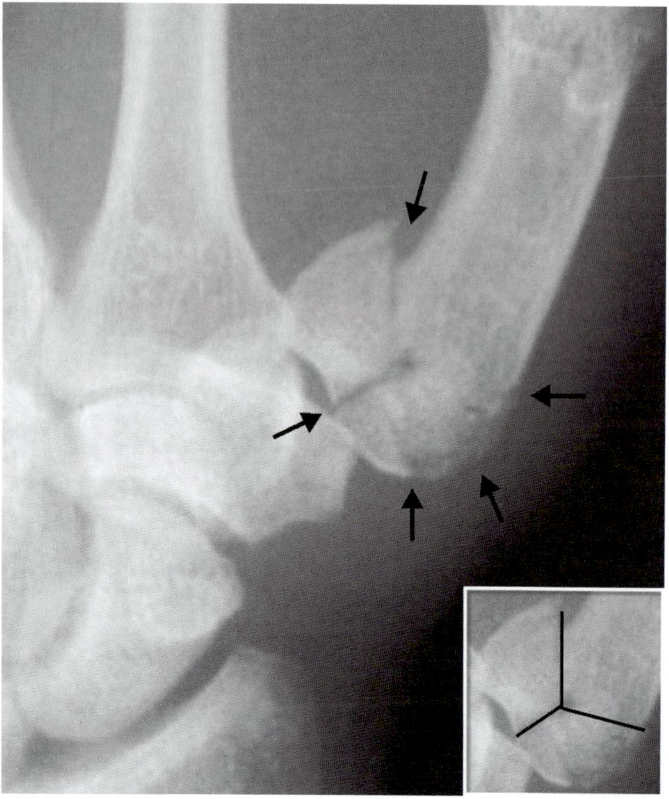

IV-41

ROLANDO FRACTURE 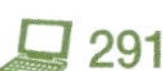 291

AP radiograph of the left wrist shows a comminuted intra-articular fracture of the base of the first metacarpal. Arrows indicate fracture lines. Rolando fracture is an intra–articular fracture of the base of the first metacarpal bone, which is characterized by the presence of a T- or Y-shaped comminuted fracture line (see the bottom-right illustration).

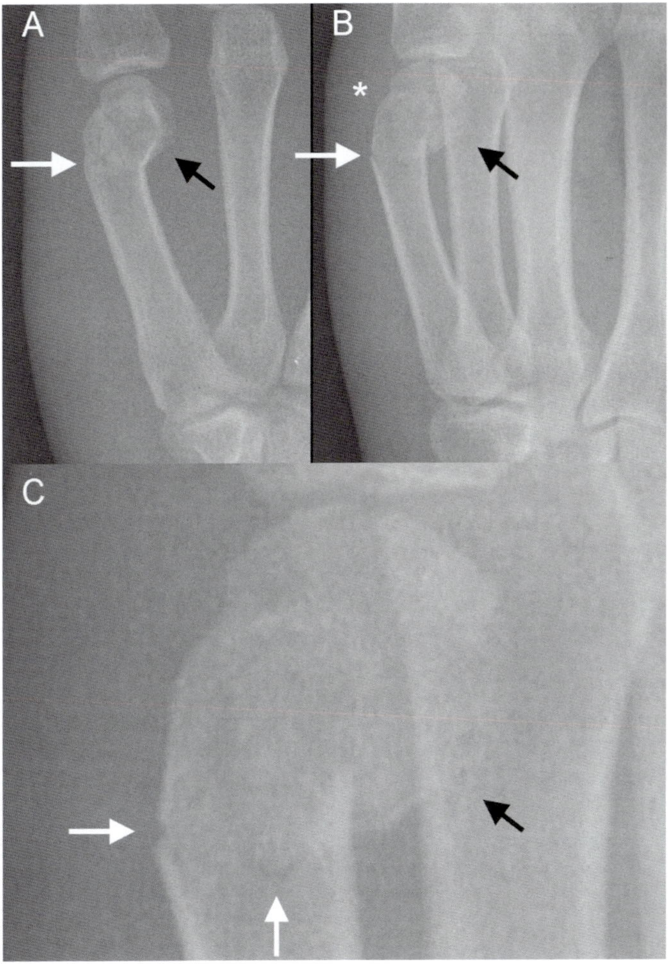

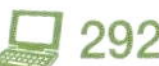

IV-42

■ BOXER FRACTURE   🖥 292

AP (A, C) and oblique (B) radiographs of the left hand show an acute fracture of the distal metaphysis of the fifth left metacarpal (white arrows). The distal fragment is slightly angulated radially and anteriorly (black arrows). There is an associated soft tissue swelling around the fracture (B, asterisk).

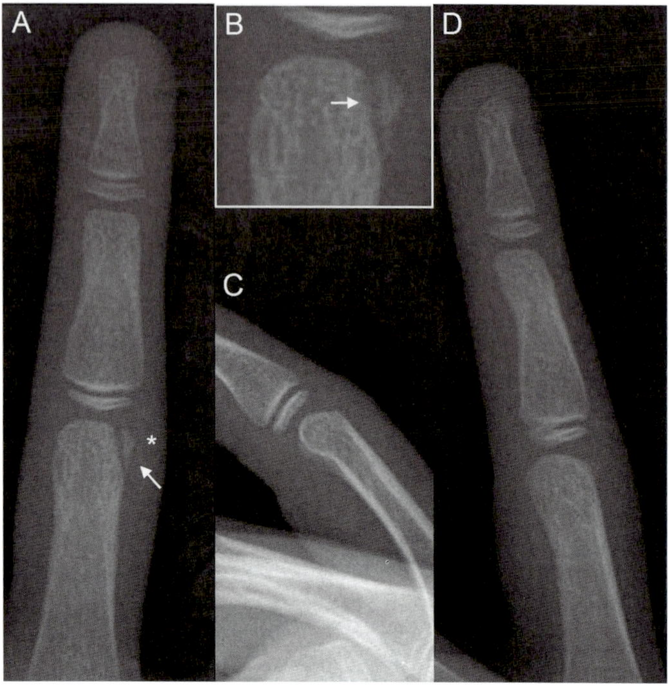

IV-43

▪ INTRA-ARTICULAR CORNER FRACTURE 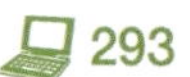 293

AP (A, B), lateral (C), and oblique (D) views of the fourth left finger show a minimally displaced intra-articular oblique corner fracture of the fourth proximal phalanx head on the ulnar side (arrows, B = magnification). There is minimal associated soft tissue swelling (asterisk).

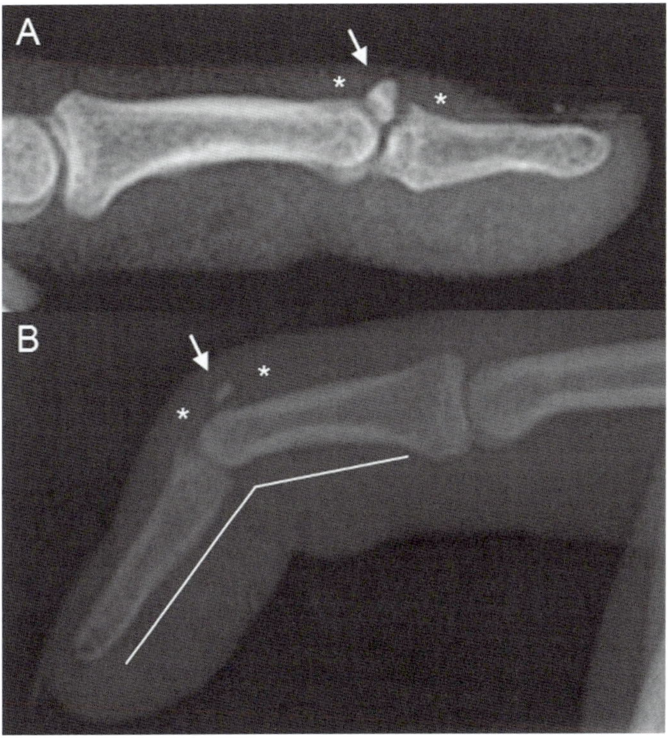

IV-44

■ MALLET FINGER 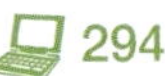 294

A: lateral radiograph of the left fifth finger shows an intra-articular dorsal fracture of the distal fifth phalanx (arrow). Mild associated soft tissue swelling is also noted (asterisks).

B: another lateral radiograph of the right fifth finger of a different patient shows an avulsion injury at the posterior base of the distal phalanx where the extensor tendon inserts (arrow). There is mild associated soft tissue swelling (asterisks). Please notice a resultant flexion deformity at the distal interphalangeal (DIP) joint (indicated by white angle lines).

5. Pelvis and Hip

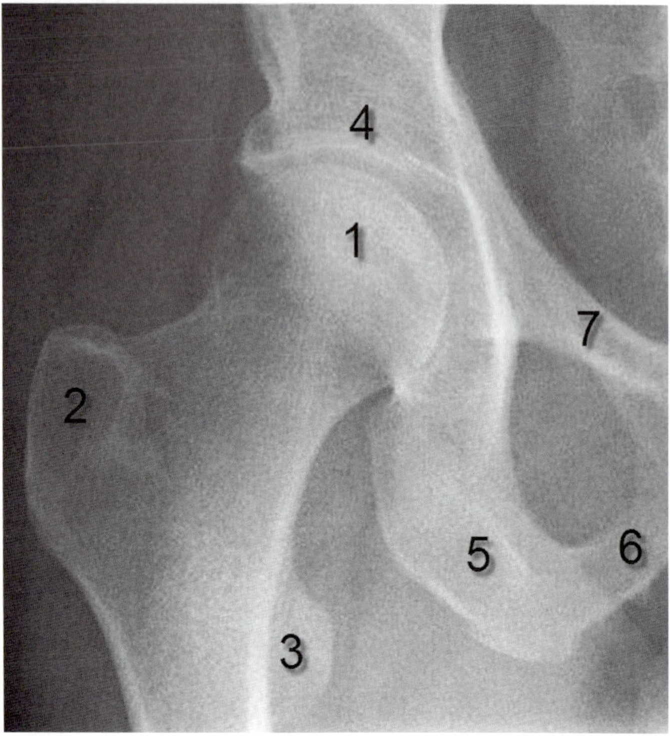

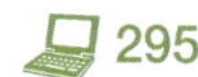

IV-45

■ NORMAL HIP ANATOMY   295

Normal anatomy of a right hip on AP view
1. Femoral head
2. Major/greater trochanter
3. Minor/lesser trochanter
4. Acetabulum
5. Ischium
6. Inferior pubic ramus
7. Superior pubic ramus

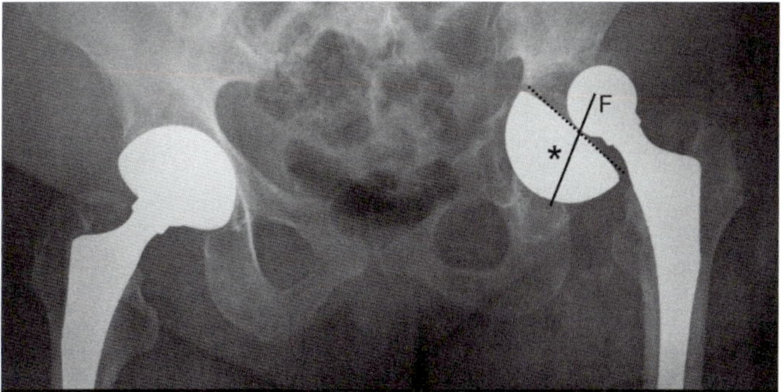

IV-46

DISLOCATED HIP PROSTHESIS WITH A MALROTATED ACETABULAR COMPONENT 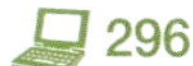 296

The AP radiograph of the pelvis shows dislocation of the left total hip implant with cephalad migration so that the cup faces superolateral. The full black line indicates the normal position of the inferior surface of the acetabular component; the dotted line indicates the current position. Compare with the correct position and alignment of the right hip prosthesis. No fracture or signs of implant loosening identified. F = head of the femoral component, * = acetabular component.

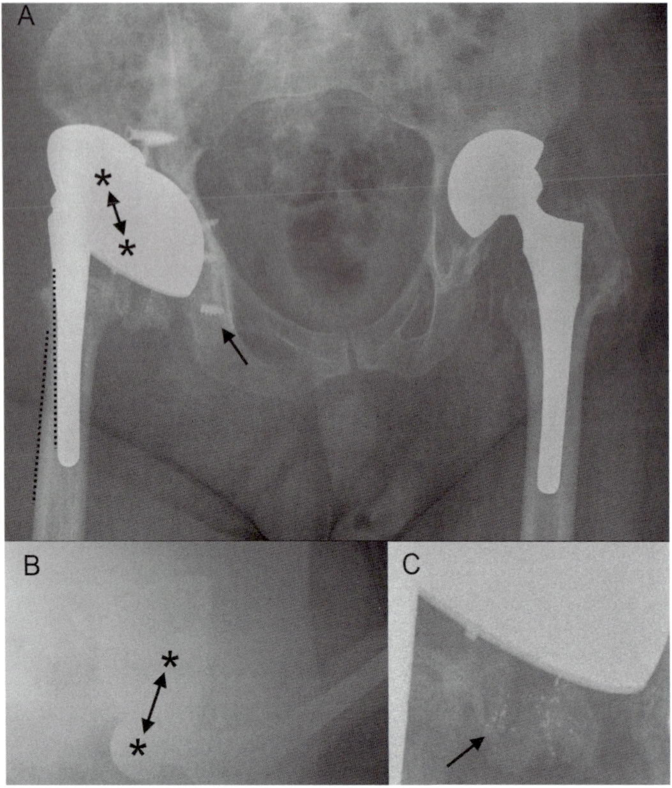

IV-47

■ HIP DISLOCATION WITH PARTICLE DISEASE 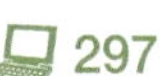 297

Frontal radiograph of the pelvis (A) and the crosstable view of the right hip (B) demonstrates a right total hip prosthesis of which its femoral component has been dislocated superiorly and posteriorly in relation to its acetabular component. The asterisks indicate the current position of the femoral head and its proper position. Double lines demonstrate the shift in position. Also noticed is malposition of the acetabular component with inferior angulation. A few acetabular screws have been broken (black arrow). The femoral stem is furthermore in malalignment with the femoral shaft (indicated by dotted lines). Magnification (C) demonstrates clusters of heavily dense material adjacent to the hip joint, representing particle disease, which is ultimately the reason for the failure of the prosthesis.

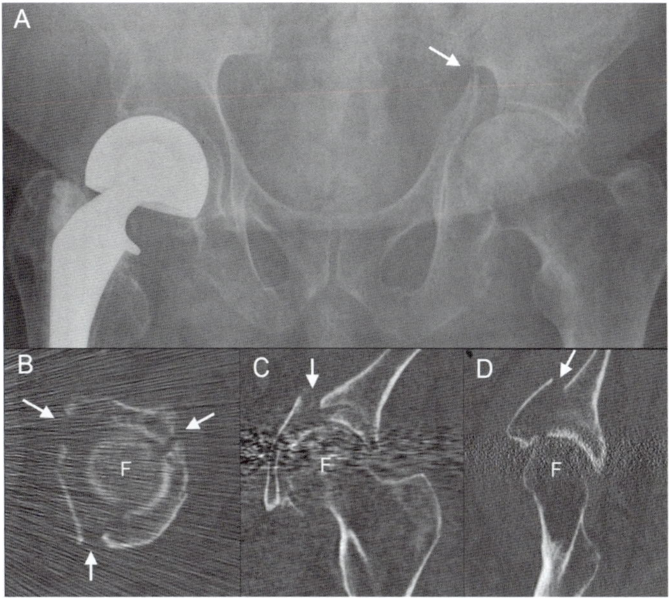

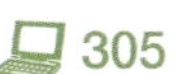

IV-48

■ ACETABULAR FRACTURE 🖥 305

The AP radiograph of the pelvis (A) demonstrates a fracture of the left acetabulum (arrow). Femoral head is in situ. CT of the left hip in bone window in axial (B), coronal (C), and sagittal (D) planes show additional fracture lines through the anterior and posterior columns of the left acetabulum. The femoral head (F) is normally located in the acetabulum. Linear streaking (or beam hardening) artifact is seen on the CT images from the right hip prosthesis.

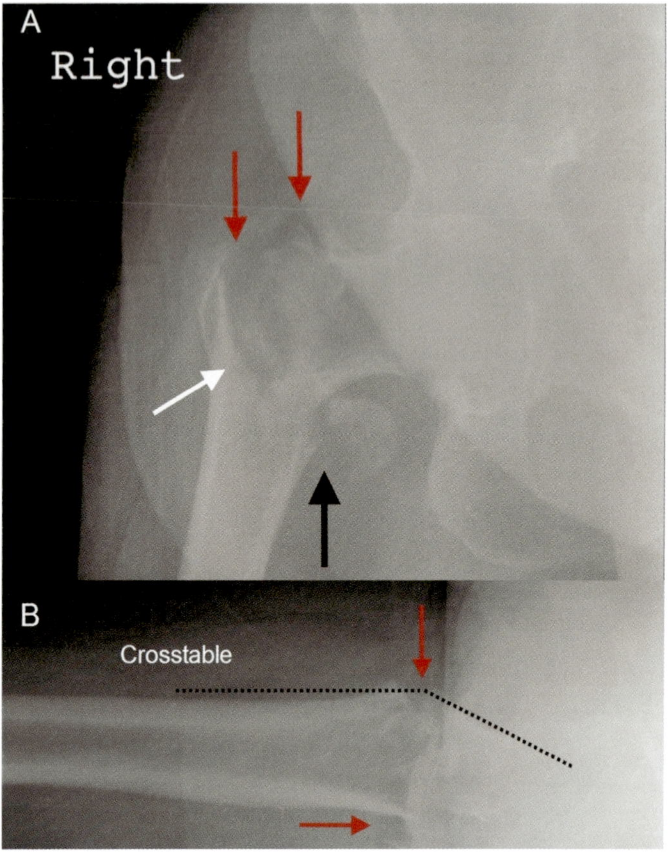

■ COMMINUTED INTERTROCHANTERIC FRACTURE

306

Frontal (A) and crosstable (B) right-hip radiographs show a comminuted intertrochanteric fracture (white arrow) with avulsion of the lesser (black arrow) and greater (red arrows) trochanters, superior migration, and moderate varus angulation. The crosstable lateral examination (B) demonstrates mild posterior angulation (indicated by the angle line).

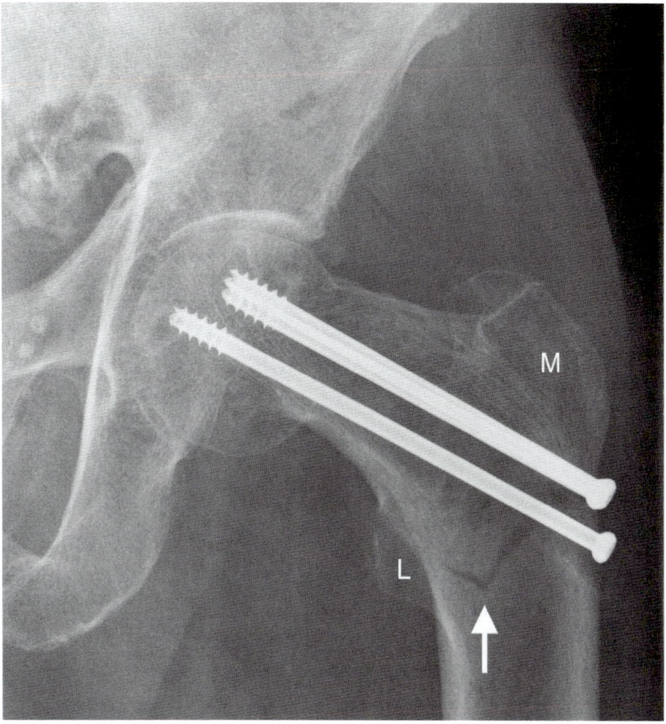

IV-50

▪ SUBTROCHANTERIC FRACTURE  307

This frontal radiograph of the left hip of a patient who underwent previous screw fixation of the femoral head demonstrates an oblique lucent line (arrow) traversing from just below the major trochanter (M) toward the inferior margin of the lesser trochanter (L), without reaching the medial femoral cortex, compatible with an incomplete subtrochanteric fracture.

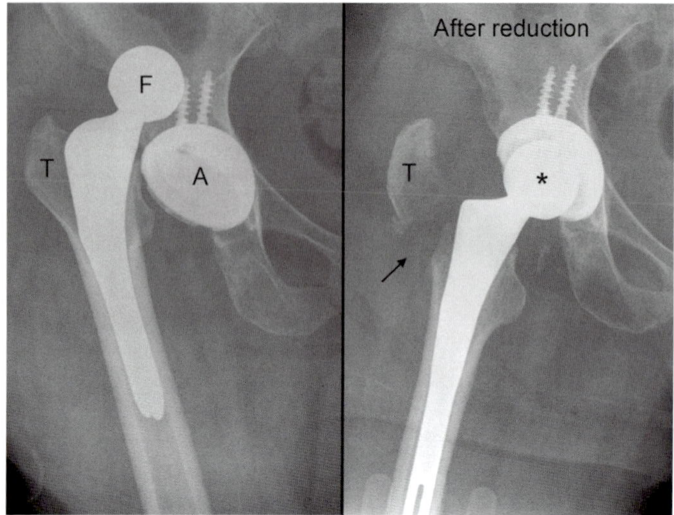

IV-51

■ MAJOR TROCHANTER FRACTURE
AFTER HIP REDUCTION

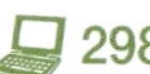 298

The AP radiograph of the right hip demonstrates a hip dislocation with superior dislocation of the femoral component (F) from the acetabular component (A, left image). The right image demonstrates status post successful reduction of the hip (asterisk). However, now a complete fracture of the major trochanter (T) is noticed, with the fracture fragment being avulsed superolaterally. This shows the importance to check radiographs after any relocation procedure – not only to confirm the proper relocation, but also to rule out potential complications of the manipulation.

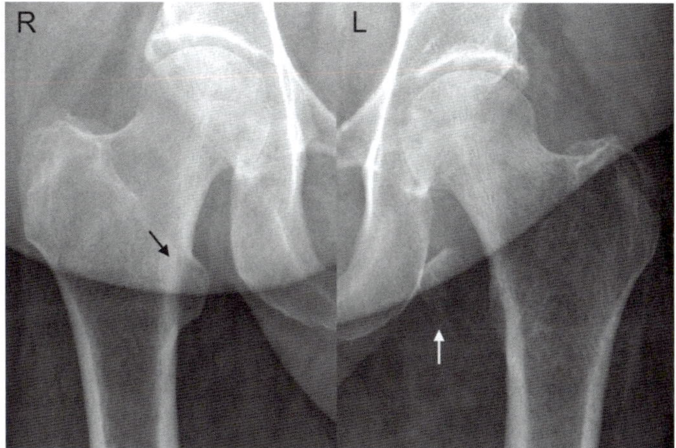

IV-52

LESSER TROCHANTER AVULSION FRACTURE – PATHOLOGIC

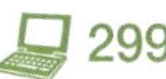 299

AP radiograph of the pelvis shows an avulsion of left the lesser trochanter to the level of the ischial tuberosity (white arrow). Lesser trochanteric fractures do not usually occur – even after trauma – unless there is another pathology involved. Such an avulsion should raise the suspicion for a neoplastic process. And indeed this patient had a breast metastasis in that location which caused the pathologic fracture. Compare the normal right lesser trochanter on the contralateral side (black arrow).

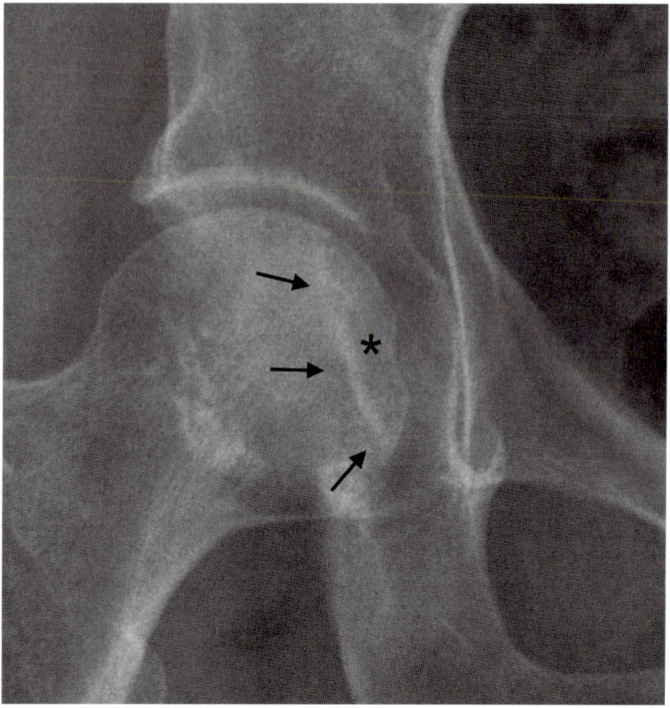

IV-53

■ AVASCULAR NECROSIS OF THE HIP – THE CRESCENT SIGN

📖 300

The AP radiograph of the right hip demonstrates a subchondral lucency (asterisk) with a crescent shaped rim of sclerosis (crescent sign, arrows) within the femoral head, consistent with avascular necrosis. The hip joint appears maintained, without signs of femoral head collapse. The crescent sign is consistent with subcortical infarction.

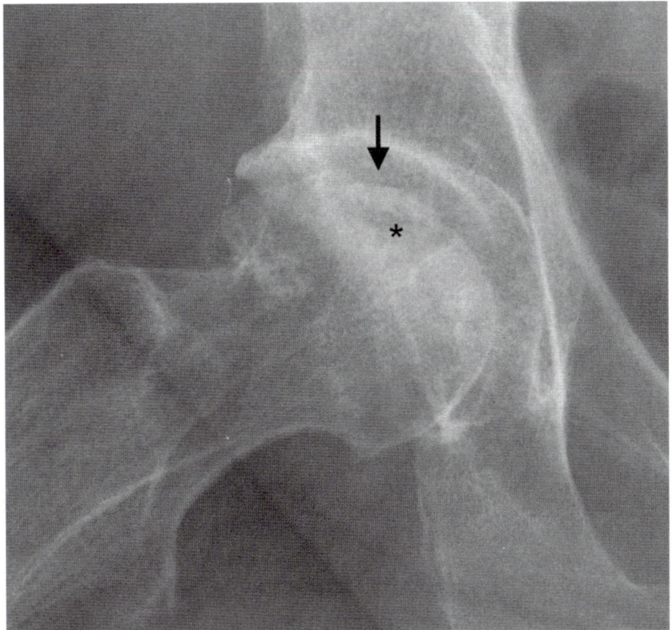

IV-54

▨ AVASCULAR NECROSIS OF THE HIP – WITH FEMORAL HEAD COLLAPSE ⌨ 301

The frogleg view of the right hip shows subchondral lucency (asterisk) of the femoral head and irregularity of the articular surface with collapse and fragmentation of the femoral head (arrow).

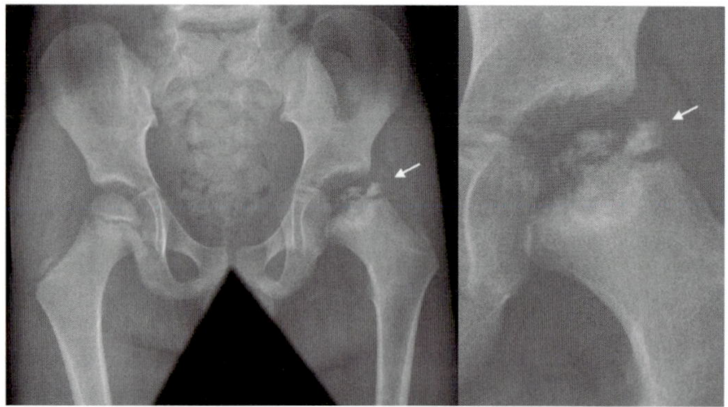

IV-55

■ LEGG–CALVE–PERTHES DISEASE 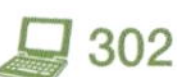 302

Frontal radiographs of the pelvis demonstrate sclerosis and fragmentation of the left proximal femoral epiphysis (arrows) in this young boy, compatible with advanced stage of Legg–Calve–Perthes disease.

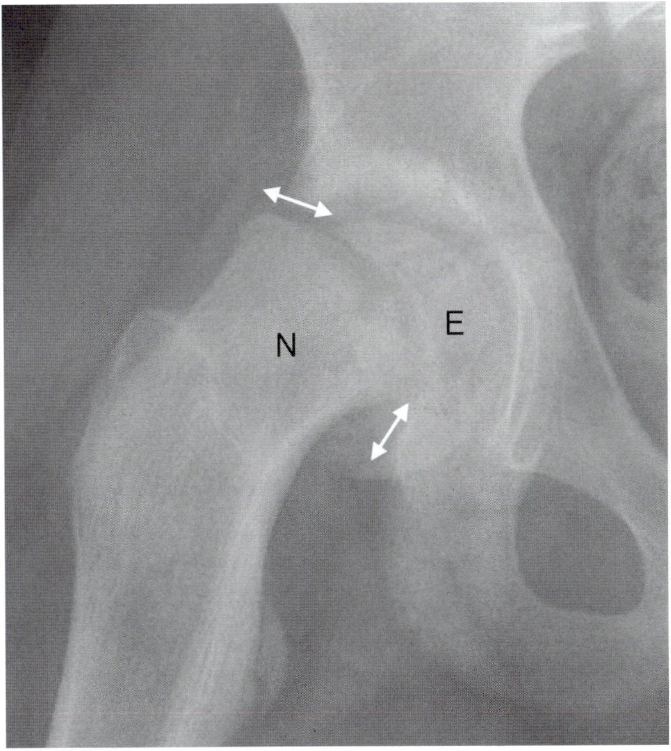

IV-56

SLIPPED CAPITAL FEMORAL EPIPHYSIS (SCFE)

 303

AP radiograph of the right hip demonstrates posteromedial displacement of the right femoral epiphysis (E). N = femoral neck.

Complication of SCFE is avascular necrosis of the femoral head. Radiographic classification predicts outcome and guides therapy: SCFE type I is <33% displacement, type II is 33–50% displacement, and type III is >50% displacement.

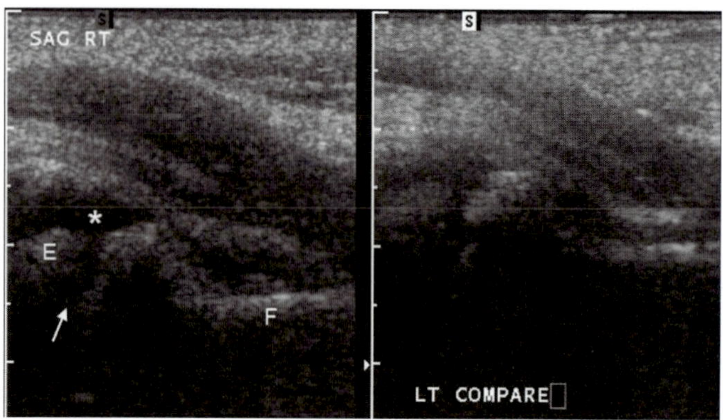

IV-57

■ SMALL HIP EFFUSION

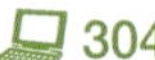 304

A grayscale ultrasound image in a sagittal plane (high frequency linear transducer was used) in a 2-year-old girl with hip pain shows a small amount of fluid in the right hip joint (asterisk). The comparison image of the left hip joint on the right demonstrates no fluid. F=femur, arrow=growth plate, and E=epiphysis.

6. Lower Extremities

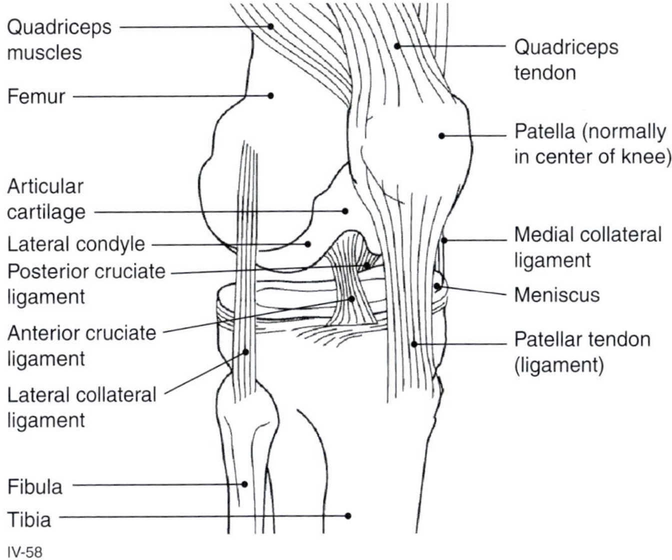

◼ KNEE ANATOMY – DIAGRAM   💻 309

Knee anatomy – diagram

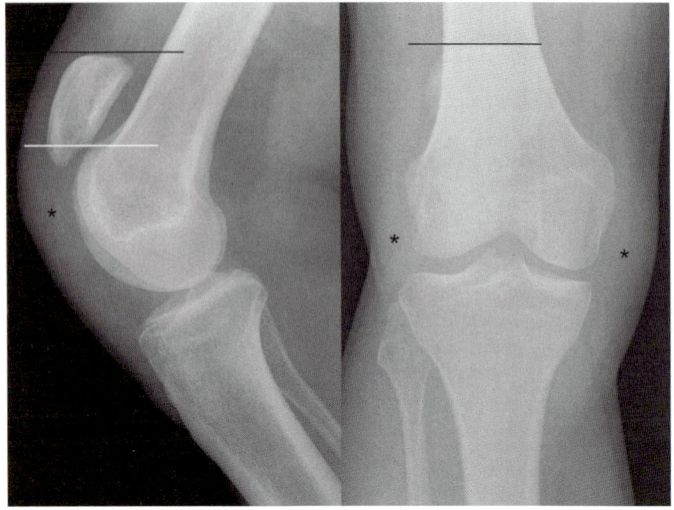

IV-59

PATELLAR DISLOCATION – SUPERIOR (PATELLA ALTA)

🖥 310

Lateral and AP radiographs of the right knee demonstrate a high riding patella in relation to the femoral condyle (patella alta). The black line indicates current position of the superior margin of the patella; the white line indicates the normal position (when the knee is flexed). Associated joint effusion and soft tissue swelling are also shown (asterisks). The cause of the superior patellar dislocation in this case was patellar tendon rupture.

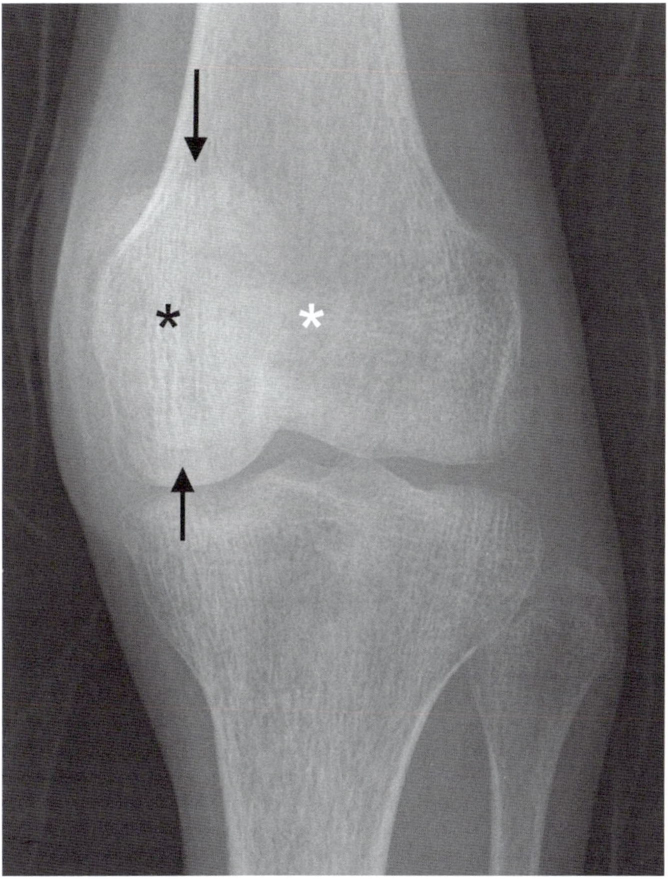

IV-60

■ PATELLAR SUBLUXATION – LATERAL 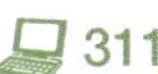 311

The AP radiograph of the left knee demonstrates abnormal position of the patella, which is located too far medially (black asterisk=center of patella), compatible with lateral patellar subluxation. The white asterisk indicates the normal location of the patellar center.

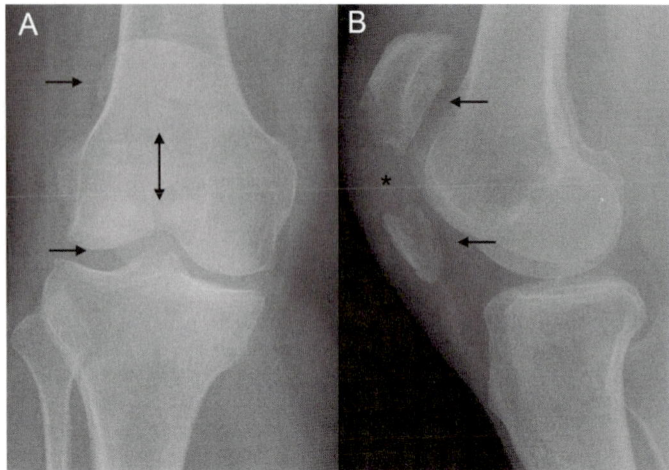

IV-61

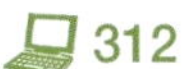 PATELLAR FRACTURE   312

AP (A) and lateral (B) radiographs of the right knee demonstrate a complete acute horizontal fracture of the patella with vertical dissociation (double arrow) of both fracture fragments (arrows) of about 3 cm. There is also associated soft tissue edema around the patella (asterisk).

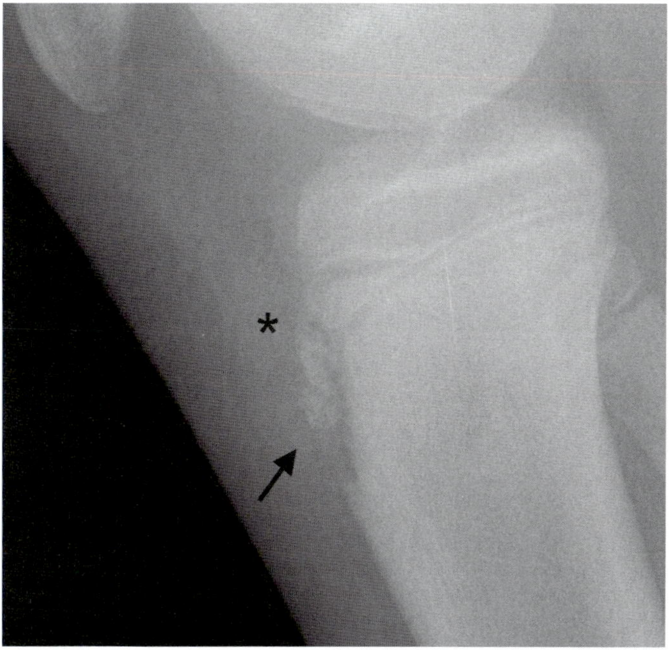

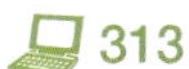

IV-62

OSGOOD–SCHLATTER DISEASE   313

The lateral radiograph of the left knee demonstrates fragmentation of the tibial tubercle (arrow) and indistinct margins of the distal patellar ligament (asterisk). These changes in this 12-year-old boy who presented with pain over the tibial tubercle are consistent with Osgood–Schlatter's disease. No acute fracture or dislocation is identified.

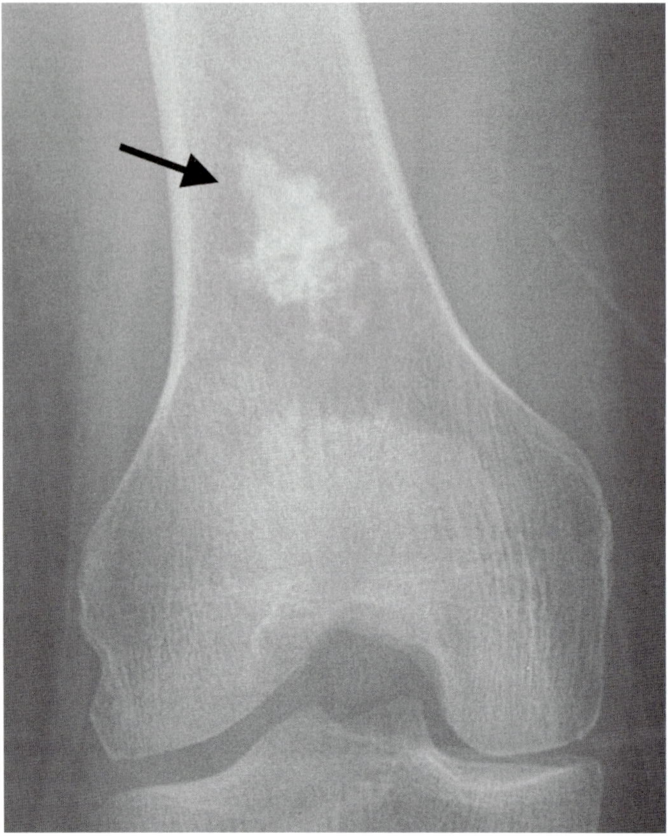

IV-63

◼ ENCHONDROMA   🖥 308

The AP radiograph of the right knee shows a sclerotic focus in the distal right femur containing stippled calcifications, which is typical for chondroid matrix and compatible with an enchondroma.

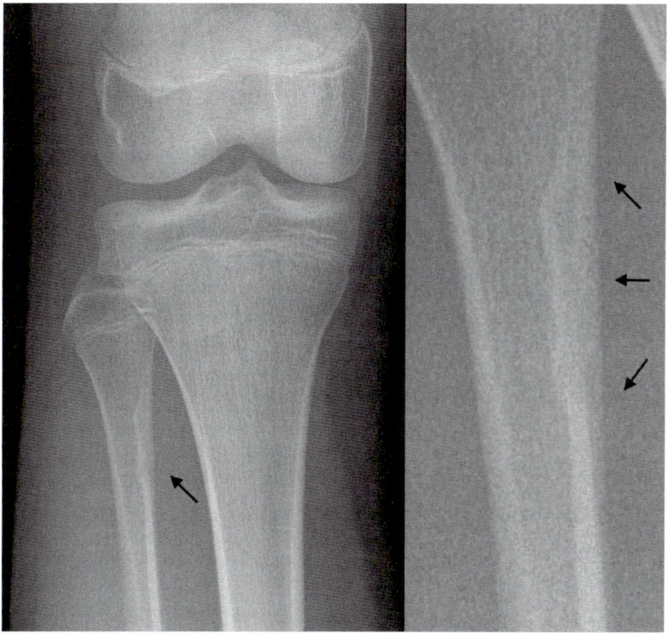

IV-64

NONOSSIFYING FIBROMA (NOF) 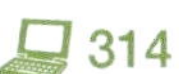 314

The AP radiograph of the right knee demonstrates an eccentric located lytic process with surrounding sclerosis involving the medial cortex of the proximal fibular metaphysis. This has a characteristic appearance for a nonossifying fibroma (NOF).

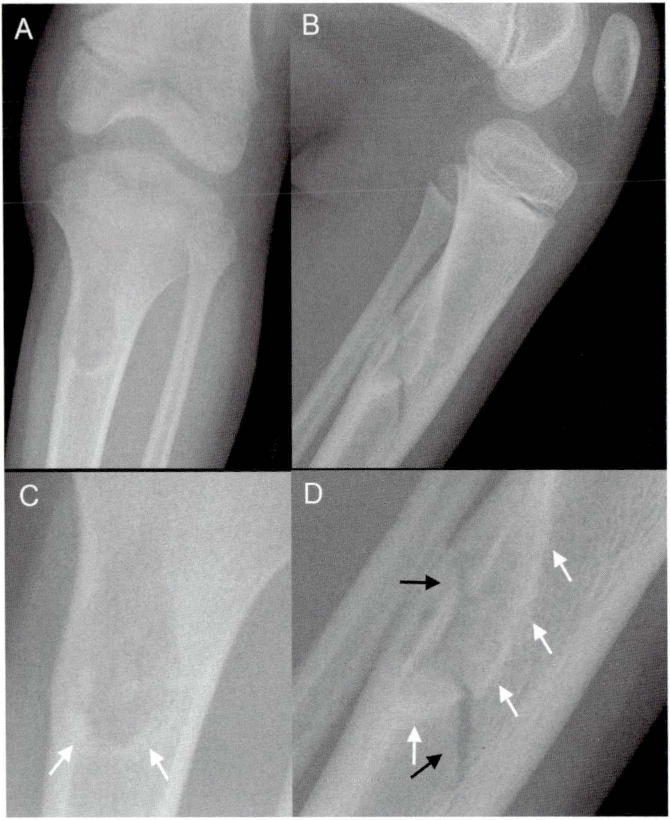

IV-65

■ PROXIMAL TIBIA FRACTURE – PATHOLOGIC DUE TO NOF

💻 315

AP (A, C) and lateral (B, D) radiographs of the left tibia and fibula demonstrate a nondisplaced pathologic fracture (black arrows) of the proximal metaphysis of the left tibia through an expansile lytic process involving the posterior cortex of the tibia. This demonstrates surrounding sclerosis (white arrows), and is characteristic for a NOF.

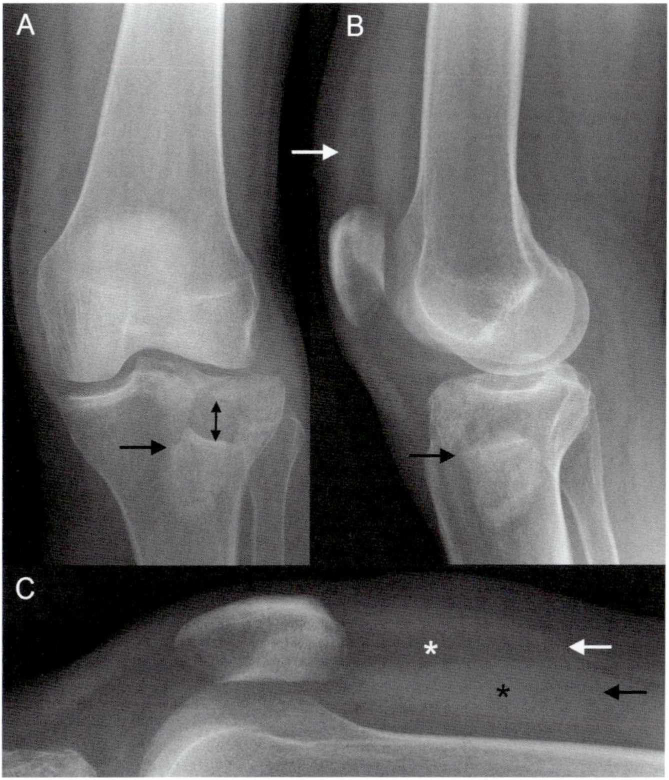

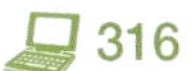

IV-66

■ TIBIAL PLATEAU FRACTURE WITH LIPOHEMARTHROSIS – RADIOGRAPH 　316

AP (A) and lateral crosstable (B, C) views demonstrate a comminuted left tibial plateau fracture. There is depression of an impacted fragment of the lateral tibial plateau (black arrows, A, B) fracture up to 1.7 cm (double arrow, A). Also noticed is a suprapatellar fat–fluid level (asterisks, C) compatible with a large lipohemarthrosis. White asterisk= fat level, black asterisk= fluid level. (Fat is less dense and lighter than water/fluid.)

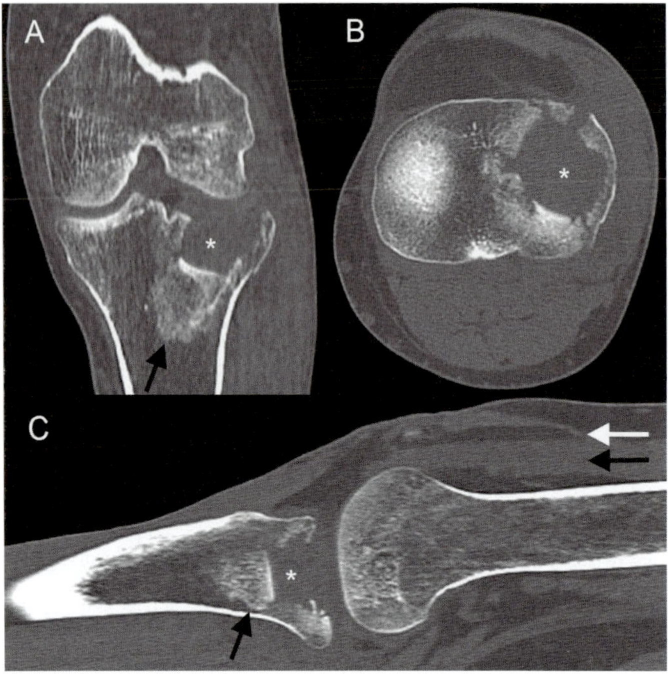

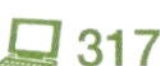

IV-67

TIBIAL PLATEAU FRACTURE WITH LIPOHEMARTHROSIS – CT

□ 317

CT of the left knee in bone window in axial (B), coronal (A), and sagittal (C) reformations demonstrate a comminuted fracture of the lateral tibial plateau (asterisk). The dominant fracture fragment involves a large portion of the lateral tibial plateau articular surface and is depressed approximately 2 cm (oblique arrows in A and C). There is a joint effusion with a fat fluid level (horizontal arrows in C) consistent with lipohemarthrosis. White arrow points to the fat level, black arrow to the fluid level.

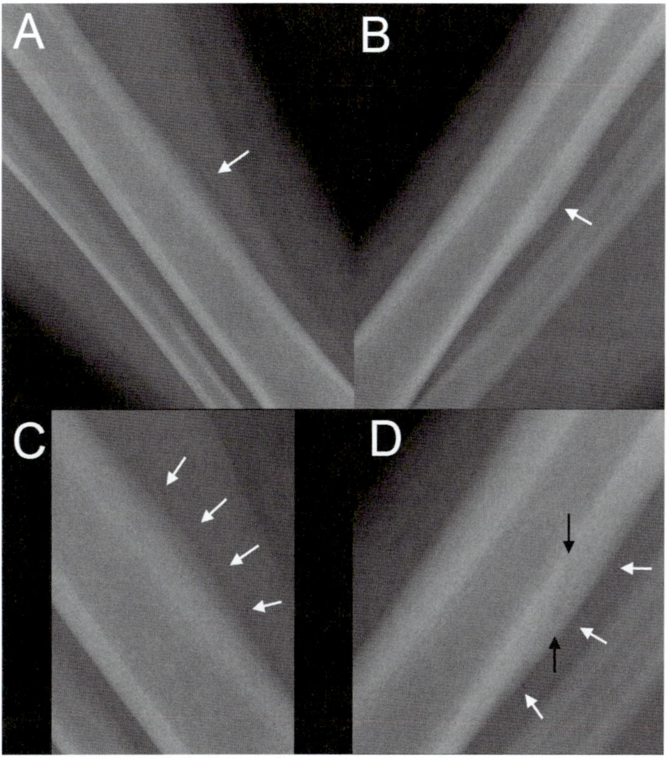

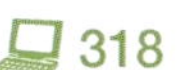

IV-68

TIBIAL STRESS FRACTURE   318

AP (A, C) and lateral (B, D) radiographs of the tibia and fibula show a subtle periosteal new bone formation at the posteromedial aspect of the right tibial shaft (A–D, white arrows). There is also an oblique oriented lucent line in the posterior cortex of the distal right tibial midshaft (black arrows), compatible with a stress fracture.

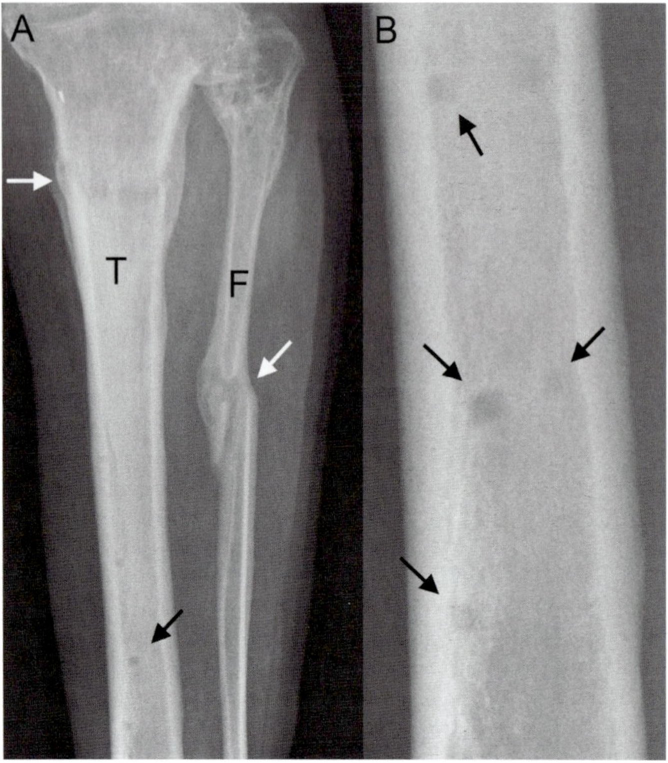

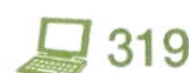

IV-69

MULTIPLE MYELOMA WITH PATHOLOGIC FRACTURES

319

The AP radiograph of the tibia (T) and fibula (F) demonstrates innumerable tiny lucencies within the mid and distal tibia (arrows, B=magnification), consistent with myeloma. There are remote fractures with posttraumatic deformity of the proximal left tibia and fibula (white arrows).

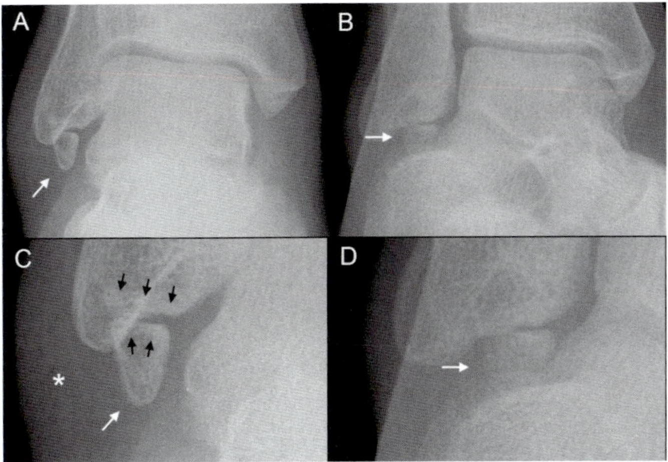

IV-70

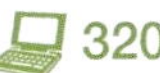 REMOTE LATERAL MALLEOLAR FRACTURE   320

AP (A, C) and oblique (B, D) radiographs of the right ankle demonstrate a prominent well corticated (black arrows) ossicle (white arrows) adjacent to the distal fibular tip consistent with a remote avulsion. There is soft tissue swelling around the ankle (asterisk).

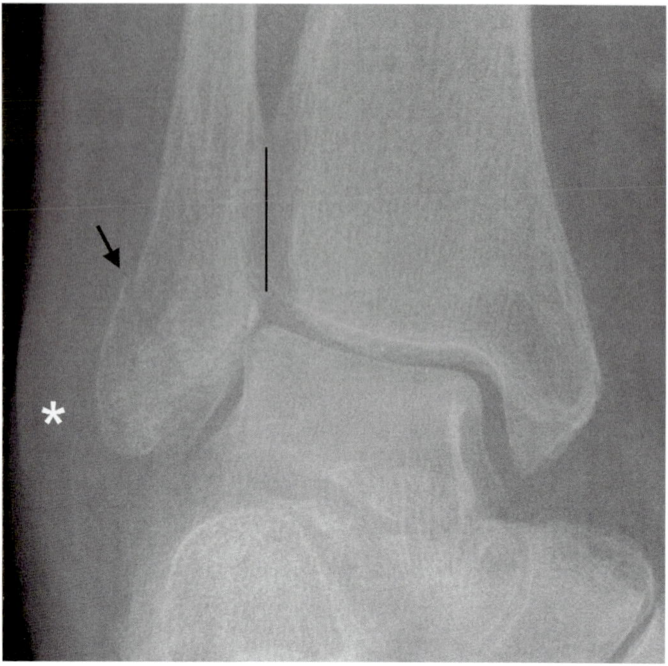

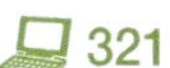

IV-71

▪ ACUTE LATERAL MALLEOLAR FRACTURE – BELOW SYNDESMOSIS   321

The oblique radiograph of the right ankle demonstrates a fracture of the lateral malleolus (arrow) with the fracture line extending below the syndesmosis (vertical line), consistent with a Weber type A fracture. There is moderate circumferential soft tissue swelling (asterisk).

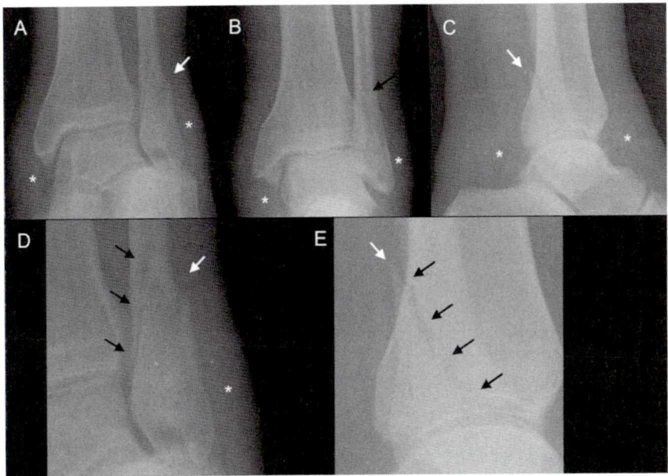

IV-72

ACUTE LATERAL MALLEOLAR FRACTURE – THROUGH SYNDESMOSIS

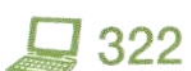 322

Oblique (A, D), AP (B), and lateral (C, E) views of the left ankle demonstrate soft tissue swelling about the entire ankle (asterisks). There is an oblique fracture through the lateral malleolus (black arrows) extending through the syndesmosis (Weber type B). The distal fracture fragment is displaced slightly posteriorly and laterally (white arrows). The ankle mortise is preserved.

ANKLE FRACTURES – WEBER CLASSIFICATION

 323

Type A
- Below level of the ankle joint
- Tibiofibular syndesmosis intact
- Deltoid ligament intact
- Medial malleolus often fractured
- Usually stable

Type B
- At the level of the ankle joint, extending superiorly and laterally up the fibula
- Tibiofibular syndesmosis intact or only partially torn, but no widening of the distal tibiofibular articulation
- Medial malleolus may be fractured or deltoid ligament my be torn
- Variable stability

Type C
- Above the level of the ankle joint
- Tibiofibular syndesmosis disrupted with widening of the distal tibiofibular articulation
- Medial malleolus fracture or deltoid ligament injury present
- Unstable: requires ORIF

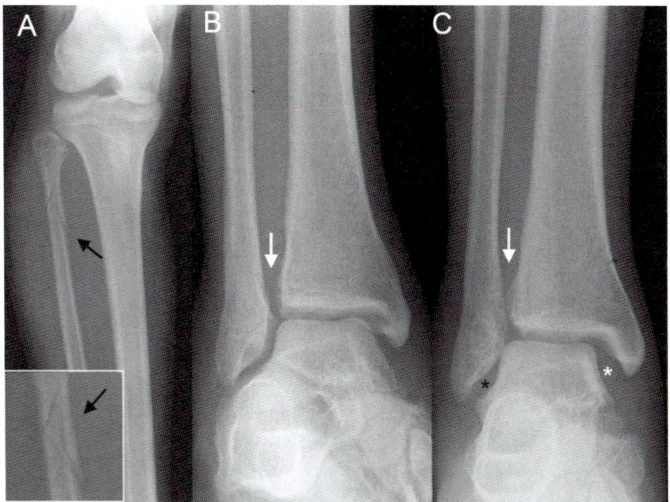

IV-73

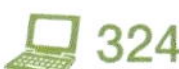 MAISONNEUVE FRACTURE 324

There is a spiral, comminuted fracture of the proximal fibula (A, black arrows). There is also widening of the distal tibiofibular syndesmosis (white arrows) and disruption of the ankle mortise with widening of the tibiotalar joint (white asterisk) and talofibular joint (black asterisk) which is compatible with a Maisonneuve fracture.

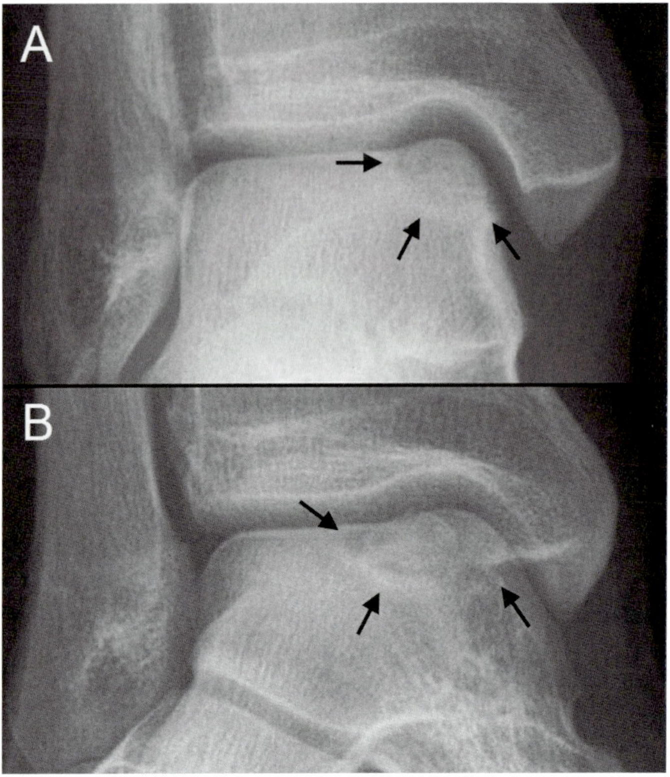

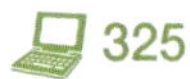

IV-74

■ OSTEOCHONDRITIS DISSECANS (OCD) OF THE TALUS

325

AP (A) and oblique (B) radiographs of the right ankle of this 15-year-old male demonstrate at the medial aspect of the talar dome a osteochondral defect and a linear lucency separating the fragment from the underlying bone. These findings are consistent with OCD. Articular surface seems to be yet intact, suggesting stability. Incongruence of the osteochondral defect with the articular surface would indicate instability.

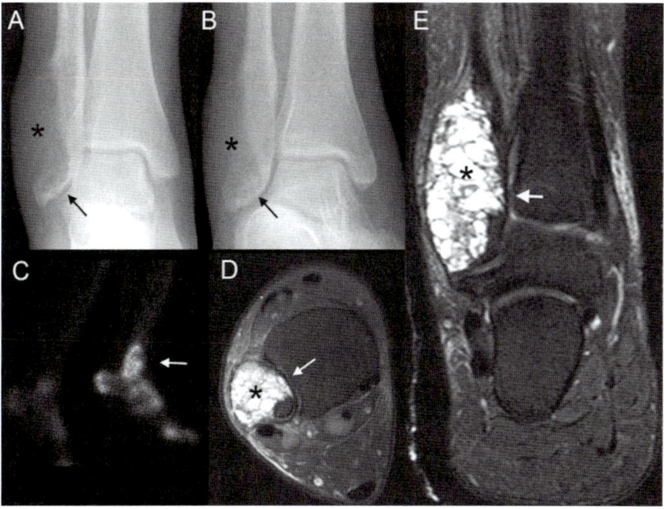

IV-75

PRIMARY BONE NEOPLASM – TELEANGIECTATIC OSTEOSARCOMA

 326

This 12-year-old girl complained about ankle pain without recalling any trauma. AP (A) and oblique (B) radiographs demonstrate an expansile mass in the distal fibular metaphysis (arrows). There is complete erosion and destruction of the cortex of the lateral metaphysis with associated soft tissue swelling (asterisk). A Tc 99m-MDP bone scan (C) demonstrates strong radiotracer uptake in the right ankle area in that location (arrow). MRI of the right ankle (fat saturated proton density) images in axial (D) and coronal (E) planes confirms a mass in the distal fibula (arrows), containing septations and fluid–fluid levels (asterisks). Biopsy confirmed a teleangiectatic osteosarcoma.

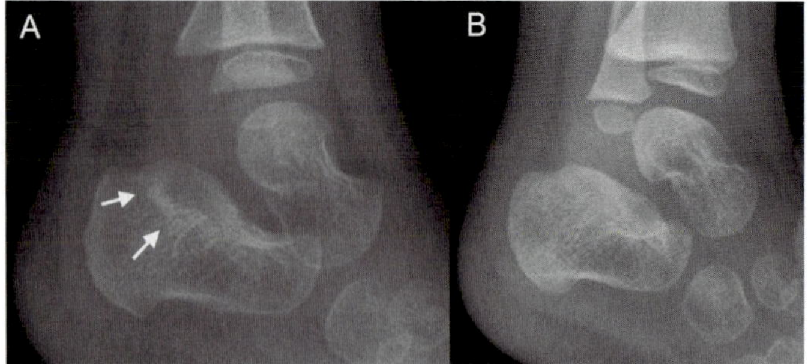

IV-76

■ CALCANEAL STRESS FRACTURE   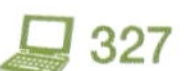 327

Lateral view of the left foot in this 2-year-old child shows a band of increased sclerosis along the superior aspect of the calcaneous (A, arrow). A previous lateral view of the left foot has been taken 3 weeks prior, which shows a radiographically normal calcaneus.

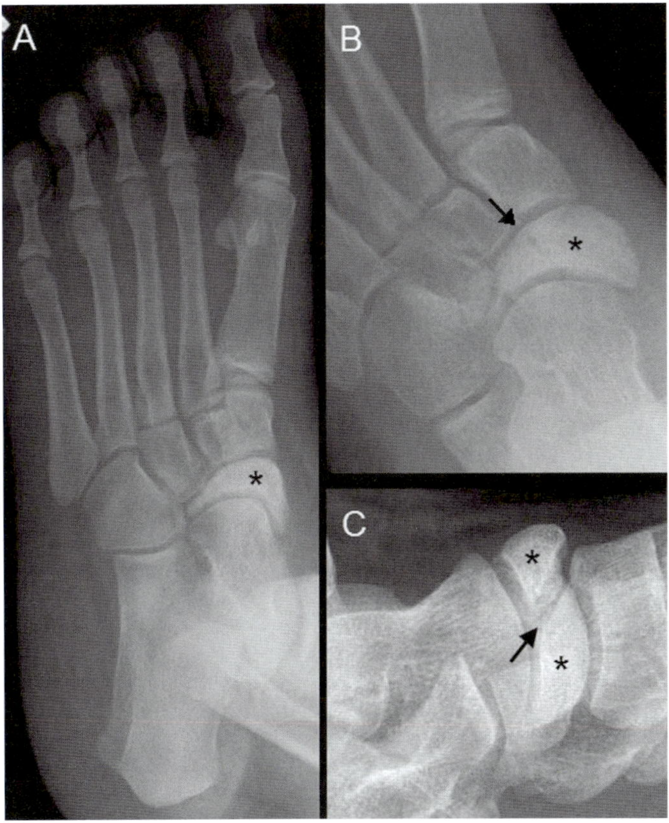

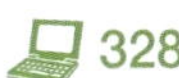

IV-77

AVASCULAR NECROSIS OF THE NAVICULAR BONE (KÖHLER DISEASE)   328

Oblique (A), AP, (B), and lateral (C) radiographs of the left foot in this 11-year-old girl show diffuse sclerosis of the navicular bone (asterisk), consistent with avascular necrosis (Köhler disease). Other radiographic findings of Köhler disease include flattening of the navicular bone and fragmentation. A nondisplaced navicular fracture is also seen (arrow).

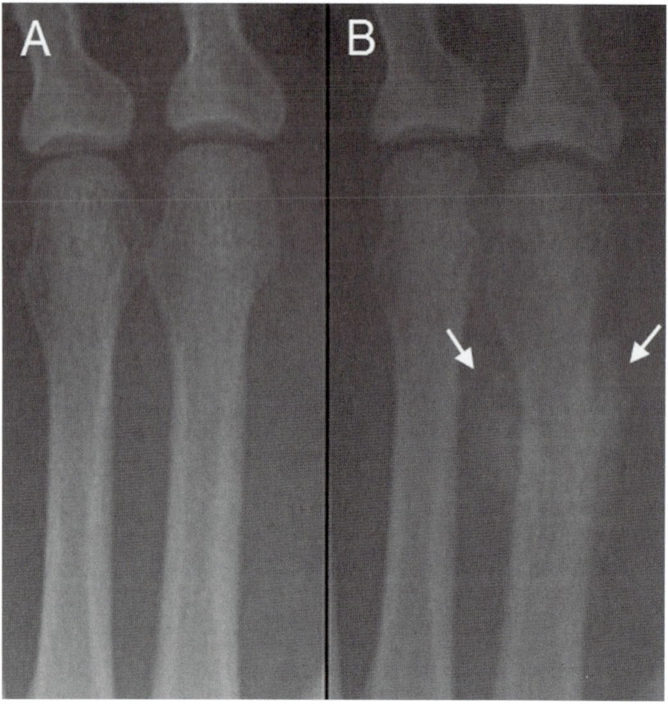

IV-78

METATARSAL STRESS FRACTURE (MARCH FRACTURE)

329

AP radiographs of the right foot demonstrate a normal second and third metatarsal in this active runner with foot pain (A). A follow up radiograph was obtained a few weeks later (B), which shows marked periosteal bone reaction at the distal shaft of the second metatarsal (arrows). Early radiographs may be negative in stress fractures and up to 50% of stress fractures are never observed on plain films at all. Stress fractures of the second or third metatarsals rarely require surgical intervention.

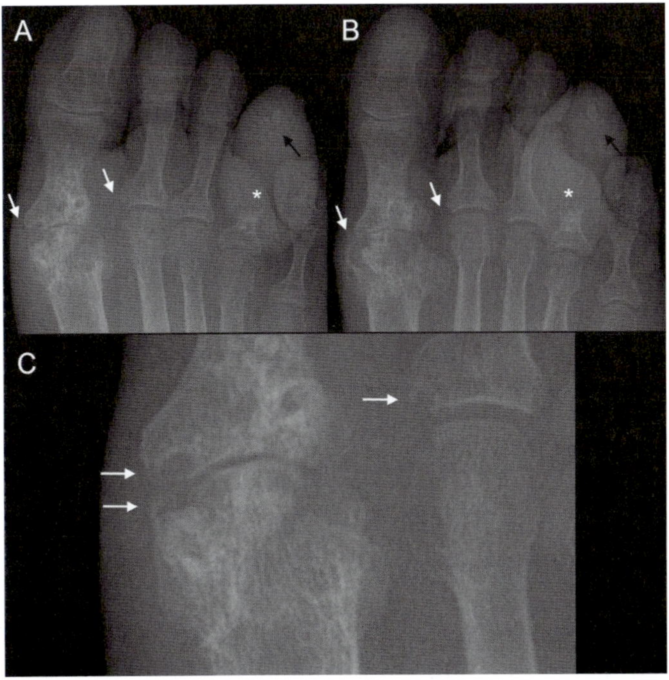

IV-79

TOPHACEOUS GOUT  330

AP (A, C) and oblique (B) radiographs of the right foot demonstrate multiple erosions with sclerotic and overhanging margins at the first and second metatarsophalangeal (MTP) joints (white arrows). The fourth digit is markedly swollen with erosive destruction of the distal aspect of the proximal fourth phalanx (asterisk), complete destruction of the middle, and near complete destruction of the distal phalanx with only a few bony fragments remaining (black arrows). These features are typical for tophaceous gout.

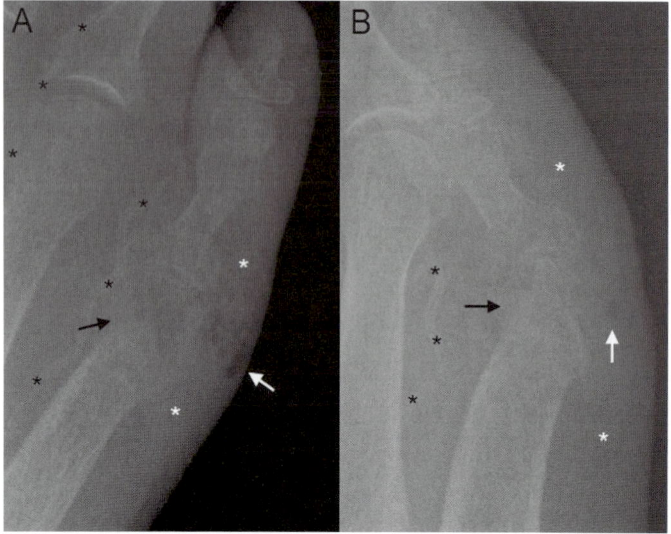

IV-80

■ METATARSAL OSTEOMYELITIS
AND GAS GANGRENE

 331

AP (A) and oblique (B) radiographs of the right foot show generalized osteopenia. There is soft tissue gas (white arrows) and swelling (white asterisks) adjacent to the fifth metatarsophalangeal joint, with poor definition of the distal aspect of the fifth metatarsal (black arrows). Findings are that of gas gangrene and osteomyelitis. Please also note advanced vascular calcifications (black asterisks) – an indicator of impaired vascular supply and risk factor for infection/osteomyelitis.

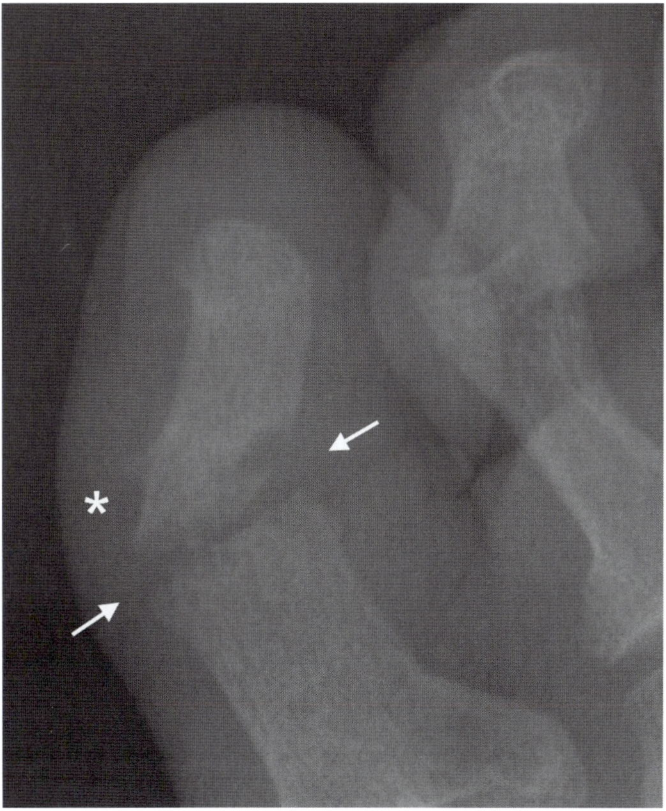

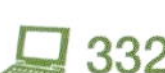

IV-81

SEPTIC ARTHRITIS GREAT TOE 332

The oblique radiograph of the right foot shows an abnormal joint space at the interphalangeal joint of the first toe, with bony destruction on both sides of the joint (arrows) and associated soft tissue swelling (asterisk), compatible with septic arthritis.

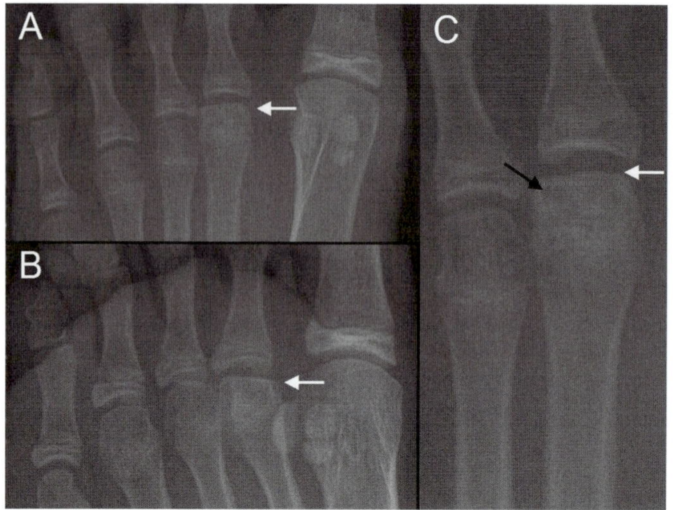

IV-82

■ FREIBERG INFRACTION  333

AP (A) and oblique (B) radiographs of the left foot demonstrate mild deformity of the second metatarsal head with scattered cystic changes (black arrow) and flattening (white arrows) of the subchondral bone (C = magnification). These radiographic findings are consistent with Freiberg infraction. Remaining bony structures appear intact. Joint spaces are maintained.

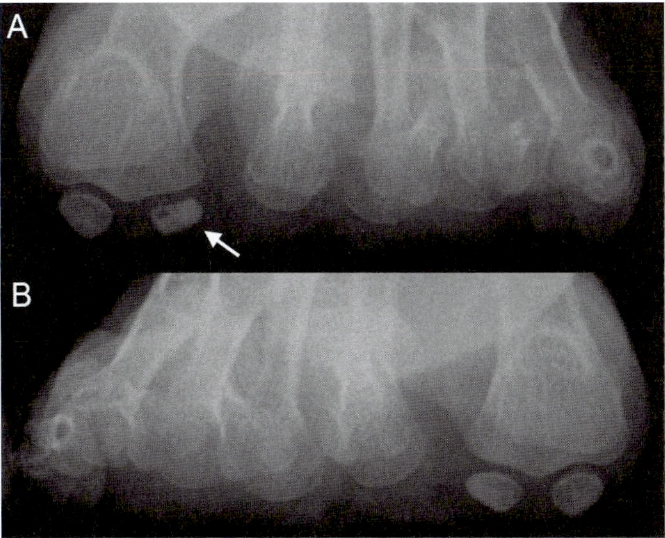

IV-83

SESAMOID AVASCULAR NECROSIS  334

The sesamoid view of the left foot (A) demonstrates a small and dense lateral sesamoid bone (arrow). Please compare with the normal sesamoid bones of the other foot (B).

References

There are many freely available high quality review articles available about specific topics discussed in this book. These selections of references are only references to high quality journal articles that are freely and directly available.

How to get access to these articles?
Each reference has a so-called PMID at the end. Please use that number and go on the following hyperlink by exchanging "PMID" with that respective number: *http://www.ncbi.nlm.nih.gov/pubmed/PMID*

That hyperlink provides the abstract and further links to direct access to these full text articles.

1. Pieroni S, Foster BR, Anderson SW, Kertesz JL, Rhea JT, Soto JA. Use of 64-row multidetector CT angiography in blunt and penetrating trauma of the upper and lower extremities. Radiographics. 2009 May–Jun;29(3):863–876. PMID: 19448121

2. Sawyer JR, Kapoor M. The limping child: a systematic approach to diagnosis. Am Fam Physician. 2009 Feb 1;79(3):215–224. PMID: 19202969

3. Fayad LM, Johnson P, Fishman EK. Multidetector CT of musculoskeletal disease in the pediatric patient: principles, techniques, and clinical applications. Radiographics. 2005 May–Jun;25(3):603–618. PMID: 15888612

4. Potok PS, Hopper KD, Umlauf MJ. Fractures of the acetabulum: imaging, classification, and understanding. Radiographics. 1995 Jan;15(1):7–23. PMID: 7899615

5. Kaewlai R, Avery LL, Asrani AV, Abujudeh HH, Sacknoff R, Novelline RA. Multidetector CT of carpal injuries: anatomy, fractures, and fracture-dislocations. Radiographics. 2008 Oct;28(6):1771–1784. PMID: 18936035

6. Gottsegen CJ, Eyer BA, White EA, Learch TJ, Forrester D. Avulsion fractures of the knee: imaging findings and clinical significance. Radiographics. 2008 Oct;28(6):1755–1770. PMID: 18936034

7. Fishman EK, Horton KM, Johnson PT. Multidetector CT and three-dimensional CT angiography for suspected vascular trauma of the extremities. Radiographics. 2008 May–Jun;28(3):653–665. PMID: 18480477

8. Pecci M, Kreher JB. Clavicle fractures. Am Fam Physician. 2008 Jan 1;77(1):65–70. PMID: 18236824

9. De Filippo M, Sudberry JJ, Lombardo E, Corradi M, Pogliacom F, Ferrari FS, Bocchi C, Zompatori M. Pathogenesis and evolution of carpal instability: imaging and topography. Acta Biomed. 2006 Dec;77(3):168–180. PMID: 17312988

10. Ebrahim FS, De Maeseneer M, Jager T, Marcelis S, Jamadar DA, Jacobson JA. US diagnosis of UCL tears of the thumb and Stener lesions: technique, pattern-based approach, and differential diagnosis. Radiographics. 2006 Jul–Aug;26(4):1007–1020. PMID: 16844929

11. Castillo M. Imaging the anatomy of the brachial plexus: review and self-assessment module. AJR Am J Roentgenol. 2005 Dec;185(6):S196–S204. PMID: 16304040

12. Miller-Thomas MM, West OC, Cohen AM. Diagnosing traumatic arterial injury in the extremities with CT angiography: pearls and pitfalls. Radiographics. 2005 Oct;25 (1):S133–S142. PMID: 16227487

13. Blake SP, Connors AM. Sacral insufficiency fracture. Br J Radiol. 2004 Oct;77(922):891–896. PMID: 15483007

14. Brunner LC, Eshilian-Oates L, Kuo TY. Hip fractures in adults. Am Fam Physician. 2003 Feb 1;67(3):537–542. PMID: 12588076

15. Clavero JA, Alomar X, Monill JM, Esplugas M, Golanó P, Mendoza M, Salvador A. MR imaging of ligament and tendon injuries of the fingers. Radiographics. 2002 Mar–Apr;22(2):237–256. PMID: 11896215

16. Glass RB, Norton KI, Mitre SA, Kang E. Pediatric ribs: a spectrum of abnormalities. Radiographics. 2002 Jan–Feb;22(1):87–104. PMID: 11796901

17. Diel J, Ortiz O, Losada RA, Price DB, Hayt MW, Katz DS. The sacrum: pathologic spectrum, multimodality imaging, and subspecialty approach. Radiographics. 2001 Jan–Feb;21(1):83–104. PMID: 11158646

REFERENCES

Book references

This is a selection of recommended textbooks covering either general radiological principles or specific topics discussed in this book.

General

1. Christian FJ. Clinical Emergency Radiology; 1st edition. Cambridge University Press, Cambridge. September 2008. ISBN: 0521870542

2. Jorge AS, Brian L. Emergency Radiology: The Requisites; 1st edition. Mosby, St. Louis, MO. April 2009. ISBN: 0323054072

3. David TS, Earl R. Emergency Radiology; 1st edition McGraw-Hill Professional, New York. September 1999. ISBN: 0070508275

4. Torsten M, Emil R. Pocket Atlas of Radiographic Positioning; 2nd edition. Thieme, New York, NY. January 2009. ISBN: 3131074426

5. Ralph W, Jack W, Mukesh MGH, John WC, Stephen EJ, Jay WP. Primer of Diagnostic Imaging; 4th edition. Mosby, St. Louis, MO. November 2006. ISBN: 0323040683

Thoracic

6. Theresa C McLoud. Thoracic Radiology: The Requisites; 2nd edition. Mosby, St. Louis, MO. April 2010. ISBN: 0323027903

7. Richard W, Charles BH. Thoracic Imaging: Pulmonary and Cardiovascular Radiology; 1st edition. Lippincott Williams & Wilkins, Philadelphia. September 2004. ISBN: 078174119X

8. Lawrence RG. Felson's Principles of Chest Roentgenology; 3rd edition. Saunders, Philadelphia, PA. December 2006. ISBN: 1416029230

9. Jannette C, Eric JS. Chest Radiology: The Essentials; 2nd edition. Lippincott Williams & Wilkins, Philadelphia. September 2007. ISBN: 0781763142

Musculoskeletal

10. Manaster BJ, David AM, David GD. Musculoskeletal Imaging: The Requisites; 3rd edition. Mosby, St. Louis, MO. November 2006. ISBN: 0323043615

Neuro

11. David MY, Robert DZ, Robert IG. Neuroradiology: The Requisites; 3rd edition. Mosby, St. Louis, MO. April 2010. ISBN: 0323045219

12. Ric H, Anne GO, Jeff R, Andre M. Diagnostic and Surgical Imaging Anatomy: Brain, Head and Neck, Spine; 1st edition. Lippincott Williams & Wilkins, Philadelphia. June 2006. ISBN: 1931884293

Abdominal

13. William D. Middleton, Alfred B. Kurtz. Ultrasound: The Requisites; 2nd edition. Mosby, St. Louis, MO. December 2003. ISBN: 0323017029

14. Dunnick NR, Carl MS, Jeffrey HN, Stephen EA. Textbook of Uroradiology; 4th edition. Lippincott Williams & Wilkins, Philadelphia. October 2007. ISBN: 0781767504

15. Ronald Z. Genitourinary Radiology: Radiology Requisites; 2nd edition. Mosby, St. Louis, MO. April 2004. ISBN: 0323018424

16. Richard MG, Marc SL. Textbook of Gastrointestinal Radiology; 3rd edition. Saunders, Philadelphia, PA. October 2007. ISBN: 1416023321

INDEX